War Against the People

War Against the People

Israel, the Palestinians and Global Pacification

Jeff Halper

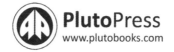

PlutoPress
www.plutobooks.com

First published 2015 by Pluto Press
345 Archway Road, London N6 5AA

www.plutobooks.com

British Library Cataloguing in Publication Data
A catalogue record for this book is available from the British Library

ISBN   978 0 7453 3431 8   Hardback
ISBN   978 0 7453 3430 1   Paperback
ISBN   978 1 8496 4972 8   PDF eBook
ISBN   978 1 8496 4974 2   Kindle eBook
ISBN   978 1 8496 4973 5   EPUB eBook

This book is printed on paper suitable for recycling and made from fully
managed and sustained forest sources. Logging, pulping and manufacturing
processes are expected to conform to the environmental standards of the
country of origin.

Typeset by Stanford DTP Services, Northampton, England
Text design by Melanie Patrick
Simultaneously printed by CPI Antony Rowe, Chippenham, UK
and Edwards Bros in the United States of America

Contents

Part VI   Domestic Securitization and Policing

List of Figures and Tables

Figures

Tables

Acronyms

AAM	Air-to-Air Missile
ABM	Anti-Ballistic Missile
AEW	Airborne Early Warning system
AIFV	Armored Infantry Fighting Vehicle
AIPAC	the American-Israeli Public Affairs Committee
APC	Armored Personnel Carrier
APAM	Anti-Personnel/Anti-Material munition
ATT	Arms Trade Treaty to promote transparency and accountability in the arms trade, signed but not ratified by Israel
BANG	Bits, Atoms, Neurons and Genes, a branch of nanotechnology, including nanoweapons
BMS	A Battle Management System that links soldiers, their field commanders and Command Post staff
BRICS-MINT	Counterhegemonic bloc: Brazil, Russia, India, China, South Africa, joined by Mexico, Indonesia, Nigeria and Turkey
C⁴ISTAR	Capabilities built into high-tech weapons: command, control, communications, computers plus Intelligence, Surveillance, Target Acquisition and Reconnaissance
CAR	Central Asian Republic
CEV	Combat Engineering Vehicle
COIN	Counterinsurgency operations
COMINT	Communication Intelligence
CQC	Close Quarter Combat, especially in urban warfare
DARPA	The Pentagon's Defense Advanced Projects Agency, "turning science fiction into reality"
DASH	Elbit's Display and Sight Helmet, part of its HMD (Helmet-Mounted Display) and HUD (Head-Up Cockpit Display) system
DIME	Dense Inert Metal Explosive, a bomblet that has a relatively small but highly destructive blast radius

	based on exploding such chemically inert materials as tungsten above the heads of targets, and incinerates them
ELINT/ESM	Electronic Intelligence and Electronic Support Measures
EMP	Electromagnetic Pulse bomb strike capability creating a short, focused and highly destructive burst of electromagnetic energy
EO	Electro-optically guided weapons
EW	Electronic Warfare
FMF	Foreign Military Financing (US)
GMTI	A Ground Moving Target Indicator
HELWS	High-Energy Laser Weapon System
IAF	Israeli Air Force
IAI	Israel Aerospace Industries
ICBM	Intercontinental Ballistic Missile
IDF	Israel Defense Force
IHL	International Humanitarian Law
IMI	Israel Military Industries
IMINT	Image Intelligence
INSAT	Nano-satellites launched for testing new industrial components under real outer-space conditions
ISR	Intelligence, Surveillance, Reconnaissance
JDAM	Joint Direct Attack Munitions
LASHAB	The Hebrew acronym for *l'khima al shetakh banui* or "warfare on built-up terrain"
LEEP	Law Enforcement Exchange Program, in which the private Jewish Institute for National Security Affairs brings American law enforcement officials to Israel and vice versa
LEO	Low Earth Orbiting satellite
MALE UAV	Medium-Altitude Long-Endurance drone
MARS	Multi-purpose Aiming Reflex Sight
MARV	Miniature Autonomous Robotic Vehicle
MAVs	Micro-Air Vehicles, also called entomopters; bug-sized devices that fly
MID	Militarized Interstate Disputes

MIRV   Multiple Independently-targetable Reentry Vehicle,
                    ballistic warheads that can be dispensed and aimed
                    against multiple targets

MISSILE Complex   A combined system of Military, Internal Security,
                    Surveillance, Intelligence and Law Enforcement, the
                    key elements of pacification

MPRS   Multi-Purpose Rifle System, which uses the same
                    technology as fire control systems of advanced
                    tanks, making any assault rifle a much diversified
                    weapon system

NBC   Nuclear, Biological, Chemical forms of weapons

NBIC   Nanotechnology, Biotechnology, Information
                    technology and Cognitive science, emerging fields
                    of nano research, including weaponry

OIC   Organisation of Islamic Cooperation

OPSAT   A next-generation optical observation satellite for
                    reconnaissance purposes, developed by IAI's MBT
                    Space Division

OPT   Occupied Palestinian Territories

PGS   Prompt Global Strike Mission, an effort to develop a
                    system that can deliver a precision conventional
                    weapon strike anywhere in the world within one
                    hour

QDR   Quadriennial Defense Review, the Pentagon's report
                    every four years of its policies, strategies and plans

QHSR   Quadriennial Homeland Security Review, also a
                    Pentagon report published every four years of its
                    Homeland Security policies, strategies and plans

QME   Qualitative Military Edge

RCWS   Remote Controlled Weapon Station

RMA   Revolution in Military Affairs, network-centric
                    warfare

RPV   Remotely Piloted Vehicles

SALW   Small Arms and Light Weapons

SAM   Surface-to-Air Missile

SAR   Synthetic Aperture Radar, a type of radar that
                    creates 2D or 3D images of an object, primarily
                    landscapes

SIBAT	The marketing arms of the Israeli Ministry of Defense; published the *Israeli Defense and Homeland Security Directory*
SIGINT	Signal Intelligence
SIPRI	Stockholm International Peace Research Institute, provides data and analysis on conflict, armaments, arms control and disarmament
SWAT Teams	Special Weapons and Tactics, law enforcement units, which use military-style light weapons and specialized tactics in high-risk operations that fall outside of the capabilities of regular, uniformed police
TA	Target Acquisition
UAS	Unmanned Aerial Systems, UAVs plus ground stations and other system elements
UAV	Unmanned Aerial Vehicle, or drone
UACV	Unmanned Aerial Combat Vehicle
UGV	Unmanned Ground Vehicle
USV	Unmanned Surface Vehicle
WINBMS	Weapon-Integrated Battle Management System

Introduction: How Does Israel Get Away With It?

This book began with a question that many activists like myself have asked over the years: How does Israel get away with it? In a decidedly post-colonial age, how is Israel able to sustain a half-century occupation over the Palestinians, a people it violently displaced in 1948, in the face of almost unanimous international opposition? Why, indeed, does the international community tolerate an unnecessary conflict that not only obstructs efforts to bring some stability to the wider Middle East, a pretty important geo-political region in which the United States and Europe are fighting a number of wars, but one that severely disrupts the international system as a whole?

Various common-sense explanations have been put forth, primarily the clout wielded by the Jewish and Christian fundamentalist communities in the US. The perception that Israel is one of "us," a white Global North nation fighting Muslim terrorism and sharing "our" moral values, plays a role as well. During the Cold War, when Israel was already a major regional military power, the case was made that Israel served US interests. "A part of the Nixon Doctrine," Chomsky reminds us,

> ... was that the U.S. has to control Middle East oil resources—that goes much farther back—but it will do so through local, regional allies, what were called "cops on the beat" by Melvin Laird, Secretary of Defense. So there will be local cops on the beat, which will protect the Arab dictatorships from their own populations or any external threat. And then, of course, "police headquarters" is in Washington. Well, the local cops on the beat at the time were Iran, then under the Shah, a US ally; Turkey; to an extent, Pakistan; and Israel was added to that group. It was another cop on the beat. It was one of the local gendarmes that was sometimes called the periphery strategy: non-Arab states protecting the Arab dictatorships from any threat, primarily the threat of what was called radical nationalism—independent nationalism—meaning taking over the armed resources for their own purposes. Well, that structure remained through the 1970s.[1]

Support for Israel gained new traction after 9/11, when it was argued that Israel provided critical support in America's War on Terror.

All this might partially explain continued American support for Israel, but even here is an enigma: America's continued role as Israel's main patron appears to actually conflict with its wider interests in the Middle East. In 2006, the Iraq Study Working Group co-chaired by former Secretary of State James Baker stated flatly:

> The United States will not be able to achieve its goals in the Middle East unless the United States deals directly with the Arab-Israeli conflict … To put it simply, all key issues in the Middle East—the Arab-Israeli conflict, Iraq, Iran, the need for political and economic reforms, and extremism and terrorism—are inextricably linked.[2]

A few years later, in March, 2010, General David Petraeus, then head of the Central Command whose area of responsibility includes the Middle East, North Africa and Central Asia, testified before the Senate Armed Services Committee that

> The enduring hostilities between Israel and some of its neighbors present distinct challenges to our ability to advance our interests in the AOR [Area of Operations]. Israeli-Palestinian tensions often flare into violence and large-scale armed confrontations. The conflict foments anti-American sentiment, due to a perception of U.S. favoritism for Israel. Arab anger over the Palestinian question limits the strength and depth of U.S. partnerships with governments and peoples in the AOR and weakens the legitimacy of moderate regimes in the Arab world. Meanwhile, al-Qaeda and other militant groups exploit that anger to mobilize support. The conflict also gives Iran influence in the Arab world through its clients, Lebanese Hizballah and Hamas.[3]

And the pattern goes on. In 2013 the Obama Administration declared Israel a "major strategic partner," even as the Israeli government was deliberately and with open disdain torpedoing Secretary of State Kerry's peace initiative.

And Europe? Can we explain the EU's consistent up-grading of its relations with Israel, including the funding of major Israeli weapons projects through its Horizon 2020 program, solely by guilt over the Holocaust? Can that explain NATO's designation of Israel as a major non-NATO ally? How to explain Israel's acceptance into the OECD, the exclusive club of advanced economies, despite a human rights record that should have excluded it?

How, indeed, do we explain the ever-closer relations of many countries to Israel that traditionally supported the Palestinians? India and China, which until the 1990s did not even have diplomatic ties with Israel, are now among its chief trading partners, particularly in the military and security sectors. In 2007 Israel became the first country outside of Latin America to be affiliated with MERCOSUR, the continent's emerging common market.

What is the genuine *quid pro quo*, the Big Reason for supporting Israel even among countries with no Jewish or Christian Zionist lobby? No less to the point, why did Israel itself reject the two-state solution? The intractable enmity of the Arab world changed dramatically with the peace agreement with Egypt in 1979, the PLO's acceptance of the two-state solution in 1988, the Oslo negotiations of the 1990s and a subsequent peace agreement with Jordan, all culminating in the Arab Peace Initiative of 2002. Even today, amidst the meltdown in the Middle East, the Palestinian Authority and the Arab League still seek a two-state solution that would leave Israel intact and secure, and Egypt remains Israel's best friend (after the American Congress). How do you explain Israel's rejection of these opportunities? It cannot be explained by security. On the contrary, the IDF would have remained as strong as ever, the only major concession being a measly 22 percent of the country with little if any security value.

I began to look outside the box of the Occupation itself. I noticed that Israel has diplomatic relations with 157 countries, and virtually all the agreements and protocols Israel has signed with them contain military and security components. I also noted that Saudi Arabia no less had initiated the Arab League's Peace Initiative in 2002, despite an almost atavistic rejection of Israel's religious ideology. From those tiny threads, it dawned on me that when military relations are mixed into the diplomatic stew, new, surprising and seemingly impossible constellations emerge. As I began to trace Israel's military relations more closely, another picture emerged in which Israel was actually a regional hegemon accepted as such—or at least related to as such—by the other countries of the region and beyond. Israel's position in the world could not be explained by normal international relations; again, most countries strongly *oppose* its Occupation policies. Nor could lobbies or the Holocaust explain it.

Israel, it seemed, was succeeding in parlaying its military and securocratic prowess into political clout, in pursuing what I now call *security politics*. The Occupied Palestinian Territories, I now understood, did not pose a financial burden on Israel or an unwanted source of insecurity and conflict. Indeed, the opposite was the case. Without an occupation and an interminable conflict, how would Israel sustain its strong international standing? The Occupation represents a *resource* for Israel in two senses: economically, it provides a testing ground for the development of weapons, security systems, models of population control and tactics without which Israel would be unable to compete in the international arms and security markets, but no less important, being a major military power serving other militaries and security services the world over lends Israel an international status among the global hegemons it would not have otherwise. Israel is a small country scrambling to carve out a niche in the transnational military-industrial complex. Where would it be without the Occupation and the regional conflict it generates?

Looking out of the box even further, I saw that Israel would be an ideal vehicle for entering a world of military systems I knew nothing about—C⁴ISTAR-capable weapons, full-spectrum dominance, COMINT/SIGINT/OSINT/HUMINT, phased-array radar, avionics, electro-optically guided missiles, ground moving target indicators, securocratic systems of control—and the science behind it, literally "rocket science." It's a world with a tremendous impact on our lives, much of it obvious. Politically, armed forces determine the power of countries, classes and cliques to rule violently over lives, lands and resources. Economically, militaries and domestic security constitute a 2.25 *trillion* dollar a year industry. Socially, wars, soldiers and police militarize our cultures, as does the very presence of arms. Some 875 *million* "small arms" are found in the world, 650 million (almost 75 percent) among civilians, 40 percent of those (270 million) in the hands of Americans.⁴

But this global pacification industry, as I call it, threatens us in fundamental ways not immediately obvious. As this book will show, global systems of control and the weapons that comprise them are becoming totalizing in their power, their development carried out by the brightest scientific minds in cutting-edge labs supported by hundreds of billions in corporate and government funds. GNR, the fusion of genetics, nanotechnology and robotics into lethal, self-replicating nanowarriors endowed with enhanced artificial intelligence, is a leading field in military research, yet how many peace and human rights activists—including me—even understand its implications? What do we know about the military or security, or, for that matter, about modern weapons and tactics? Speaking for myself, I couldn't have told you the difference between a howitzer and a mortar, and the intricacies of C⁴ISTAR systems still baffle me. To be sure, a vast literature on weapons, war and policing is available, but it is not very critical (the writings of P.W. Singer, Jeremy Scahill and a few others aside). And how many of us spend much time in the "Military History" section of the bookstore? The militaries of the world and the technologies of control they are spawning hardly register on our low-tech radars.

Critical analysts and activists, to be sure, regularly point to the deleterious effects of militarism (less so policing), but we have little idea of how securitization actually works. Few of us have military or police backgrounds, and most of us come out of the social sciences or humanities, not the "hard" sciences. C.P. Snow's "two cultures" have come home to roost. We of the social sciences have little if any idea of what is being cooked up by the mad scientists of our defense-related universities and corporate research centers, while they, unencumbered by the problematics of progressive political analysis or social movements, pursue research or commercial projects with little concern over how their research or products will be used.

This book attempts to bridge these gaps, while pushing global pacification into the center of left politics. It deserves to take its place alongside other key transnational movements of counterhegemony such as transnational labor, feminism and the environment.⁵ Because securitization represents the enforcement arm of transnational capitalism, ensuring the smooth flow of capital and resources while addressing "challenges" to its hegemony, I begin by placing the pacification industry in its global context, that of the capitalist world-system. Within that framework I examine how "hegemony," a fluid, seemingly benign and unobtrusive form of domination, aspires to securitization and pacification. In order to "nail down" this slippery yet vital force at different levels of the world-system—the ruling "core," a semi-periphery of relatively strong states and the peripheries—I identify several fundamental "hegemonic tasks," each calling for a different constellation of military, security and police structures, together with appropriate weapons and systems of control. Since my analysis revolves around pacification, I focus in particular on "securocratic wars."

This book, then, sets out to address six major concerns.

First, to lay out the aims and structure of the global pacification industry and how it operates through securocratic wars. This I do in Chapter 1.

Second, to examine "security politics" and its role in international affairs. I begin with the questions, "How does Israel get away with it?" and "Why does Israel *want* to get away with it instead of obtaining peace and security?" Taking as my vehicle for examining the global pacification system a small but pivotal military power, Israel, I show, through its need to strategically "niche-fill", the contours of the world's arms and security industries. Chapters 2 and 3 examine Israel's place in the wider scheme of global pacification.

Third, to survey some of the major weapons systems Israel develops, deploys and sells to the powers of the core and semi-peripheries, weapons inspired by the Pentagon's overall aspiration to "Full-Spectrum Dominance and Control." This I do in Chapters 4–6. My survey of Israeli weapons systems may strike you as somewhat descriptive and "catalogue-like," but that's because it's necessary to lay out in some technical detail the weapons systems and technologies arrayed against us. How, exactly, do they control us, and where are weapons systems going?

Fourth, to examine Israel's model of securocratic control, which I call its Matrix of Control over the Palestinians. This I do in Chapters 7 and 8. In Chapters 9–11, I go on to examine how Israel applies its Matrix and its weapons of suppression to countries on the peripheries of the world-system where the hegemons' need for control is more of a securocratic than military nature.

Fifth, to explore how the ruling political and corporate classes within the core use Israeli weapons and tactics to maintain their own hegemonic positions at home, the subject of Chapter 12.

Finally, after raising the alarm as to the technologies and method of pacification available to the world-system's hegemons, I offer suggestions as to how left and progressive activists can take the information and analysis I offer here and begin to integrate them into a more effective movement of resistance and counterhegemony.

This work is the product of an "activist-scholar." Researching and writing a book such as this with minimal institutional support—including limited access to online resources—is not easy. In my case, the author is engaged full-time in running a grass-roots political organization (ICAHD, the Israeli Committee Against House Demolitions), resisting the Israeli Occupation "on the ground" (where the IDF often disrupts my work calendar), advocating for a just resolution of the Israeli–Palestinian conflict (I am completing this manuscript on a month-long speaking tour of Canada—in the winter!) and, always, scrambling for funds. But being "on the ground" is also a powerful place to be in terms of generating questions and issues that might not penetrate the university. Indeed, this project began in the ICAHD office in Jerusalem in a wide-ranging series of conversations with

Jimmy Johnson, now an activist in Detroit whose own writings on the arms industry have provided useful analysis for me and others.

I wish to acknowledge the readiness of Roger van Zwanenberg of Pluto Press in London to publish this work and the financial support the project received from the Pluto Educational Trust (PET). Appreciation also to David Shulman and the people at Pluto Press for shepherding this book through. Prof. Colin Green provided generous financial and logistical support for a two-month research stay in London. There John Chalcraft and Jonathan Rosenhead at LSE greatly facilitated my "guerilla research" and Brunel professor Mark Neocleous introduced me to the Anti-Security Project, which helped me flesh out the concept of "pacification." Colin also arranged for me to spend time with Desmond Travis, my first opportunity to try out my ideas on a professional military person. On a subsequent trip to Ottawa, another member of the Anti-Security Project, Prof. George Rigakos, kindly invited me to speak at a seminar sponsored by Carleton University's Department of Law and Legal Studies.

In Israel, I had the pleasure of getting to know Leila Stockmarr, a doctoral student at the London School of African and Oriental Studies (now known as SOAS) doing her dissertation on the private security industry of Israel. We spent hours sharing our analyses and attending the ISDEF International Defense and Security Expo in Tel Aviv. I also shared my analysis with Yotam Feldman, whose provocative film "The Lab" presages what I've written here; Prof. Eyal Ben-Ari who has written extensively on the IDF, and Elisha Baskin, who directs a critical Israeli arms monitor site *Hamushim* ("Armed"). Mandy Turner, director of the Kenyon Institute in Jerusalem and the source of extremely useful feedback and sources, chaired the session "Global Militarism and Violence in the 21st Century" at the ISA conference in San Francisco, the first time I presented my findings in an academic setting.

As the research began to take shape, I had the opportunity to discuss over several days a wide range of issues connected to world-systems analysis with Prof. Tom Reifer of the University of San Diego. Shir Hever, a long-time political colleague with whom I had discussed the project at various stages of its development, read the manuscript and kindly spent a day with me sharpening the analysis and sharing his valuable insights. Aneta Jerska, Coordinator of the European Coordinating Committee on Palestine (ECCP) and also, with me, a founding member of The People Yes! Network, has been instrumental in "translating" the information and analysis of this book into a website and other effective advocacy materials.

Otherwise, my work has been sustained by people close to me. Linda Ramsden, the director of ICAHD UK, has been a source of organizational, financial, political and moral support, a person who genuinely believed in the project and a key strategizer on how to move it forward after this book. My mentor, Anthropology Professor Emeritus Stan Newman, shared his sharp street-wise insights, analyses and criticisms, including his experiences as a policeman in Israel. And, as usual, my wife Shoshana enabled and critically enriched this work. My "kids," Efrat, Yishai and Yair, always keep me politically honest and up-to-date. (Yishai is a senior editor of the *Ha'aretz* website in English, an invaluable resource). My grandchildren, Zohar, Alex and Nora, are the ones for whom I write, the ones that will inhabit the world of nanoweapons my "Sixties" generation has left for them. And, finally, I extend thanks to my "students," the thousands of people who have heard my talks on one or another aspects of this research, for whom I'm grateful for the feedback and pushback, and to Richard Barnes for his keen proofreading.

Part I

The Global Pacification Industry

1

Enforcing Hegemony: Securocratic Wars in Global Battlespace

We are witnessing today the rise of a new kind of war, "securocratic war." For centuries, as transnational capitalism steadily expanded over the entire world, corporate and political elites have had to secure their hegemony against endemic resistance. At the dawn of the twentieth century, which marked the high point of classical imperialism, the gap between the per capita GDP of the poorest and richest nation was a ratio of 22:1; by 2000 it stood at 267:1.[1] While a few get rich and a substantial middle class arises primarily in the Global North, the experience of the vast majority of people worldwide becomes one of impoverishment, marginality, exploitation, dislocation and violence. This "surplus humanity," increasingly alienated from even its own resources and cultures, inhabits what Mike Davis calls "a planet of slums."[2]

Under capitalism, accumulation of resources, capital and profits by some comes at the expense of many others. The Global North, sometimes called "the West," lies at the "core" of this world-system. It is here that the transnational corporate class is concentrated, and from here it coordinates the management of globalized circuits of resource flow, globalized production, marketing, financing and, in the end, capital accumulation. As such, the transnational capitalist class represents a hegemonic power within hegemonic powers, capable of mobilizing the power of core states and supranational institutions when necessary to protect and advance its interests.[3]

The "core" of the world-system, the Global North, both dominates world politics and economy and stands in fundamental opposition to the countries and peoples of its peripheries, the so-called "developing world" or "Third

World." Occupying a kind of middle ground are the stronger states of the semi-periphery, particularly those of the BRICS/MINT bloc: Brazil, Russia, India, China and South Africa, followed by Mexico, Indonesia, Nigeria and Turkey.[4] The division is not strictly geographical by any means. Elites allied to those of the core—what I call lower-level hegemons—are found in "core nodes" of global commodity chains throughout the world. By contrast, the poor and marginalized of the Global North constitute extensions of the peripheries into the core itself.

Once the capitalist system had spread throughout the world eliminating all competing systems, it could no longer expand and, taking the form of endocolonialism, began feeding off itself. Eventually, this gave rise in the mid-1970s to the virulent neoliberalism we know today, characterized by what Harvey has termed "accumulation by dispossession."[5] Under this totalizing form of transnational capitalism,

- Land is commodified and peasant populations forcefully expelled. In cities this takes the form of gentrification, the displacement of poor and working-class populations by real estate developers.
- Rights to the commons, once public or indigenous lands accessible to all, are suppressed as their assets, including natural resources, become the property of the state or commercial interests, often ruining the environment as well.
- Property rights and public services are privatized. Once commonly used, collectively owned, or the products of small-scale tenure, they become the exclusive province of states, corporations and wealthy individuals.
- Unions and other forms of social solidarity are weakened or destroyed as labor is commodified. Production is outsourced to the cheap unprotected labor of the periphery. More humane alternative forms of production and consumption, whether indigenous or cooperative, are suppressed. Impoverishment, job insecurity (even of the middle classes) and huge income gaps come to characterize the world-system.
- Social services and welfare are reduced or removed, basic public services such as education and health care are under-funded, and government policy, embedded in public-private "partnerships," comes to reflect corporate interests.
- Exchange and taxation are monetized, particularly concerning land, but extending into all areas of life, including cultural production.

- Various forms of exploitation and usury come to dominate social and economic relations. Poorer countries are forced into debt, thereby leveraging them into the neoliberal system and into economic and political dependency upon the core. By the same token, the credit system extracts maximum capital from families and individuals while locking them into a consumer economy. Even criminal activities such as the slave trade, and particularly traffic in women, assume unheard-of proportions and economic/political clout.

- Though promoting electoral regimes and an abstract commitment to "democracy," neoliberal regimes actually distance the people from exercising any democratic control over state policies.

- Cultural identities, histories, symbols and communities are destroyed or appropriated, a form of cultural genocide. Atomized individuals are idealized as the most fitting expression of "freedom." Basic social solidarity is destroyed.

And in order to enforce accumulation by dispossession,

- Core militaries, security agencies, police forces and prison systems assume a central role. They not only secure vital resources and transportation routes between the peripheries and the core, but also protect the ruling classes and their middle-class allies from endemic unrest and resistance. And not only in the core: core-supplied militaries and security forces play an instrumental role in shoring up comprador elites of the peripheries—client-state leaders, local strongmen and warlords, even selected non-state actors such as the Taliban at particular times and other useful "insurgents." True to the spirit of accumulation, these securitization agents also constitute an enormously profitable industry.[6]

"Securing insecurity," then, has always been capital's overriding preoccupation, and accumulation by dispossession was and continues to be a violent process. In the history of accumulation, noted Marx in *Capital*, "it is a notorious fact that conquest, enslavement, robbery, murder, in short, force, play the greatest part."[7] Inevitably, the process of coercing core capital accumulation out of Europe's far-off colonies gave rise to an integrated "military-capitalist complex."[8] By the mid-sixteenth century, Spain and Portugal were using the term "pacification" to gloss their conquests.[9] The place we have now reached, where post-war capitalist endocolonialism has morphed into neoliberalism, has brought the issue of pacification back as the dominant force of capitalist rule, far more totalizing than conventional inter-state warfare. For neoliberal securitization is indeed total, constituting nothing less than "pure war" and the endless preparation for war.[10] It has given rise to human-security states driven by the quest for total security, their security logic resting on what Glover calls "the logic of 'The War on ____ [poverty, crime, drugs, terrorism, etc.].'"[11]

The new forms of war police these endemic insecurities. Despite their different names—"securocratic wars,"[12] "wars amongst the people,"[13] "resource wars,"[14] or counterinsurgencies[15]—they share a common goal: pacification in the name of enforcing the hegemony of transnational capital. Pacification of the world-system as a whole, of its peripheries, even of its victims in the core. Pacification that secures the world-system against threats from counterhegemons (including you and me if the reactions to the anti-globalization or Occupy movements are an indicator), or from anti-systemic forces.

Members of the Anti-Security Project advocate for re-appropriating the term "pacification" as a way of exposing the seemingly self-evident justifications of "security."[16] "Security" is something we all want but, asks Rigakos plaintively, do we really want to be pacified?[17] Pacification, he continues,

> ... uncovers what security seeks to mask: that the entire premise of security is based first and foremost on the security, extension and imposition of property relations and that these property relations are the manifestations of brute force ... Pacification, therefore, is not passive. Security pretends to be. To study pacification makes it clear that we are studying the fabrication of a social order.[18]

The very term "pacification" raises a slew of critical questions. *Who* is being pacified, and *by whom? Why* are they being pacified and *what* are they resisting—or are perceived as resisting? *Whose interests* are being served by pacification and to what ends? And *in what ways* are we being pacified?[19] These are the sorts of questions this book is trying to address.

A Global Pacification System

I have already suggested *why* we are being pacified: to ensure the hegemony of transnational capital over the entire world-system. *Who* is pacifying us is more complex. The short answer would be the core hegemons, although their hegemony is dispersed and shared among a number of actors: the transnational elites themselves, both economic and political, acting through their corporations and states, the latter charged with advancing the interests and capacities of the business sector while protecting its circuits of production and marketing; supranational institutions such as the World Bank, the IMF, the WTO, the OECD, the EU, various "free trade" pacts, world courts and, if necessary, NATO—all backed up by a military-industrial complex that provides the *how* of pacification even as it feeds into the core's industries.

This is not to imply that a closed and limited set of individuals runs the global system in some conspiratorial form, or that disagreement and even conflicts do not exist among the core hegemons. Indeed, deep-seated differences and divergent interests can be found within their ranks. It does imply, however, a certain identifiable logic running through the political economy of the world-system, one that gives coherency and direction to the agency of the dominant transnational actors. That logic trickles down to groups and individuals in society through institutions, laws, cultures, ideologies and religions, shared experiences, framings, education and other channels. Together they form a total system of social control, what Foucault calls "governmentality," which has both local and global expressions.[20]

The best way to portray the underlying logic of the capitalist world-system, the policies and practices imposed by core power, the unseen but disciplining hand of governmentality and the dynamic skein of relationships that actually comprises the world-system's workings at all its levels is through the concept of hegemony. Like "pacification," "hegemony" is not a common term, perhaps because it represents fluid, often elusive social relations, which is precisely what gives it the ability to capture the fluid agency of power among so many actors at different levels of the world-system. It is the agent of governmentality, enforcing those norms and behaviors, but also relations of power, through which the transnational elites and their lower-level allies run the world-system.

Another reason why hegemony is so elusive is that it hides its coercive governmentality behind a benign façade of consensus, democracy and seemingly technical but necessary laws and regulations. Hegemony implies hierarchy and domination, of course, but also indirect rule—even the ability to deny one is actually calling the shots. This is crucial when trying to dominate a world otherwise characterized by great geographical, historical, cultural and ideological diversity, when class, religious, gender, ethnic and national divisions constantly engender multiple sources of opposition, resistance and counterhegemony. Hegemony is thus a social structure, an economic structure and a political structure which lays down general rules of behavior for states and for those forces of civil society that act across national boundaries—rules which support the dominant mode of production.[21]

But it can also be enforced. When the ruling classes feel their domination being threatened or challenged, they have at their disposal powerful instruments of outright coercion: armies, paramilitaries, special forces, security agencies, the police and prison services. In particular, their dominion depends on how well they execute three overarching "hegemonic tasks":

1. Core hegemons must be able to maintain their overall domination over the world-system despite challenges from potential counterhegemons (China in particular, but also the emerging bloc of BRICS/MINT countries) and forces seeking to dismantle the capitalist world-system entirely, such as the Islamic State or anti-globalization movements, as well as confronting other systemic threats such as the effects of climate change or new military technologies.
2. Core hegemons must be able to maintain their hegemony over the peripheries, whether directly or though support for "pliant" comprador elites.
3. The ruling political and corporate classes of the core and semi-periphery must be able to maintain their hegemony within their own countries.

Each of these three tasks requires a different form of hegemony, which in turn requires expedient forms of pacification. Together, they constitute a Global Pacification System (Figure 1.1).

Hegemonic Task 1: Maintaining Overall Core Hegemony

This first hegemonic task falls primarily although not exclusively on the shoulders of the United States, the current world power. Seeking, as hegemons do, "consensual" governmentality rather than direct rule, the United States projects an image of "soft power" (freedom, democracy, rock music and Hollywood) backed, however, by intimidating military power.[22] "Projecting power" and "global reach"—two flagship Pentagon terms—

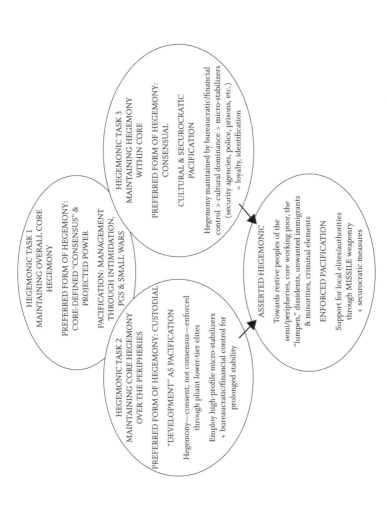

HEGEMONIC TASK 1
MAINTAINING OVERALL CORE HEGEMONY

PREFERRED FORM OF HEGEMONY: CORE-DEFINED "CONSENSUS" & PROJECTED POWER

PACIFICATION: MANAGEMENT THROUGH INTIMIDATION, PGS & SMALL WARS

HEGEMONIC TASK 3
MAINTAINING HEGEMONY WITHIN CORE

PREFERRED FORM OF HEGEMONY: CONSENSUAL

CULTURAL & SECUROCRATIC PACIFICATION

Hegemony maintained by bureaucratic/financial control > cultural dominance > micro-stabilizers (security agencies, police, prisons, etc.) = loyalty, identification

HEGEMONIC TASK 2
MAINTAINING CORE HEGEMONY OVER THE PERIPHERIES

PREFERRED FORM OF HEGEMONY: CUSTODIAL

"DEVELOPMENT" AS PACIFICATION

Hegemony—consent, not consensus—enforced through pliant lower-tier elites

Employ high-profile micro-stabilizers + bureaucratic/financial control for prolonged stability

ASSERTED HEGEMONIC

Towards restive peoples of the semi/peripheries, core working poor, the "lumpen," dissidents, unwanted immigrants & minorities, criminal elements

ENFORCED PACIFICATION

Support for local elites/authorities through MISSILE weaponry + securocratic measures

Figure 1.1   The global pacification system

broadcast the US's "hard power," the willingness to use military might as the "enforcer of last resort."

Towards this end, the Pentagon has divided the world into six military commands, and despite the unlikelihood of major interstate warfare, continues to spend inordinate amounts on its military. After reaching a low point in weapons production in the late 1990s, military spending rebounded, spurred by the Global War on Terror and the Iraq War. By 2011, the US defense budget had risen to $708 billion, the highest since World War II and a third more than it was at the height of the Vietnam War in 1968.[23] Despite the profits it generates for the arms industry, spending at that level has proven difficult to sustain. In February 2014, Secretary of Defense Chuck Hagel announced reductions of more than $75 billion over two years in the Pentagon's 2015 budget. While this reduced the military to its smallest size since before World War II—440,000 active duty soldiers, down from 520,000—a concomitant increase in Special Operations forces to 69,700 in anticipation of "asymmetrical" threats[24] shows that the commitment to global domination still exists. And while the Obama Administration plans to cut military spending to 2.3% of GDP in 2024, the lowest allocation in the post-World War II era,[25] the US still accounts for the lion's share of global military spending. Of the $1.75 trillion spent on the world's militaries in 2013, the Pentagon's budget accounted for 36 percent of the total—$640 billion—while core spending in general reached 50 percent of the world's military spending. (By contrast, the main counterhegemonic powers—Russia, China and Brazil—together accounted for only 17.6 percent.) In 2013, the US sold $61.5 billion in arms to other countries—nearly 30 percent of all weapons sales around the world. Factoring in NATO, the core's share of military spending went from a 49 percent share to 70 percent.[26]

Why such a heavy investment by the US and its core allies in weaponry designed to meet seemingly outdated "traditional challenges" of interstate warfare? Why did Britain spend more than $57 billion on arms and the military in 2010, the fourth largest military budget in the world, when its own Strategic Defence Review of 1998, since reiterated in various defense papers, concluded that "There is no direct military threat to the United Kingdom or Western Europe. Nor do we foresee the re-emergence of such a threat"?[27]

Placed in the context of preserving core hegemony, new generations of major platforms must be regarded first and foremost as "hegemonic weapons," less for use in actual fighting (they have proven largely inappropriate for asymmetrical warfare) than for intimidation. This is reflected in the remarks of Defense Secretary Robert Gates:

> What all these potential adversaries—from terrorist cells to rogue nations to rising powers—have in common is that they have learned that it is unwise to confront the United States directly on conventional military terms. The United States cannot take its current dominance for granted and needs to invest in the programs, platforms, and personnel that will ensure that dominance's persistence.[28]

Preserving the US as "the only nation able to project and sustain large-scale operations over extended distances" lies, then, at the base of American military strategy.[29] Thus, even if the relative strength of Euro-American hegemony appears to be on the decline, the absolute structural strength of their combined armed forces is assured with the deployment of advanced weapons systems based on precise "full-spectrum" military capabilities able to respond quickly anywhere in the world. The rationale of the Prompt Global Strike (PGS) capability echoes the hegemonic goals of the first task:

> A war can be won without being waged. Victory can be attained when an adversary knows it is vulnerable to an instantaneous and undetectable, overwhelming and devastating attack without the ability to defend itself or retaliate. What applies to an individual country does also to all potential adversaries and indeed to every other nation in the world.[30]

In the Pentagon's view, China is the only "rising power" of the semi-periphery that might challenge core hegemony.[31] And yet China is focused primarily on defending what it considers its own strategic hinterland, and that mainly against US incursions.[32] Although China is steadily modernizing its armed forces, hoping to become a major military power by 2050, its military spending ($216 billion in 2014) constituted only a third of that of the Americans.[33] China's goal in its incremental military build-up seems to be similar to that of the US—projecting power so that conflicts may be resolved in its own interests—but without the active hegemonic policies and practices of the American military, which maintains some 1,000 military bases in 174 countries and has eleven aircraft carrier battle groups circling the planet (no other potential adversary has more than one). China publicly states that it harbors no hegemonic designs or aspirations for territorial expansion.[34] Russia, the only other country able to mount a major military challenge to Euro-American hegemony but whose military expenditure is just a sixth of the American's, is virtually dismissed by the Pentagon.[35] It's worth noting that despite increases in Russian and Chinese military spending, the combined 2014 defense budgets of the top six NATO countries is three times that of Russia and China together.[36]

The countries of the core and semi-periphery possess enough deterrent power that wars between them are non-existent. Conventional interstate warfare may still be the form of war for which most militaries prepare, but the last war that pitched roughly equal state militaries against each other was the Iraq–Iran War, fought back in 1980–88, and before that, the "Yom Kippur War" of 1973.[37] Indeed, no first- or second-rate powers have engaged in more than border skirmishes with each other since World War II.[38]

Hegemonic Task 2: Maintaining Core Hegemony Over the Peripheries

Given the unlikelihood of major interstate warfare, military confrontations today fall mainly into the second task of global pacification: maintaining core hegemony over the peripheries of the world-system. For most of the so-called Third World, until recent years that relationship could best be described as "custodial": their sovereignty was contingent at best on the political, financial and military support of the core hegemons or their supranational surrogates. In the best of times, these regimes were shored up through "development" programs, ensuring, however, that the rulers have the military power to fend off challengers and the securocratic power to keep the population in line—as long as they cooperate in looting their own countries and maintaining a modicum of "stability." Hence the term "comprador elites." Not seeking outright domination or control, all Capital wants is to ensure the smooth flow of resources from the periphery to the core, as well as access to its cheap labor.[39] Custodial hegemony has been characterized as "military humanism,"[40] or as Empire Lite.[41]

Indeed, Duffield contends that "development has always been linked with what we now understand as counterinsurgency."[42] The vulnerable peripheries are the location of "small wars," "limited wars," "asymmetric wars," "resource wars," or "high-/low-intensity operations," beginning with the colonial wars of the 1960s and those accompanying the struggles of the Eastern European countries to free themselves from Soviet rule and continuing through the current campaign against ISIS. The aims of these small wars are limited and their impact localized. The "small wars" of the second half of the twentieth century, most often fought by third- and fourth-rate armed forces, were no less deadly or destructive, however, than previous inter-state ones.[43]

The decline of interstate wars has been countered by the rise of wars involving semi-state or non-state actors. For the most part, the major powers have stayed out of them, at best supplying arms but not taking sides as long as their interests are not greatly compromised. Kaldor describes localized identity wars as "new wars,"[44] although the looting of territories cursed (it seems) with valued resources often lay behind them. "When we speak of wars in the last third of the twentieth century," Tabb points out

> ... we are talking about civil wars. Between 1965 and 1999, if we look at those wars in which more than a thousand people were killed a year, there were seventy-three civil wars, almost all driven by greed to control resources—oil, diamonds, copper, cacao, coca, and even bananas ... countries with one or two primary export resources have more than a one-in-five chance of civil war in any given year. In countries with no such dominant products there is a one in a hundred chance ... Resource wars with their devastating impacts on civilians have become the norm ... Africa bleeds because of its abundant wealth.[45]

Civil wars generated by artificial states imposed on peoples from the colonial times often pit semi-legitimate state authorities against revolutionaries or "insurgents" of various kinds. Indeed, given the excesses and authoritarianism of many states of the periphery, small wars against rivals shade into generalized and endemic securocratic war against the restive population as a whole. What stands out in the shift from interstate to "new" wars is not the degree of bloodshed but whose blood is shed. Kaldor points to the dramatic reversal in the ratios of civilian to military casualties between the old and "new" wars. At the beginning of the twentieth century, 85–90 percent of casualties in war were military. That fell to half in World War II. By the late 1990s, 80 percent of war casualties were civilian, and by the turn of the twenty-first century, each and every conflict produced more than a million refugees and displaced persons.[46]

Only when these localized conflicts threaten the regional hegemony of one major power or another, or spill over in ways that threaten the smooth functioning of the world-system itself, do they assume the proportions of counterhegemony, however, thereby triggering intervention of outside powers. The Taliban in Afghanistan have defeated a number of world powers in succession. Forces of political Islam throughout the Middle East, North and West Africa and the Caucasus are extending into sub-Saharan Africa, as well as into Europe and as far as western China. The Pentagon's preoccupation with "asymmetrical" conflicts stems from the constant need to smooth out rough spots that may interfere with the global circulation of resources and goods, as well as to counter any counterhegemonic movement that may endanger key parts of the world-system. The attacks of 9/11 also exposed the vulnerability of the core countries themselves. In fact, the ability of "insurgents" in Iraq, Afghanistan, Pakistan, Yemen, Somalia, North Africa and elsewhere to hold their own against the core's vastly superior weaponry and forces while succeeding in disrupting life in the core itself has transformed counter-insurgency into a generalized securocratic campaign. The Pentagon's Quadrennial Defense Review (QDR) of 2006 was entitled *The Long War*, a phrase meant to replace "the War on Terror." It asserts that

> Since 2001, the U.S. military has been continuously at war, but fighting a conflict that is markedly different from wars of the past. The enemies we face are not nation-states but rather dispersed non-state networks. In many cases, actions must occur on many continents in countries with which the United States is not at war. Unlike the image many have of war, this struggle cannot be won by military force alone, or even principally. And it is a struggle that may last for some years to come ... .[47]

The militaries of the US and their partners have been deployed in recent years mainly to carry out regime change, nation building and counter-insurgency, invading countries enjoying only contingent sovereignty with impunity. This reorientation of the core's armed forces from inter-state warfare to counter-insurgency and urban warfare is described by the Pentagon as a new "global military force posture."[48] It is geared towards contending with "hybrid warfare" that pits conventional military forces against "a combination of state and non-state actors ... that simultaneously and adaptively employs a tailored mix of conventional, irregular, terrorism and criminal means or activities in the operational battlespace."[49] Hybrid threats include "rogue states" (a highly subjective and tendentious term, to say the least), semi- or non-state actors such as Chechnyan or Tamil fighters, Hezbollah, al Qaeda, the Taliban, Hamas in Gaza and, most recently, ISIS, Mexican or Colombian drug cartels and other highly organized criminal networks, plus even more "hybrid" forces of regular and irregular soldiers, gangs and ethnic groups ravaging the Congo and West Africa. The picture, however, is far more complicated. One could argue that the greatest source of counterhegemony in the world-system—indeed, the major threat to the world-system dominated by the Global North—is Saudi Arabia and the Gulf States, supposed allies and the source of much of its energy, yet suppliers of military wares, finances and radical Islamic ideology to Sunni jihadists. It is worth noting that in 2014 Saudi Arabia spent $81 billion on its military, as much as Russia, and its purchase of more than $6 billion in military hardware makes it the world's largest importer of arms; the UAE spent $23 billion more.[50] Saudi Arabia may not be a rogue state but something even less controllable: an entity that employs state mechanisms to pursue proxy wars far beyond its borders.[51] Iran, too, plays a similar role in Shi'ite insurgencies, though its defense budget is only around $10 billion.[52]

Here, radical Islam intersects with failed custodial hegemony. The 2006 QDR tellingly identifies rising conflict zones as North Africa, the Horn of Africa and South East Asia—all areas identified by Klare as future arenas of resource wars and all areas in the grip of Islamic insurgencies.[53] Not that all of the endemic conflicts on the periphery arise from religious or political ideology, as Kaldor reminds us. "With coldblooded lucidity," writes Davis, American war planners

> ... now assert that the "feral, failed cities" of the Third World—especially their slum outskirts—will be the distinctive battlespace of the twenty-first century. Pentagon doctrine is being reshaped accordingly to support a low-intensity world war of unlimited duration against criminalized segments of the urban poor.

As global poverty becomes urbanized, so, too, does war; Davis terms it "the urbanization of insurgency."[54]

Hybrid wars pose threats to militarily stronger countries since non-state actors, mobile, not confined to a particular battlefield or locale and able to access a wide range of weapons, can reach their population centers far from the actual scenes of conflict. "While it is clear that the United States will dominate conventional adversaries for the foreseeable future," writes General James Mattis, Commanding General of the US Marine Corps Combat Development Command,

> ... our conventional superiority creates a compelling logic for states and non-state actors to move out of the traditional mode of war and

seek some niche capability or some unexpected combination of technologies and tactics to gain an advantage [in] a projected world of more unconventional adversaries. Of course, the greatest probability is the rise of so called irregular challengers. Irregular methods—terrorism, insurgency, unrestricted warfare, guerrilla war, or coercion by narco-criminals—are increasing in both scale and sophistication and will challenge U.S. security interests globally.

We expect future enemies to look at the four approaches [catastrophic, traditional, disruptive and irregular] as a sort of menu and select a combination of techniques or tactics appealing to them … This unprecedented synthesis is what we call Hybrid Warfare.[55]

Hybrid war, a form of what the British general Rupert Smith calls "war amongst the people," therefore has strong securocratic elements. One side of the "hybrid" equation may be conventional military force, but the other is securocratic, the threat posed to societies from "below." "Our opponents," writes Smith

… are formless, and their leaders and operatives are outside the structures in which we order the world and society. They are the "insurgents" in Iraq, the "terrorists" in the Philippines or the Israeli-occupied territories, or the armies of the "war-lords" in Afghanistan and Africa … The threats they pose are not directly to our states or territories but to the security of our people, of other peoples, our assets and way of life. They are of and amongst the people—in the flesh and in the media—and it is there that the fight takes place.[56]

In these conflicts, that admittedly can't be won and which entail prolonged periods of occupation, core militaries are by necessity being "policized."[57] A corollary to this is the militarization of the security services and police forces of the dependent states of the periphery. Human-security states have always been the norm in the semi-periphery and peripheries of the world-system where fragile regimes strive to keep order over societies whose social and economic fabric has been fundamentally disrupted by neoliberal policies of "development." They preside over ethnic and religious polyglots characterized by wide disparities of wealth, high levels of endemic violence and "uninsured lives" lacking any safety net whatsoever, and are driven by the logic of securitization.[58] This warehousing of "bare lives" in countries barely sovereign is, as Duffield contends, a recipe for unending war.[59] When "development" fails to create a state system capable of providing for the basic needs of its people, and when in fact a government must assert its authority to make up for a loss of popular support, the result is enforced pacification, securocratic repression carried out jointly by the military, Presidential Guards and elite or special ops units, paramilitaries, security services and the police. Indeed, says van Creveld, most of the world's armed forces are fielded by countries that have no need for them other than internal security or enforced comprador hegemony.[60]

Hegemonic Task 3: Ensuring the Control of Transnational Elites of the Core and Semi-Periphery Over Their Own Societies

Securocratic pacification has become increasingly evident among the core states themselves as the ruling classes impose neoliberal regimes of austerity and declining social services over the middle and working classes. In order to counter growing employment insecurity and to deflect attention from the effects of underemployment extending into the middle class, even as income disparities balloon to unprecedented proportions, the ruling classes have focused public attention on security threats, thus opening the way to securitization as a kind of pacification. Pacification in the core societies has its own particular colorization: it is packaged in as "consensual" a form as possible, in keeping with the ethos of core-state democracy.

The assertion of hegemony begins, then, with the "soft power" of consensus in the Gramscian sense of "cultural hegemony," domination through fostering a popular identification of the people with the values, symbols and agendas of the ruling classes—patriotism, religion and sports being among the most powerful. The more successful the fabrication of consensus, the more social control can devolve to agencies that merely "maintain social order," the classic definition of the police. Ideally, the role of domestic security agencies, the police, the judicial system, the prisons, the social welfare system and other agents of discipline becomes so self-evident and routine that they are generally perceived as little more than necessary mechanisms of regulation. Where they truly discipline and punish—among marginalized minorities, the working poor or unemployed, unwanted immigrants, criminal elements and dissidents—is kept out of the public eye or, if visible, is lauded as "defending the public."

When consensus weakens, however, hegemony must be asserted more broadly. In what is actually class-based securocratic war, the authorities' efforts to ensure the "security" of the public conceals a deeper agenda of "securing the insecurities" inherent to capitalism itself.[61] Core countries drift towards becoming "securocratic states," or "human-security states",[62] and Tasks 2 and 3 merge to a certain degree: "The crossover between the military and the civilian applications of advanced technology—between the surveillance and control of everyday life in Western cities and the prosecution of aggressive colonial and resource wars—is at the heart of … the new military urbanism" writes Graham:

> Policing, civil law enforcement, and security services are melding into a loosely, and internationally, organized set of (para)militarized "security forces." A "policization of the military" proceeds in parallel with the "militarization of the police" … "High intensity policing" and "low intensity warfare" threaten to merge … Western security and military doctrine is being rapidly reimagined in ways that dramatically blur the juridical and operational separation between policing, intelligence and the military; distinctions between war and peace; and those between local, national and global operations. [Wars] become both boundless and more or less permanent.[63]

And then there is the economics of it all. A prescient President Eisenhower addressed the dangers of the emerging military-industrial complex in the US already in the 1950s, but by the 1970s the neoliberal program of using government to protect and advance corporate interests, particularly through policies of privatization and outsourcing, had introduced strong economic incentives into the development, spread and use of military systems.[64] The same can be said of Homeland Security. Klein notes that the global homeland security industry was economically insignificant before 2001; by 2007 it was a $200 billion sector. By 2013, it had grown to $415.5 billion and, driven by the threat of cross-border terrorism, cybercrime, piracy, the drug trade, human trafficking, internal dissent and separatist movements, is expected to gross $544 billion by 2018.[65] Klein points out that when the Bush Administration seized on the opportunity offered by 9/11 to launch a multi-pronged "War on Terror," it made it "an almost completely for-profit venture, a booming new industry that has breathed new life into the faltering U.S. economy."[66] The threats proved congenial not only to the time-tested strategy of harnessing fear as a pretext for protecting privilege, but 9/11 became a means to mobilize Gramscian consensus around patriotism, identity with the neocon's political agenda abroad and the ability to impose strict control *á la* the PATRIOT Act at home. There is even an official Department of Homeland Security Industry Day held annually in Washington.

Phase 4: Securitization

In terms of the global pacification, Hegemonic Task 1 remains the overarching one for the transnational elites and their allies. Maintaining hegemony over the world-system has its impact. Producing major weapons platforms for core armies devours massive financial resources and distorts major economies. It also provides technology for lesser systems of securitization. It is a form of pacification not directly felt by people, however. Big Power "projection of power" does its job without major interventions. The fall of the Soviet Union shows how it can work effectively without firing a shot. How the core militaries will react to the next major hegemonic challenge, especially if it threatens the current system of Euro/American-centric capitalism, remains to be seen. For the moment, what concerns us particularly are wars associated with Tasks 2 and 3, whose success is measured by how well they have securitized a society, that of adversaries or the hegemon's own, militarily or through effective policing.

All wars have securocratic dimensions, of course, beginning with the immediate securing of the terrain after a battle or advance; so do police actions. In military terms, securitization comprises "Phase 4" warfare. After the first three phases of any war—defining its goals, determining its operational requirements, and initiating decisive operations—Phase 4 calls for planning and engaging in post-conflict stability operations as antagonists transition from warfare to peace and civilian government control.[67] While Phase 1 may be more or less thought out, the history of wars, the vicissitudes of battle and the degree to which victory is achieved, invariably center on Phases 2 and 3. And since wars are supposed to end with victory, least thought is given to Phase 4. The victors dictate the terms; the vanquished have little choice but to submit. The US had no plan whatsoever for post-conflict Iraqi stabilization, relying on overwhelming "Shock and Awe" of Phase 1 to do the trick.[68]

As warfare moves from conventional interstate war to "hybrid wars" ("wars amongst the people") and on to "securocratic wars" fought by domestic security and police forces against those who may challenge the hegemonic order (Figure 1.2), Phase 4 "stability operations"—

securitizing—becomes the primary common denominator. Securitization and ultimately pacification underlie what I call the MISSILE Complex, the integrated use of the Military, Internal Security, Surveillance, Intelligence and Law Enforcement.

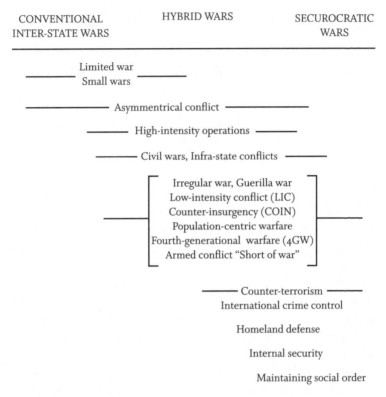

CONVENTIONAL   HYBRID WARS   SECUROCRATIC
INTER-STATE WARS   WARS

Limited war
Small wars

Asymmentrical conflict

High-intensity operations

Civil wars, Infra-state conflicts

Irregular war, Guerilla war
Low-intensity conflict (LIC)
Counter-insurgency (COIN)
Population-centric warfare
Fourth-generational warfare (4GW)
Armed conflict "Short of war"

Counter-terrorism
International crime control

Homeland defense

Internal security

Maintaining social order

Figure 1.2   Phase 4 "Stabilizing operations" and securitization

Wars of securitization are total and perpetual. What is more, when they are waged by core powers, they are waged in the name of liberal, universal values, making it difficult to even identify them as wars representing particular interests, another advantage of hegemony even in its asserted forms. Securocratic warfare is fought in the name of everyone, its seemingly self-evident assaults are assaults on everyone's enemies—the "War on ... " phenomenon. Ironically, securocratic warfare is liberal warfare; it claims to fight for perpetual peace and universal human emancipation: the good of the world-system, the good of liberal civilization and, indeed, the good of the human species being identified with the need to pursue a (capitalist) world order that is totally securitized.

"Liberal imperialism" acts out of the assumption that deviation from liberal norms poses a danger not only to the world-system it dominates, but to no less than life itself. This is what justifies "asymptomatic intervention," preventive measures at home and pre-emptive war abroad. War is thus rendered endemic, since it is neither possible nor desirable to end the "permanent emergency" which threatens to make life in the core ungovernable. In fact, the emergency governs. Pacifying humanity becomes the only way to remove war, but that endeavor itself becomes a violent, never-ending, totalitarian project—war with unlimited means to unlimited ends. Liberal capitalism, then, spawns a manner of global rule shaped by an inherent commitment to war and constant preparedness for war. It's a supreme irony, say Dillon and Reid, that "The martial face of liberal power is directly fueled by universal and pacific ambitions."[69]

The "template" that people are expected to internalize constitutes Foucault's governmentality, a "technology of domination" that creates and enforces a self-regulating global order seemingly without overt sources of sovereignty and power. Liberal capitalism thus promotes such "universal" values as individualism and individual responsibility, a better life through hard work, self-reliance, liberal democracy ("freedom"), human emancipation ("civilization," "our way of life"), inalienable human and civil rights, personal security, perpetual peace and, of course, the economic rationality of the market, whereas in reality they arise from the dictates of the capitalist workplace and market. When "soft power" proves inadequate, however, the core acts to *enforce* them, if not through the implementation of international law or appeals to supra-national regulators, then through unilateral wars and policing operations "for the public good."

Again, wars of securitization are total, a country's entire territory treated as an unrestricted battlespace extending across urban areas, regions of operations, the entire planet and on into cyberspace, the electromagnetic sphere and space itself. The Pentagon defines "battlespace," the limitless battlefield of post-modern war, as

> … the environment, factors, and conditions that must be understood to successfully apply combat power, protect the force, or complete the mission. This includes the air, land, sea, space, and the included enemy and friendly forces; facilities; weather; terrain; the electromagnetic

spectrum; and the information environment within the operational areas and areas of interest.[70]

The concept came into use with the introduction of "network-centric warfare" in the mid-1990s. "The new way of warfare exhibited over the last decade [the 1990s]," write military analysts Bowie, Hafa and Mullins,

> ... is not compatible with the clash of interstate armies that prevailed during the Cold War. Indeed, as opposed to the Eurocentric vision of warfare encompassing large armies and vital interests, the strategic center of gravity has moved to uncertain threats emanating from Asia ... Meanwhile, enemies of the future could include rogue states, nonstate actors, and possibly a peer competitor, all poised to undermine the use of force by the United States, with the objective of exploiting sensitivities to casualties, international public opinion, and battlefield vulnerabilities ... Militarily, there has been a dramatic trend away from scripted plans and operational orders to a fluid, nonlinear, and adaptive battlespace in which targets are generated while attack platforms are en route. Factors that account for this approach to target generation begin with requirements for extended reach in recent operations. Added to the tyranny of distance is the elusive nature of enemy forces and sketchy target sets characterized by fleeting opportunities, which are masked by deception.[71]

Battlespace, says Gray,

> ...is now three-dimensional and ranges beyond the atmosphere. It is on thousands of electronic wavelengths. It is on the "homefront" as much as on the battlefront ... Battle now is beyond human scale—it is as fast as laser beams; it goes 24 hours a day. It ranges through the frequency spectrum from ultralow to ultrahigh, and it also extends over thousands of miles ... Civilians, and nature itself, are usually more threatened than the soldiers are.[72]

Wars of securitization fought in an undifferentiated battlespace thus bring together "foreign" and domestic" spaces, both monitored in parallel by high-tech satellites, drones, "intelligent" CCTV, "non-lethal" weaponry, data mining and biometric surveillance.[73]

Nothing in principle now stands in the way of the core hegemons imposing a global order of their own, while securocratic wars in an undifferentiated global battlespace provide the vehicles of global pacification. When we critically employ the concept "pacification," writes Neocleous,

> … we are compelled to connect the police power to the war power. Indeed, as a *critical* concept "pacification" insists on conjoining war and police in a way which is fundamentally opposed to the mainstream tendency that thinks of war and police as two separate activities institutionalized in two separate institutions (*the* military and *the* police). This ideological separation…has imposed on scholars a banal dichotomy of "models," such as the "criminological model" versus the "military model" … the "militarization of the police" and the "policization of the military" or the coming together of "high intensity policing" with "low-intensity warfare." Such models obscure the unity of state power … "Pacification" is intended to grasp a nexus of ideas—war-police-accumulation—in the security of bourgeois order.[74]

Part II

A Pivotal Israel

2

Why Israel? The Thrust Into Global Involvement

How does Israel manage to constantly augment its international clout even as it pursues unpopular policies towards the Palestinians, policies that ultimately disrupt the entire Middle East and beyond? "Normal" diplomacy offers little insight into that puzzle. I began, therefore, to explore a less visible, parallel kind of diplomacy that I call "security politics": how a country parlays military prowess into political gain. In Israel's case, it leverages the development and sales of sophisticated weapons systems, military technologies, surveillance and security systems and counter-terrorist tactics into political influence, a "value-added" to normal international relations. If this is the basis of security politics, then it is by nature clandestine. Conducted by small, closed groups of political, economic and military elites representing interests hidden from public view, security politics circumvents formal channels of decision making and avoids parliamentary or public oversight. Security politics constitutes the dark underbelly of "normal" politics—a "shadow world" described in great detail by Feinstein[1] and Scahill.[2] It involves a wide array of actors—armies, paramilitaries, security firms, corporations, law enforcement agencies, criminal cartels and gangs—all of whom sell and exchange weaponry worth hundreds of billions of dollars, much of that for purposes the public would be unlikely to support. The goals of normal international relations, pursuit of a country's national interests, are fairly straightforward, although different governments may define their interests in different ways. Security politics adds to this two other elements: the role played by arms in helping allies or clients maintain power and assert their hegemony, and the role of profit.

Security politics have been noticed by others. Schelling uses the term "the diplomacy of violence,"[3] Dror speaks of "security statecraft,"[4] Abadi talks of "garrison state diplomacy,"[5] Perera offers "Uzi diplomacy,"[6] while Klieman refers to "weapons trade diplomacy" or simply "arms diplomacy."[7] For a small country like Israel, where its ability to compete in the global arms market, to harness military sales in order to develop technologies that are key to other areas of its economy, to obtain that political clout which comes from military parity with the Big Boys and to perpetuate its Occupation, security politics are key (Figure 2.1).

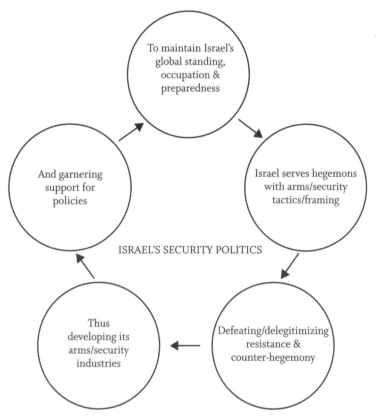

Figure 2.1   Israel's security politics

The need to pursue an aggressive security politics is what thrusts Israel into wide-ranging global involvement unusual for such a small country. Without an Occupation, Israel would have neither the drive nor the conditions by which to develop, deploy, test and export world-class weaponry and models of control; true, it would still need a military given the array of hostile forces in its region, but not one so exaggerated in power (nuclearized, for example), or demanding such aggressive international arms diplomacy. Without the Occupation to defend, without the claim to land and control beyond its recognized borders that the Occupation engenders, and without the military and securitization prowess Israel thereby acquired and needs to constantly nurture, it would resemble Finland or Vietnam: small countries facing significant military challenges yet able to balance military preparedness (symbolically at least) with the security afforded by broader diplomatic and military alliances.

A Nation-in-Arms: The Military Way

Now it could be argued that the pursuit of security politics, and certainly broader national interests, is not unique to Israel, which is by no means the only country, even the only small country, to engage in security politics or invest heavily in arms. Holland and Belgium do as well. Nor is it the only one threatened by, or that thinks it is threatened by, implacable enemies. In few countries, however, does the military play such a dominant role in government, the economy, the cultural life of its people, or in its international relations. Israel expends about $15 billion a year on its military, between 6.5–8.5 percent of its GDP.[8] Finland, by contrast, with a comparable GDP, spends $3.8 billion annually on defense (1.3 percent of its GDP). Morocco, engaged in a long war in the Western Sahara, spends $3.4 billion (3.4 percent), while Uganda, locked into prolonged external and internal warfare, spends only $3.4 million (2.3 percent). Even the US, by far the largest spender on its military, devotes only 4.3 percent of its GDP for defense (though that added up in 2011 to a staggering $708 billion). Venezuela under Hugo Chavez, bloated with oil revenues and rapidly modernizing and upgrading its armed forces, spent only $3.2 billion (1.4 percent) on its army. Israel, with the world's fifteenth highest defense budget, spends far more on its army than Iran, North Korea, Pakistan, or Egypt.[9]

On the surface, there seems good reason for this military build-up. Israel is by far the most conflict-prone state in modern history. It has fought six or seven interstate wars, three major Palestinian uprisings (the Revolt of 1936–39 and two Intifadas), has been involved in over 166 dyadic militarized interstate disputes (MIDs) that involved the threat, the display, or the use of military force against another state, and engaged in a violent military action of some magnitude against its neighbors, including the Palestinians of the Occupied Territories, during each and every year of its existence.[10] For the seventh year running, it has been named the "most militarized nation in the world" by the 2014 Global Militarisation Index (Singapore, whose army Israeli built, is ranked second).[11]

The assumptions that often justify such a preoccupation with security and the military—that the conflict has been thrust upon Israel and that its wars and continued suppression of the Palestinians arise out of *ein breira*, "no choice"—are questionable. Until the Syrian civil war and the rise of ISIS led to a general meltdown in the Middle East, Israel, despite its conflict with the Palestinians, enjoyed relative peace with the Arab world— *de jure* in regard to such key states as Egypt and Jordan, *de facto*, with many nuances such as informal security ties, economic representations and similar foreign policy goals, in its relations with the others. Despite the enmity of Hezbollah and Iran, the only obstacle to Israel's achieving security and acceptance in its region and beyond is its ongoing Occupation. In fact, since 1988 if not well before the Palestinians have been willing to recognize Israel within the 1967 borders, in return for a small state of their own. Israel's acceptance of the Arab Peace Initiative would have normalized its relations altogether.

So why, then, does not Israel move to end its conflicts with the Arab and Muslim worlds, in particular by ending its Occupation? Why did it not agree to a two-state solution back in 1988? Most pointedly, why does it *choose* to be the most militarized state in the world? Every ongoing event and short-term development offers compelling specific reasons for one action or another. Stepping back, however, reveals a longer-term political logic: Israel lives and has always lived in a state of deep cultural militarism. Ben-Eliezer describes the collective state of mind wherein Israelis came to view organized violence as the optimal solution for their political problems: the "Military Way." Emerging at the very start of the Zionist project in the 1880s, it crystallized over the decades into a deeply rooted feeling that military actions are legitimate, reasonable and desirable ways of dealing with "the Arabs"; indeed, it is the only way the Israeli–Arab conflict can be controlled and managed. Encapsulated in symbols, narratives, rituals, holidays, educational curricula and political discourse internalized by generations of Israeli Jews and reinforced by nearly universal military service, cultural militarism has become part of the natural order in Israel. Having military control over one's permanent enemies is preferred and is actually far less threatening than the alternatives: a dubious political solution involving existential compromises and the prospect of an Arab demographic takeover.[12]

With the establishment of Israel in 1948, militarism was officially entrenched in Israeli culture and policy making. The army became the primary instrument of nation building. Identification with the IDF would define and mobilize "Israeli-ness," not least among the young and the immigrants. For Ben-Gurion, Israel as "a nation-in-arms" should foster "a desire to fight and an ability to fight. In order to want to fight, there must be a nation, and we are not [yet] a nation."[13] Blurring distinctions among army, politics and society was considered, then, a *good* thing.[14] Cultivating the idea that Israel's wars are forced upon it *ein breira*, that "the few are pitted against the many," Israel's military culture keeps its populace in a constant state of mobilization.[15] In the end, a nation-in-arms comes to have "a large compulsory draft, a large reserve military with great involvement in wars and the preparation for them, a war industry and a war economy, and a national culture that sanctifies the military solution to political problems and that places the military and the soldier at society's center."[16] IDF Chief of Staff Yigael Yadin provided the quintessential expression of "positive militarism": "Every [Jewish] citizen is a soldier on eleven months' annual leave."[17]

The conquest of the rest of Palestine in 1967 only confirmed in the eyes of many Israelis the necessity and efficacy of militarism in determining political realities.[18] Indeed, while a two-state solution could have been achieved on terms extremely favorable to Israel at virtually any time from 1967 until the present (Arafat approached the US Administration already in 1973 in hopes of negotiating a solution), it instead *chose* the path of domination and pacification. Reiser attributes this to "the centrality of security" in Israeli political thought;[19] Maoz points more critically to an Israeli "proclivity to amass and use excessive military force despite diminishing threats."[20] Security, he goes on to say,

> ... has consistently dominated foreign policy. In virtually every major decision process, security considerations supersede diplomatic considerations ... The dominance of the security establishment in Israeli political affairs [derives from] the excessive involvement of former military personnel in almost every aspect of Israel's political, social, and economic life. An "old boys' network" was formed within the Israeli political elite, composed of former generals who have entered political life across the entire left-right continuum ... this network is characterized by a shared set of basic political and military beliefs— which largely follow Ben-Gurion's strategic philosophy.[21]

Central to Israel's security thinking are two fundamental assumptions: Arabs understand only force and, overall, they will never truly accept an Israeli state. Peace making, in this conception, actually weakens Israel's security by projecting weakness. "The basic belief is that the world does not function according to principles of justice and morality," says Peri. "Thus, the diplomatic method, negotiations, compromise, and reconciliation solutions are not really effective. What is effectual in the international arena is power ... Reality is shaped by the use of force, and if diplomacy does not achieve national goals, war is not a choice to be decried."[22]

Israel's emergence as a major military power took place already in the early 1950s, when France began supplying not only sophisticated arms but arms technology, some of which Israel still employs. This enabled Israel Military Industries (IMI, or *Ta'as*) to make major advances in the development and sales of arms by the mid-1950s. Israel was taken seriously enough as a military power that in June 1956, the French government agreed to provide it with a massive shipment of modern armaments, including Mystère IV jets, Super-Sherman tanks and tank transports, trucks, armored personnel carriers and ammunition, in return for Israeli participation in the planned joint attack on Egypt. (Besides being able to purchase first-line offensive weapons from France, heavy weaponry also arrived from the US, Britain and West Germany, the latter funding much of Israel's ability to purchase or acquire arms and grow its military industry through its massive reparations and restitutions.) When Israel took an active military role in attacking Egypt alongside Britain and France in the Sinai Campaign of 1956, its first conventional war, it took its place among the Global North countries fighting Soviet inroads, a pretext for its involvement in countering other attempts of Middle Eastern countries to self-determination, in Iran most visibly, but elsewhere as well.

The alliance with France lasted until 1967 when, post-Algeria, France began seeking renewed influence in the Middle East, finally breaking with Israel during the Six Day War. By this time, however, Israel had acquired capabilities in aeronautics, missilery and nuclear technology and the required infrastructure to develop its own arms industry, and was looking to diversify its sources of military supplies.[23] In fact, the shift to the next, and current, hegemonic protector, the United States, had been taking place from the early years of the Kennedy Administration, whose sale of the Hawk surface-to-air missile system proved the breakthrough that made other transfers of sophisticated weapons to Israel possible.[24]

In 1970, the US signed with Israel the Master Defense Development Data Exchange Agreement, the greatest transfer of US technology to any other country ever undertaken—a massive "giveaway" of American military technology, according to Neff.[25] It was made through what are called Technical Data Packages, a vast complex of blueprints, plans and types of materials required to actually construct weapons. Over the next eight years, more than 120 such packages were given to Israel. This massive infusion of technology, coupled with the 1975 Memorandum that gave Israel the access to American military technology necessary for establishing its own sophisticated arms industry, massively boosted Israel's economy. By 1981, Israel had emerged from being a technologically backward arms importer of modest weapons to the seventh largest exporter of military weapons in the world, with overseas sales of $1.3 billion. Klieman noted:

> The Americans have made virtually all their most advanced weaponry and technology, meaning the best fighter aircraft, missiles, radar, armor, and artillery, available to Israel. Israel, in turn, has utilized this knowledge, adapting American equipment to increase its own technological sophistication, reflected tangibly in Israeli defense offerings.[26]

Following the fall of the Shah's regime in Iran in 1979, a loss to both the US and Israel, the Reagan Administration signed another Memorandum of Agreement, this time expanding Israel's ability to compete with US companies for defense contracts on over five hundred items, from bombs and grenades to electrical components and parts for airplanes and tanks. Israel was not only competing with US firms, but the American government promised to purchase $200 million worth of Israeli weapons—all part of a $3 billion package of military aid, including the funding of Israel's redeployment from the Sinai to the Negev.[27] That was followed in turn by the Strategic Memorandum of 1981.

In 1983, following Israel's invasion of Lebanon and the Soviet Union's re-arming of Syria, the US fundamentally altered its relationship with Israel to the latter's benefit. In the context of the Cold War, the Reagan Administration redefined the axis of power in the Middle East as itself and Israel against the Soviet Union and Syria. Israel received close to $3.5 billion in military aid, most of it a grant, but more significant was the decision to integrate it into the US global defense system.[28] A Joint Political Military Group, the Defense Policy Advisory Group and the Strategic Dialogue Group were established to discuss shared threats and develop joint strategies. The two countries' navies and air forces held joint maneuvers and the US began to stockpile military equipment to which

Israel would have access in time of need. Israel was exempted from the requirement of spending Foreign Military Funds (FMF) exclusively in the US; 15 percent could be used to fund or purchase Israeli-made weaponry (such as the Lavi jet fighter and the Merkava tank). By 1982, the US was funding 37 percent of the Israeli defense budget.[29]

Despite such massive Big Power investments in Israel's arms industry and the high degree of technological capacity that country demonstrated, producing large platforms upon which other major arms producers derive their prestige, clout and much of their profit proved beyond the economic means of such a small state, as attempts to manufacture the Kfir and Lavi jet fighters, the Arava and Westwind planes and Sa'ar missile boats demonstrated. The fact that Israel produces several series of spy satellites and the rockets needed to launch them into space, together with a number of missile and anti-missile systems and the Merkava tank, nevertheless testifies to the country's technological capabilities, albeit supported with massive funding from abroad.[30]

It was that technological capacity which enabled Israel to move on to the next stage of its arms strategy, shifting from arms independence to niche-filling—developing and marketing technologically advanced sub-systems, or "add-on" technology.[31] Not only did this shift prove economically more do-able, but it proved no less effective as an approach to security politics, especially as weapons systems became more technologically sophisticated. By producing "dual-use" technologies of equally vital applicability to military and civilian markets, Israel was able to subsidize its arms manufacture with an economy of scale based on exports. Encouraged and facilitated by R&D grants from the Ministry of Trade and Industry, and boosted by privileged access to US, German and French military technology, by 1999, 39 percent of IAI's revenues came from the civilian sector, as did 38 percent of Elbit's.[32] The end of the Lavi project in 1987 marked that shift. Still, the launch of Israel's first satellite in 1988 demonstrated its continued ability to develop, manufacture and field major platforms, albeit with substantial foreign aid and access to military technology.

The shift away from "weapons independence" and self-sufficiency also reflected lessons learned in the cancellation of the Lavi fighter aircraft project. The cost of the project was one consideration. No less significant was the great opposition it aroused in the US. The Americans feared that the technology built into the Lavi would compete with that of American arms manufacturers themselves. Moreover, the Lavi project risked transferring sensitive technologies to foreign countries, especially if Israel sold the jet fighter, as it intended to do.[33] Israeli decision makers began to understand that competing with the US carried risks and was better packaged as niche-filling. The shift meant that henceforth the Israeli arms industry would supply the IDF with cutting-edge technological solutions for force multiplication, much easier to market abroad.

The development, deployment and export of conventional weapons systems and their high-tech components represent only one aspect of the Military Way; it has always been complemented by counter-insurgency, war amongst the people, stemming from Israel's prolonged conflict with the Palestinians and the need to garner support for its occupation policies. Already in 1909, soon after the Palestine Office of the World Zionist Organization began purchasing land, mainly from absentee landlords in Beirut, the first Zionist paramilitary unit was established. Described as more of a gang than an army, *Hashomer* (The Guard) was hired to evict the Arab tenant farmers who had long farmed those lands and to protect the Jewish settlers who replaced them.[34] Dressed in flamboyant costumes mixing Bedouin, Circassian and Cossack motifs, The Guard went far beyond passive protection. Taking as its battle-cry the motto "In blood and fire Judea shall rise again!", it was the first to take the military road, initiating reprisal raids when the Arabs tried to resist.[35]

The Guard's activities mark the beginning of the Israel–Arab conflict; indeed, it pioneered tactics that still stand at the heart of Israeli military thinking. "Escalation domination," for example, the intentional use of disproportionate force to intimidate the enemy, played a prominent role in both the Second Lebanon War and the 2014 assault on Gaza, now called respectively the Dahiya Doctrine and the Hannibal Procedure. The long-standing policy of "cumulative deterrence," the use of limited yet persistent force over time to instill fear and "respect" for the Jewish settlers, had its roots more than a century ago as well.[36] Such militaristic approaches characterized the struggle with the Palestinians leading up to the establishment of the state,[37] the early years of fighting the fedayun or "infiltrators" in the 1950s[38] and, since 1967, in establishing by force Israeli control over the Occupied Palestinian Territories (OPT).

Israel's export of its doctrines and tactics of counter-insurgency, including its ubiquitous weapons of suppression, the Uzi above all, has been well documented in a spate of books appearing first in the 1980s: Israel Shahak's *Israel's Global Role: Weapons for Repression*, the first critical study of Israel's security politics,[39] Steve Goldfield's *Garrison State: Israel's Role in U.S. Global Strategy*,[40] Bishara Bahbah's *Israel and Latin America: The*

Military Connection,[41] Milton Jamail and Margo Gutierrez' *It's No Secret: Israel's Military Involvement in Central America*,[42] Binyamin Beit-Hallahmi's *The Israel Connection: Who Arms Israel and Why*,[43] Flapan's *The Birth of Israel: Myths and Realities* (1987), and Andrew and Leslie Cockburn's *Dangerous Liaison: The Inside Story of the U.S.-Israeli Covert Relationship*,[44] among others. Three more recent publications that nevertheless rely mainly on data from the 1980s are Thomas's *The Dark Side of Zionism: Israel's Quest for Security Through Dominance*,[45] IJAN's *Israel's Worldwide Role in Repression*,[46] and Almond's article "British and Israeli Assistance to U.S. Strategies of Torture and Counterinsurgency in Central and Latin America, 1967–96: An Argument Against Complexification."[47] "Perhaps because we are so immersed in our perpetual struggle here in Israel and the occupied territories," Shahak mused, "we tend to forget that in recent years, the State of Israel has also assumed an additional task of great magnitude: to be an ally and arms supplier to the most contemptible and hated regimes in the world."[48]

Beit-Hallahmi is less sparing:

> Mention any trouble spot in the Third World over the past 10 years, and, inevitably, you will find smiling Israeli officers and shiny Israeli weapons on the news pages. The images have become familiar: the Uzi submachine gun or the Galil assault rifle, with Israeli officers named Uzi and Galil, or Golan, for good measure. We have seen them in South Africa, Iran, Nicaragua, El Salvador, from Seoul to Tegucigalpa, from Walvis Bay to Guatemala City, from Taipei to Port-au-Prince, Israeli citizens and military men have been helping, in their own words, in "the defense of the West".[49]

Alongside weaponry and Israeli military "trainers," Israel offers a model of securocratic control that I call the Matrix of Control. The Matrix had already emerged in 1948 when a military regime was imposed over the country's Palestinian citizens. Ended in 1966, it was immediately transferred onto the OPT the very next year. Over the past half-century, it has been refined into an effective model of securitization. For the first twenty years, Occupation was known as the "easy" or "enlightened" occupation, when the IDF faced few security threats and little resistance. With the outbreak of the First Intifada in 1987 and the beginning of the Oslo peace process in 1993, the Matrix further refined its model of control by outsourcing much of the military control of the OPT to a Palestinian Authority, which operates under clear IDF directives, as well as by establishing massive "facts on the ground," that prejudice any negotiations and render Israeli control irreversible. The attacks of 9/11, the Bush Administration's declaration of war on "global terror" and the American-led invasion of Iraq in 2003 have all foisted Israel's extensive experience in dealing with Palestinian "terror" into demand. Exporting the Matrix has become central to Israel's security politics, offering as it does an effective model of counterinsurgency, stabilization and long-term pacification.

Moreover, freed from the constraints of the Oslo peace process by a supportive Bush Administration and its Global War on Terrorism, Israel was able to unleash the full force of its military against the Palestinians' "infrastructure of terrorism." Operation "Defensive Shield," launched in March 2002, effectively ended Palestinian resistance in the West Bank. The Military Way seemed vindicated—and, indeed, universalized. Terrorist insurgencies regarded by Western militaries as "unwinnable wars" can be defeated, Israel argues, in a way crucial for its security politics, by conventional armies. We will show you how.[50]

Table 2.1 summarizes the evolution of Israeli security politics.

Table 2.1   The evolution of Israel's security politics

1882–Present:	The Military Way
1948–Present:	A Nation-in-arms seeking a big power patron (France: Early 1950s–1967; US: 1967–the present; NATO)
	The early version of the Matrix of Control developed through the Military Government imposed on Palestinian citizens of Israel (1948–1966)
1967–1990s:	Surge in military growth of industry for conventional "arms independence" (Kfir & Lavi jet fighters; Arava and Westwind planes; Sa'ar missile boats, etc.)
	Last Israeli–Arab conventional war (1973)
	Israel passes on captured Soviet arms to West
	Israel engages in counter-insurgency in Third World, often as American surrogate
	"Lazy" Occupation until First Intifada (1987); consolidation of the Matrix of Control as a securocratic model
1990s:	Post-Soviet downturn in world/Israeli arms industry First Intifada, Oslo and the outsourcing of the Occupation to the PA
2000–Present:	New surge in arms production, but strategic and do-able "niche-filling" shift to OPT as a laboratory and a source
	Second Intifada (2001) and development of weapons of scrutinization

Arms And Israeli Security Politics

In his book *Israel's Global Reach: Arms Sales as Diplomacy*, published in 1985 when Israel's arms exports were a sixth of what they are today, the Israeli military scholar Aaron Klieman spelled out clearly the logic of Israel's security politics. Arms sales, he wrote at that time

> ... represent a central component of Israel's external relations, defense posture, and foreign trade ... the manufacture and transfer of Israeli arms can be expected to figure prominently in the search for security, economic viability, and also as an independent course of diplomacy ... [In addition to bolstering Israel's overall military might,] weapons transfers outside of Israel are presented as serving, directly or indirectly, at least four additional military and defense functions. These are: (a) strengthening the Israeli army's immediate, intermediate, and longer-range preparedness goals; (b) enhancing Israeli deterrence capability by projecting a positive image of strength; (c) fitting into a wider strategic perspective; and (d) doubling as a tool of diplomacy through supporting countries friendly to Israel ... .[51]

Klieman then identifies five major ways in which arms diplomacy contributes to Israeli security politics: arms as influence and prestige, Israeli arms and their connection to Western security and American interests in particular, arms as independence, arms as military contacts, and arms as commerce. (He also mentions arms and "the Jewish factor," but that's less relevant for us here.)[52] Let's follow his useful framework for charting our initial discussion of Israeli security politics.

Arms as Influence, Arms as Prestige

"Arms diplomacy" has a compound effect on normal diplomatic relations. Trade in arms alone might not have a direct policy impact; looking at the rupture in relations between Israel and Turkey, two longstanding military partners, it may not even prevent a rupture of relations with a close ally. It does, however, enhance bilateral political relationships, creating attachments and vital joint interests that may well be parlayed into broader political support. Being able to parlay Russia's influence over Iran, Syria and perhaps even Hezbollah is one reason Israel has worked to strengthening its military ties with Moscow. "We obviously gained greatly from Russia's decision to cancel a huge S300 PMU contract with Iran," said a senior official of Israel's Ministry of Defense, referring to the $800 million contract for surface-to-air missiles signed in 2007, but terminated in 2011 after intense Israeli lobbying with Russia.[53]

Israel, says Klieman,[54] "does subscribe to the commonly accepted thesis that friends can be won and nations influenced to some degree by indirect, day-to-day access by providing some of their security needs." Military relationships have "given Israel some small but crucial influence over events in many areas where other instruments of foreign policy do not work." Kumaraswamy agrees:

> More than six decades after its founding, arms sales remains Israel's most effective foreign policy instrument. Its close ties with countries are often measured by the depth of military-security ties. This was true for countries as diverse as Turkey, Singapore, South Korea, South Africa (during apartheid), and India since 1992. Despite being dependent on the US, Israel has emerged as a key player in the international arms market, especially in areas such as high-tech weaponry, upgrading, intelligence gathering, surveillance, and counter-terrorism.[55]

Indeed, in the US, by far Israel's most important patron, the arms industry represents the most important special interest pressing for strong US support of the Israeli government:

> The military-industrial complex has a considerable stake in encouraging massive arms shipments to Israel and other Middle Eastern US allies and can exert enormous pressure on members of Congress who do not support a weapons-proliferation agenda,…particularly when so many congressional districts include factories that produce this military hardware.
>
> The arms industry contributes more than $7 million each election cycle to Congressional campaigns, twice that of pro-Israel groups. In terms of lobbying budgets, the difference is even more profound: Northrop Grumman alone spends seven times as much money in its lobbying efforts annually than does AIPAC and Lockheed Martin outspends AIPAC by a factor of four. Similarly, the lobbying budget of AIPAC is dwarfed by those of General Electric, Raytheon, and Boeing and other corporations with substantial military contracts.[56]

Israel's close military/political relations with Washington carry other benefits as well. Israel is uniquely situated to act as a mediator between the major military powers and lesser ones seeking to benefit from its privileged contact, positioned in particular "intermediately between the Western superpower and skittish developing countries."[57] Israeli diplomats "are not above suggesting the purchase of its military goods as an acceptable and fair *quid pro quo* for using the near legendary strength of the pro-Israeli lobby in the Congress and its influence with the American Jewish community on behalf of the arms client."[58] El Salvador hoped its close ties with Israel would induce the pro-Israel lobby in the United States to lend a "discreet hand" in congressional debates to push for higher U.S. military aid levels. So, too, did the Chilean regime hope that published photos of General Pinochet with high-ranking Israelis such as former Chief of Staff Mordechai Gur, who visited Chile during the *junta*, would help make it more palatable.[59]

"Arms as influence" shades into a less tangible form of influence, which Klieman calls "arms as prestige." "Being associated with the international traffic in weapons," observes Klieman

> ... does confer certain positive symbolic benefits, especially for a small state like Israel for whom power is a function of reputation, of how it is perceived by others ... Arms are a signal to friends and enemies alike of Israel's strength and determination to act in defense of its vital interests ... They suggest that it pays to be on good terms with Israel; that Israel has something more tangible than moral support to offer governments prepared to deal with it; that it has global reach ... Such triumphs of Israeli statecraft as the resumption of diplomatic relations with Zaire, Liberia, and Sri Lanka [to which today we might add Brazil, India and China] ... are attributable in large part to the interest these countries have in gaining military support from Israel.[60]

Klieman mentions the interest and visibility generated by Israel's participation in international trade fairs as a tangible expression of arms-as-prestige. "Success in this arms market," he suggests

> ... confirms not only that Israel is a reality of international life but that it is also a factor to be reckoned with in world as well as in regional politics. Here again, the symbolic importance is inestimable given Israel's continuing diplomatic struggle for legitimacy and international recognition.[61]

Indeed, the increasing number of subsidiaries opened by Israeli arms companies abroad, to the degree that they provide local leverage for Israeli firms, contribute as well to Israel's arms-as-influence.

Arms, Western Security and the United States

Israel's national security doctrine rests on a fundamental tenet: the country's security and perhaps its very existence depends on cultivating special relations with a superpower, meaning, since 1967, the United States.[62] By the time American Secretary of State Dulles visited Israel in 1953, Ben-Gurion made it clear that Israel stood as a western bastion in the Middle East; indeed, Israel saw itself as part of the West, not of the Middle East. When its special relationship with France ended in 1967, Israel shifted its strategic partnership to the US, together with its western allies and, of course, NATO. Israel's stellar performance in the 1967 war and its readiness to transfer captured Soviet arms and technology to the West convinced the Johnson Administration to sell Israel additional Hawk missiles and Phantom fighters, marking the true beginning of the "special relationship," and establishing the policy of guaranteeing Israel a qualitative military edge over its neighbors.[63] In 1989, the Reagan Administration conferred on Israel the status of a major non-NATO ally (MNNA). This has endowed Israel with even greater military privileges and benefits. As a MNNA, Israel is able to purchase American defense equipment on favorable financial terms and acquire restricted weaponry such as anti-tank rounds made of depleted uranium, cluster bombs and other anti-personnel weapons, used by Israel in its assaults on Lebanon and Gaza. It can bid on certain defense contracts for the repair and maintenance of military equipment outside the United States, and participate in joint training exercises. Most important for Israel, it can join in cooperative research and development projects with the Department of Defense, thus obtaining privileged access to American military technology—despite complaints that Israel illicitly profited from US technology at considerable cost to American companies and even to US security. By the early 1990s, Israel and the US were engaged in 322 cooperative ventures valued at $2.9 billion, together with 49 programs involving Israel in co-development, co-production, or research with American weapons manufacturers.[64] Crucially for Israel's economies of scale and security politics alike, its MNNA status also allows it to transfer US military technology into its own domestically produced weapons then sold to third countries, or to transfer American military technology directly to other countries (albeit in a supposedly supervised manner).

As the years passed, Israel became the largest recipient of direct American economic and military assistance, receiving as of 2014 more than $121 billion in bilateral assistance, almost all of it in the form of military aid.[65] Indeed, almost half of all American military assistance each year goes to Israel.[66] In late March 2003, just days after the invasion of Iraq, President George W. Bush approved a special grant of $1 billion on top of the $2.7 billion regular fiscal year 2003 assistance and $9 billion in economic loans guaranteed by the US government over the next three years.[67]

No less important, US policy guarantees Israel a "qualitative military edge" (QME) over all other militaries of the region. The Naval Vessel Transfer Act of 2008 defined the QME as

> ... the ability [of Israel] to counter and defeat any credible conventional military threat from any individual state or possible coalition of states or from non-state actors, while sustaining minimal damage and casualties, through the use of superior military means, possessed in sufficient quantity, including weapons ... that in their technical characteristics are superior in capability to those of such other individual or possible coalition of states or non-state actors.[68]

Any proposed arms sales to any country in the Middle East "other than Israel" must include a determination that the sale or export of the defense articles or services will not adversely affect Israel's QME.[69]

This has generated an American arms race in the Middle East of obvious benefit to the Pentagon and especially to American defense contractors, but not coincidentally to Israel as well. Between 2008 and 2012, Israel imported $1.35 billion in arms, placing it thirtieth among recipient states, with 95 percent of the weaponry coming from the US, representing approximately 6.4% of its total arms exports.[70] Still, Israel was only the fifth largest importer of military goods in its region. Saudi Arabia spent $52.1 billion on arms, the UAE $17.2 billion, Egypt $8.9 billion and Iraq $6.7 billion, compared to Israel's expenditure of $5.9 billion.[71] Nonetheless, since the QME policy requires a superiority of Israeli arms, Israel's military power and its ability to acquire cutting-edge technology constantly spirals upwards. Saudi Arabia, an American ally supposedly threatened by Iran, was allowed to purchase advanced F-15 fighters, but only after Israel was able to buy 20 new F-35 fifth-generation Lockheed Martin stealth fighters (with $2.75 billion in American military assistance).[72] Since then, Israel has purchased another 14 with an option for an additional 17, eventually bringing Israel's F-35 fleet up to two operational squadrons of 24 planes apiece.[73]

Israel, together with a handful of other countries (Egypt, South Korea, Turkey and Greece), also enjoys special "offset" arrangements, or "reciprocal purchase deals," with the Americans. That means it is able to divert funds into its own arms industry or, conversely, that American arms contractors can spend a portion of the contract in Israel instead of the US. Israeli companies also manufacture some of the major components of the F-35. In 2014, Israel Aerospace Industry (IAI) opened a production line for F-35 wings. It expects to produce 811 pairs of wings over the next 20 years. IAI will provide wings for the Israeli Air Force's 50 F-35s, as well as for the US Air Force and European customers, with the exception of Turkey. Israel's contribution to the F-35 project is valued at $4 billion.[74]

In 2007, the Bush Administration approved a 10-year, $30 billion military aid package that gradually raises Israel's annual Foreign Military Financing (FMF) grant from a baseline of nearly $2.55 billion in 2009 to approximately $3.1 billion for 2013–18 (not to mention special grants periodically awarded Israel, such as those for developing the Iron Dome rocket defense shield). In the aftermath of the 2006 war in Lebanon, four FMF arms packages, worth an estimated at $1.2 billion, replenished Israel's arsenal of missiles, munitions, bomb kits and support gear, plus hundreds of millions of gallons of fuel and an array of new munitions such as Paveway laser-guided bombs, cluster bombs (up to 4 million were dropped on Lebanese soil in 2006, 1 million of which remain unexploded), Joint Direct Attack Munitions (JDAM) kits and GBU-28 "bunker busting" bombs.[75] Indeed, under the "special relationship," the US sells Israel state-of-the-art arms often unavailable even to America's allies, or those developed in joint US-Israeli projects. The US, for example, will supply the Israel Air Force with 102 F-16s, specially designed for Israeli use (it is tellingly named the F-16I or *Sufa*, "Storm" in Hebrew). The Israeli F-16I enables Israel to carry out retaliatory strikes throughout the Middle East; it is capable of reaching targets well within Iran without having to refuel, thus boosting Israel's deterrent power.[76]

For all this, the amount of military assistance is even greater than official figures indicate. Unlike other countries, Israel receives its military aid in a single annual deposit into an interest-bearing account with the Federal Reserve Bank, the interest then used to service debts from earlier

Israeli non-guaranteed loans. Uniquely, Israel is also allowed to use 25–35 percent of the assistance package to buy arms, technology and equipment from non-American sources, including from its own domestic companies, representing a significant subsidy.[77] When, for instance, a missile defense system against rockets coming in from Gaza became a national priority, Congress budgeted more than $900 million so that Rafael, an Israel for-profit company, could develop it, allocating yet another $947 million in 2013. This, despite the fact that Israel is exporting the system for profit, one of its potential buyers being the American Army itself![78]

The War Reserves Stocks for Allies plan allows Israel to access up to $1.8 billion worth of US armored vehicles and artillery munitions stored in Israel, which it did in the 2006 invasion of Lebanon and, more recently, in Operation Protective Edge. In July 2012, President Obama signed the United States-Israel Enhanced Security Cooperation Act that, among other benefits, provides Israel with surplus weapons and equipment made available by the American withdrawal from Iraq and pushes for an expanded role for Israel in NATO. In 2014, President Obama signed into law the United States-Israel Strategic Partnership Act (approved by the House 410–1 and by the Senate unanimously), again declaring Israel a "major strategic partner" and granting it access to information, programs and joint projects in defense, intelligence, homeland security, science, trade and other areas not available to any other country, while also reaffirming Israel's QME. The Act requires the Pentagon to spell out how major weapons sales to Middle Eastern countries would alter the balance in the region and whether the US government had made any security assurances to Israel in conjunction with the sale.[79] Significantly, the bill approves the sale of military equipment to Israel that would enable it to execute an air strike on Iran, in particular advanced aerial refueling tankers necessary for Israeli fighter jets to reach targets in Iran, which had been refused to Israel by the Bush administration. This follows a proposed sale of twelve V-22 Osprey helicopters, ideal platforms for sending Israeli special forces into Iran, making Israel the first country outside the US to deploy them.[80]

Of prime importance is Israel's ability to access privileged US military technology, enter into joint military projects and serve as a major subcontractor for the Pentagon and American arms companies—crucial for a small country with limited production capabilities of its own. The degree to which Israeli military technology is integrated with that of the US and other countries—and why it is so difficult to categorize weapons system as "American" or "Israeli"—is graphically illustrated by Israel's Sa'ar-5 missile boats. From the 1980s into the early 2000s, Israel produced missile boats in its own shipyards. Construction proved too costly, however, and the Sa'ar-5 class was subcontracted to Northrop Grumman of the US, which built three corvettes: the *Eilat* and the *Lahav*, both launched in 1993, and the *Hanit*, launched in 1994. These ships, designed to remain at sea for long periods of time, are primarily deployed as command ships for task forces. They are therefore equipped with Israeli-made combat systems installed by IAI's MBT Missile Division, which specializes in integrated naval combat suites for new ships and in upgrades to existing ships, as well as in the design and production of naval attack missiles, loitering weapons systems, advanced air defense and anti-missile systems, and precision-guidance munitions. As major subcontractors, Elbit provided combat data systems, Tadiran installed communications systems and Elop, the electro-optic surveillance and fire-control system.

The *Eilat*'s anti-air/anti-surface capability is based on two Israeli-made Barak missile-launch systems, armed with 22-kg warheads and supplemented by eight launchers of Israeli Gabriel II medium-range anti-ship missiles. The ship, however, also sports two US-made Boeing Harpoon missile launchers, while its guns come from Raytheon and General Dynamics but also from the Italian firm Oto Melara. Its torpedoes come from Alliant Techsystems (ATK) of the US. The ship's sensor suite comes from Elta and its sonar array from Rafael, both Israeli companies, its search-and-attack sonar from an American company. The countermeasure systems installed on the *Eilat* are a mixture of American and Israeli technologies. Its radar warning receiver is supplied by Elisra, an Elbit subsidiary specializing in electronic warfare, its Deseaver chaff rocket launchers (which form a radar decoy screen around the vessel) are produced by Elbit, and another decoy system, the Wizard (wideband zapping anti-radar decoy), is a product of Rafael. The *Eilat* is also equipped with a naval attack helicopter—either an AS565 Panther "Eurocopter" produced by a French company or an American-made Kaman SH-2F—giving it airborne anti-submarine warfare capability.[81]

From the purely economic point of view, American military aid, while surely appreciated, accounts for only 3 percent of Israel's GDP. Its true significance lies in the privileged access it affords to American military technology, in American funding of new technologies in their expensive pre-marketing R&D phases, in the carry-over of military technologies into civilian high tech and in the guarantee of QME—all ultimately translated into Israeli security politics.[82] Beyond this material aid, the United States, of course, provides Israel with a political umbrella shielding it from international pressures. Since the 1970s, the US has vetoed Security Council resolutions critical of Israel 43 times (as of this writing), more than all other countries have used their veto on all other issues combined.[83] In the other direction, the US Administration uses Israel as a conduit when it wishes to avoid Congressional bans, embodied in the Arms Export Control Act, on selling arms to countries with serious human rights violations or, as in the case of India and Pakistan, when it wishes to avoid taking sides.

Europe may not compete with the US when it comes to supplying Israel with arms. It is, however, Israel's largest trading partner, and the fact that many "dual-use" military products cross over into civilian applications is of signal importance.[84] Israel curries military relations of greater or lesser extent with almost every European country. European arms export licenses granted to Israel in 2010 added up to $150 million, France being the largest European arms exporter to Israel, followed by Germany and, interestingly, Romania.[85] Yet export licenses do not reveal the full extent of Israeli-European military relations. Joint projects, whether in R&D or actual production, commercial sales among private companies, the shifting of products from producers to third-party licensees, military aid packages, trade in such dual use goods as computers, electronics, telecommunications, materials processing and security products, illicit and black market transactions and a general lack of transparency in reporting—all these mitigate against accurate monitoring.[86]

Between 2003 and 2007, France issued licenses worth more than $623 million for arms exports to Israel, which has turned to France to buy lasers and specialized equipment for reconnaissance that it had been unable to obtain from the US.[87] The French Air Force deploys the Harfang UAV, a medium-altitude long-endurance (MALE) drone evolved from the IAI's Heron, for strategic and theater reconnaissance, intelligence collection and communications support in Afghanistan, Libya and Mali. The French have also purchased the Heron itself from Israel in a $417 million deal, while IAI and France's Dassault aviation have formed a joint company in France that will assemble the Heron-TP and fit it with some French payloads.[88]

Germany is Israel's largest trading partner in Europe and Israel's second most important trading partner after the United States. It is virtually tied with France as Europe's largest exporter of arms to Israel, but actually moves far ahead if the transfer of six (of a projected nine) nuclear-capable Dolphin II-class submarines is added in. As in the case of other joint military projects entered into with European partners, Israel exploits the opportunity to engage in the development of platforms it could not build itself in countries whose production capacities far outweigh its own to develop sophisticated navigation, radar, EO capabilities, missile-firing systems and other high-tech capabilities they are then able to adapt to domestically produced weapons systems for export. To make this all affordable, Israel receives favorable terms of financing (two of the submarines were donated by Germany) and is able to channel a good portion of the costs through American companies, making them eligible to be paid by American foreign military aid.[89]

Italy is another major military/military technology partner with Israel. In 2012, the Alenia Aermacchi M-346, produced by the Italian firm Finmeccanica, was selected as the next-generation jet trainer for the Israeli Air Force. Thirty planes were purchased in the billion-dollar deal, including maintenance, logistics, simulators and training. To offset the costs, the Italian military agreed to buy two IAI-supplied Gulfstream AEWAC aircraft and other military wares for $750 million. In addition, the Italian company Telespazio, a subsidiary of Finmeccanica, will acquire a high-resolution optical military satellite for earth observation called OPTSAT-3000; built by Israel Aerospace Industries/MBT Space Division and worth $182 million, its services have been sold to the Italian Ministry of Defense.[90]

Israel and Italy also cooperate in cutting-edge applications of military nanotechnology—Israel being the first country to publicly acknowledge plans to develop an arsenal of nanotechnology weapons. Little noticed was the establishment in 2008 of a joint laboratory between the Weizmann Institute of Science in Rehovot and the LENS Institute for Atomic Physics in Florence, dedicated to advanced applications for both civilian and military purposes. Indeed, hidden in arms exports and joint projects is the basic research and technology transfer that underlie and enable the development of new weapons systems. The new Israeli-Italian lab was built as a "gesture" by the Italian government to mark Israel's sixtieth anniversary, and was awarded an initial endowment of €250 million, not much in terms of the arms trade but a meaningful sum when focused on the "applied" science underlying it.[91]

Much of Israel's military contribution to Romania has been in its upgrading of that country's dated Warsaw Pact arms, an Israeli specialty. And in terms of arms-as-influence, an Israeli official boasted "Whenever there is an issue about us in the EU when there is not a consensus, Romania always sides with us."[92]

Meanwhile, in 2004, Spain and Israel signed an agreement for collaboration on R&D, focusing on such areas as Future Soldier Programs,

NBC (nuclear/biological/chemical) war and composite materials. Indeed, the vast majority of defense projects between Israel and Spain include technology transfer.[93] Thus, while Rafael landed a $425 million order to supply 2,600 electro-optically guided Spike LR anti-tank missiles and 260 launchers to Spain in 2007, more to the point, since Spain is seeking to manufacture a Spanish-made missile, is Rafael's agreement to collaborate on the transfer of the Spike LR production know-how to Santa Barbara Sistemas of Spain, a subsidiary of General Dynamics.[94]

Finland is also a major arms trading partner; indeed, it is Israel's ninth largest provider of arms and ammunition and its second largest supplier of missile technology after the US.[95] The Finnish corporation Insta Def Sec Inc. had subcontracted anti-tank guided missiles to Rafael. In 2012, it signed a $30 million contract with the Israeli firm Aeronautics Defense Systems for purchase of its Orbiter 2 unmanned air system (UAS). The 55 mini-UASs will provide the Finnish armed forces with new surveillance, target acquisition and reconnaissance capability, joining nearby Poland as an Orbiter customer.[96]

As for Europe as a whole, Israel has been the main non-EU participant in the European Security Research Programme (ESRP), a joint security-oriented research program of EU members and invited non-members that lasted from 2007 to 2013. Through ESRP, Israel gained access to—and, as a project evaluator, some control over—EU defense research while expanding its contacts with European defense and security industries. Israel was involved in 17 ESRP projects and led six. ESRP was especially active in promoting drones for military and civilian purposes, particularly the use of drones in border security, an Israeli specialty. Programs not specifically military in nature have important dual-use or carry-over effects for Israel's war industry, of course. Capecon, an acronym for Civil Applications and Economical Effectiveness of Potential UAV Configurations, is a European program for developing UAVs for civilian use, in which Elbit Systems plays a key role. ESRP also funded Israeli homeland security projects.[97]

By the time the program ended, Israeli firms and research institutes had received around €634 million.[98] Despite serious disagreements over funding Israeli projects in the Occupied Territories, the EU signed with Israel for the next round of funding, known as Horizon 2020, the biggest single R&D budget in the world, which will make €80 billion of funding available over seven years (2014–20)—in addition to the private investment that this money and research will attract. Moreover, since the EU launched the dedicated "security research" component of its funding programs, funding has poured into Israel's defense and homeland security sectors.[99]

IAI has teamed up with the European Aeronautic Defense and Space Company (EADS) to develop the Harfang UAV. Considered a "European" project, Harfang is expected to become an integral part of NATO's integrated computer command, intelligence, surveillance, electronic target acquisition and reconnaissance (ISTAR) capabilities.[100] Similarly, Elbit Systems has teamed up with the British company BAE to develop and produce the THALES Watchkeeper UAV, based on Elbit's 450 Hermes medium-altitude, long-endurance (MALE) drone, projected to be *the* European-produced unmanned aerial vehicle.

NATO sets the standard for integration with the core militaries, and Israeli-produced weapons systems and components carefully meet those standards of interoperability, crucial for both their marketing and operational integration. IAI's Heron-TP unmanned air system has an edge over the American Reaper as the accepted NATO system, which would make it the choice of many European countries.[101]

Towards that end, in 1995, Israel was among the first group of nations to join NATO's "Mediterranean Dialogue." In 2004, the Atlantic Forum of Israel was established as a vehicle for promoting NATO-Israel integration. The next year, Jaap de Hoop Scheffer became the first NATO Secretary General to visit Israel. Later that year, Israel participated in several other NATO exercises, including a training mission in the Ukraine in which its ground troops joined forces with soldiers from 22 nations, and exercises for developing "anti-terror patrols" in the eastern Mediterranean. Israel even hosted a conference of air force commanders from NATO and its partners.[102] *Jane's Defense Weekly* (June 28, 2005) commented that "Israel was seeking to extend its strategic alliance with NATO beyond what is offered to its Mediterranean cooperation group, even up to full membership of NATO." And, indeed, in 2006, a US Congressional committee unanimously approved a resolution recommending upgrading Israel's affiliation to "a leading member of NATO's Individual Cooperation Program," a promotion, says the bill, that "will ultimately lead to Israel's full membership in the alliance."[103]

During two weeks in November 2013, the Israel Air Force hosted its largest international air combat exercise, Blue Flag, which included 100 aircraft of the air forces of Italy, Greece, Romania and other NATO states. Focusing on air-to-air and air-to-ground missions, Israeli officials hoped that the exercise might make Israel into a global training ground for Western air forces.

Israel cleverly frames the security challenges facing NATO members as integral to its own security politics. "Placed in their broad strategic context, the multiplicity, complexity and high-risk nature of the challenges facing NATO and its allies in Hindu-Kush's arc of instability—Pakistan and Afghanistan—are nearly identical to those of Israel," read a summary of "common threats" presented at a conference on the US-Europe-Israeli Trilateral Relationship by Israeli security think-tanks:

> Countering the possible break-out of WMD proliferation; the attempts to empower moderates and foster economic, social, and political development, *while weakening and discrediting radicals*; *waging counter-insurgency and low-intensity warfare within an opaque order of international humanitarian law that rewards terrorists*; these challenges lay bare not only common strategic challenges but also reflect the commonality and affinity of values share by Israel and its natural Western habitat—the Euro-Atlantic community—and are sufficient for a broad-based partnership between Israel and NATO.[104]

Arms as Independence

For all its identification with the West and its willingness to serve its interests (AIPAC, the American Israel Public Affairs Committee, Israel's lobby in Washington, boasts that Israel is "America's surrogate in the Middle East"), Israel has also learned that Big Powers can be fickle and unreliable. Unable to achieve the freedom of action it desired due to a lack of arms independence, Israel has turned this disadvantage to its benefit. If the US wants Israeli concessions, it will have to "pay" for them through "inducements," guarantees, arms sales and access to joint weapons projects and research. In 1975, when the Ford Administration attempted to wrest from Israel territorial concessions over the Sinai, imposing another arms embargo in the context of "reassessing" its policies in the Middle East, Israel agreed to surrender parts of Sinai in return for a Memorandum of Understanding in which the US would supply it with such sophisticated weapons systems as Pershing surface-to-surface missiles and newly manufactured F-16s.

A decade later, Israel conditioned territorial concessions to Syria on an American agreement to supply arms on a long-term basis rather than year-to-year.[105] This deal marked a shift in policy that contributed significantly to Israeli arms independence. No longer had Israel to negotiate solely the purchase of finished American systems; from here on, cutting-edge military technology would be transferred, together with the licensing needed for future Israeli export and the financing of co-production projects, all of which advanced Israel's arms industry measurably. Israel could now manufacture American-developed electronic countermeasure systems such as jamming pods, precision laser-guided weapons and ground-based surveillance units. The Culver-Nunn Amendment of that same year permitted Israel to bid for American military contracts even against American firms, as well as to share in the production of electronic countermeasure systems and aspects of McDonnell Douglas F-4 and A-4 aircraft.[106]

After this, the US tried only intermittently and without much success in using arms to pressure Israel. Carter attempted to move Israel forward on peace with Egypt by selling F-5s to Egypt and F-15s to Saudi Arabia, though he was careful to guarantee Israel's qualitative military edge by selling it even better F-15s and F-16s. In 1981, the Reagan Administration temporarily suspended arms shipments to Israel when the Begin government bombed the Iraqi reactor at Osirak, and again, a month later, when it bombed the PLO headquarters in Beirut, and yet again a few months later, when Israel unilaterally annexed the Golan Heights. But by then a pattern of rapid "suspension of the suspensions" had emerged, and Israel understood it would face no meaningful penalties by defying US policy. Indeed, yet another Strategic Memorandum accompanied the suspensions of 1981, this one expanding Israel's ability to share in American intelligence, operations, arms research and development and military trade.[107] By the mid-1970s, AIPAC had become a major force in Congress, and the Reagan Administration an unstinting friend. Israel had achieved a great measure of arms independence both in terms of access to American (and European) military technology and its own ability to produce and sell arms.

As Israel's war industry developed, however, another challenge to arms independence emerged. The requirement to secure American permission for sales of arms containing American components and technologies threatened to limit its ability to parlay arms exports into security politics, besides limiting its business relationships and therefore its reliability as an arms supplier on its own terms. This rubbed up against another basic tenet of Israel's security doctrine: "autonomy of action before alliance."[108] Israeli military and arms manufacturers, fearing the danger of being marginalized, of becoming merely sub-systems producers, of facing limitations on foreign sales and technology transfers, warned of becoming over-dependent on a single power, including their American benefactor.[109]

This double-edge to currying relations with superpowers led to the formulation over the years of yet another related security tenet: distrust of powerful allies who might prove unreliable—or striving for military self-reliance and spreading one's security politics among them.[110] If any country has taken to heart Kissinger's adage that countries don't have friends, only interests, it's Israel. Shifting alliances and interests, the aspiration to arms independence and the need to diplomatically defend unpopular policies of occupation call for security relationships that extend beyond the US and Europe to the BRICS/MINT bloc, despite the fact that they represent the main challengers to Euro-American hegemony, and on to countries of the periphery. Though cast as an American client state, Israel has political, military and economic agendas of its own, which it pursues with an effective mixture of diplomacy, security politics and PR. Its export-driven arms industry requires arms independence, even at the risk of straining relations with its closest allies. Israel therefore prefers informal ties and defense cooperation with a wide range of countries, over binding defense pacts that might constrain military production, trade and cooperation.

The tension between arms independence and international pressures has surfaced in the past. From the establishment of the state well into the 1960s, Israeli governments endeavored to develop nuclear weapons against absolute American opposition; however, it was able to recruit the active support of French, together with covert British assistance, in acquiring crucial restricted materials. Additional materials obtained from Argentina, perhaps even stolen from US nuclear facilities, and a Mossad operation in 1968 to divert 200 tons of uranium from the Congo to Israel, played their roles as well. So, too, did the immigration to Israel of some 40 top Soviet-Jewish nuclear scientists in 1989.[111]

A willingness to buck its main hegemonic patron is nowhere more evident than in Israel's military relations with China. In the 1990s, China was Israel's most important arms export market, but much of that trade involved the transfer of American military technology within "Israeli" weapons systems, and thus required US permission to export, whether overtly or as components of other systems. Thus Israel sold and transferred American technology to China in the course of helping China develop a number of surface-to-air, air-to-air and intermediate missile systems, as well as supplying advanced armor for battle tanks. Israel's Lavi fighter jet even provided the prototype for China's next-generation fighter, the J-10, even though the Lavi itself relied heavily on American technology—and, indeed, fears that Israel would transfer that technology lay behind American pressures to end the Lavi project. Nonetheless, despite an American ban on military sales to China following that country's suppression of the democracy movement in 1989 and despite an agreement with Israel not to re-export American technology, the US mostly turned a blind eye. In the Cold War context, after all, China played a role in containing the Soviet Union. Israel, said one US official, became a "back door to US technology that the United States won't sell [the Chinese]," while China looked to Israel for the arms and technology it could acquire from neither the United States nor Russia.[112]

That changed with the end of the Cold War. Now China threatened to become America's major rival for hegemony. Israel, which established formal diplomatic relations with China in 1992, threatened to upgrade China's military capacity using America's own technology. Rather than allowing that military trade to grow, the US moved to enforce its restrictions on Israeli transfer of technology and weapons systems. Matters came to a head with Israel's sale to China of Phalcon airborne warning and control system (AWACs) in 2000, based as it was on American technology, a $250 million deal Israel was forced to cancel. In 2005, the US actually imposed sanctions on Israel's defense industry, cutting off financial and technical assistance for a number of weapons systems, including the F-35 aircraft, the Arrow 2 anti-ballistic missile, and the Tactical High Energy Laser Project.[113] All this came at a steep economic and political cost to Israel. The cancellation of the Phalcon deal eroded Israel's credibility as a weapons supplier in the international arms market and laid bare Israel's susceptibility to US pressure.[114]

Nevertheless—and indicative of Israel's own security politics agenda— it has managed to remain China's second largest arms trading partner (following Russia). China is also Israel's second top export destination after the United States and the largest in Asia. In 2013, trade with China amounted to $11 billion, as Israel supplied it with radar systems, optical and telecommunications equipment, drones, flight simulators and other weapons systems and technologies, plus upgrades in target acquisition and fire control that enhance the capabilities of the older guided missile destroyers and frigates and technology it cannot acquire from either the United States or Russia.[115]

A degree of arms independence is evident in current Israeli-Russian relations as well. Given the tensions evident between the Netanyahu government and the Obama Administration and growing EU sanctions, the Israeli authorities are viewing Russia as a strategic partner of increasing importance, especially given the need to influence its policies on Iran and Syria. Although it is clear that Moscow cannot take Washington's place, Foreign Minister Avigdor Lieberman has suggested out loud that Israel is too reliant on the US. Tellingly, the Israeli government has not fully supported the US in its conflict with Russia over the Ukraine.

In the end, Israel's insistence on a modicum of arms independence has facilitated its quest for a sophisticated indigenous arms industry of its own, at times in defiance of its superpower patrons. That, in turn, has enabled it to carve out a position as a military partner on parity with others of the Global North, thereby adding to its ability to buck international pressures in political and military matters. This helps explain how Israel "gets away with it." By the 1980s, it was one of only six countries outside of North America and Europe with "across-the-board capabilities" to produce the four major weapons systems: aircraft, small naval vessels, armored fighting vehicles and missiles.[116] In 2015, the Global Firepower Index ranked Israel the world's eleventh strongest military power—and the index's measures do not include nuclear capability, which would raise Israel, the world's fourth largest nuclear power, considerably higher.[117] Considered the most powerful country in the Middle East, its QME over all its neighbors guaranteed by the US, Israel has more military aircraft than any European country and more land-based weapons (tanks, armored vehicles, anti-tank platforms, mobile rocket throwers, self-propelled guns, crew-served mortar weapons and towed artillery pieces) than any European country except Greece. The sophistication of its vessels, equipped with systems of electronic warfare and capable of launching long-range ballistic missiles armed with nuclear warheads, makes up for its shortfall in naval vessels.

Arms as Military Contacts

The ties between the world's political, economic and military establishments are many and diverse, and it is these upon which security politics is based. Weapons, Klieman observes,

> … can be a singularly serviceable tool of diplomacy in Third World countries under direct or indirect military government. Whether such regimes are desirable is a moot question given Israel's inability to determine the nature of a recipient's political system, especially where

the armed forces are already in power. Ongoing military training and assistance programs ... established personal contacts between Israeli personnel and junior officers like Idi Amin or Col. Joseph Mobutu [both of who won their paratrooper wings in Israel] with ambitions but also prospects of eventually coming to power in their countries. Even in those countries where civilian government still prevails, the military chiefs are a powerful interest group with a strong behind-the-scenes influence upon their country's budget as well as foreign policy orientation.[118]

Israel furthered these relations by exporting at a cheap rate surplus platforms, weapons systems and equipment the IDF no longer needed. "Naturally and gradually," says Eilam, "this was followed by the export of items and weapon systems developed and manufactured in Israel. In time this grew to exporting via bi-national and multinational companies, as is common practice in the modern era." He continues:

Over the years, there were quite a few cases in which defense deals preceded the establishment of political-defense relations. For example, diplomatic relations with Sri Lanka followed exports of weapon systems. Israel directed its export efforts to a range of countries, including states that were "ostracized" by the international community (Chile and South Africa); South American states suspected of drug dealing; African states connected to genocide (and even China, at least in the American version); states that were formerly hostile towards Israel (Egypt and Jordan); "wavering" states in North Africa, and the Gulf emirates.

Israel managed to establish connections with African states via supplies of arms needed by those states, for example, in exports to Uganda, Congo, Kenya, and Ethiopia. The military technology acted as an important key to relations with China, before the crisis with the United States erupted, and links with India, mainly when it was under a technological embargo (led by the United States) and was looking for a way to breach the technological obstacles that delayed its ambitious development processes. There were also the cases of Poland, which after the disintegration of the Warsaw Pact decided to realize its technological-industrial ambitions in order to find its place among Europe's industrial leaders, and Turkey, which was looking to develop its industry with the leverage of defense acquisitions, obtained courtesy of Israel.[119]

In regard to servicing almost any regime—Israel does arms and security business with some 130 countries[120]—the fact that it does not hinge its sales on a country's human rights record, as other major powers at least say they do, means that doing business with it poses no political expectations— although support for Israel in international fora is appreciated. On the contrary: "Sensitive issues of domestic jurisdiction like human rights policy … which dominate arms negotiations with the superpowers, therefore are unlikely to enter diplomatic negotiations of the terms of sale [with Israel].[121] Beit-Hallahmi is more forthright:

> What Israel has been exporting to the Third World is not just a technology of domination, but a worldview that undergirds that technology. In every situation of oppression and domination, the logic of the oppressed is pitted against the logic of the oppressor. What Israel has been exporting is the logic of the oppressor … What is exported is not just technology, armaments, and experience, not just expertise, but a certain frame of mind, a feeling that the Third World can be controlled and dominated, that radical movements in the Third World can be stopped, that modern Crusaders still have a future …
>
> The only thing that guarantees the continuing rule of the Third World oligarchies is the suppression of any spark of independence or power among their peoples. Israeli advisers have much to offer in the technology of death and oppression, and that is why they are so much in demand.[122]

Arms as Commerce

Even as it contributes to the Israeli economy, trade in arms is yet another expression of arms diplomacy. "Military sales and assistance often provide the opening wedge for a variety of other commercial contacts which would otherwise have been difficult," says Klieman pointing to the fact that arms sales to countries critical of Israel, even to those that have severed formal diplomatic relations, often grow despite the political alienation. "Trade has followed not the flag," he observes sardonically, "but, symbolically, the Uzi submachine gun."[123]

The sheer scale of arms exports is astounding for a small country, especially one that does not produce major platforms. From exporting "somewhere in excess of $1 billion" in military sales in the early 1980s it has, since 1982, been among the top twelve arms-exporting nations; in

2012, its security exports amounted to $7.4 billion, placing it among the world's ten leading defense exporters (although that declined to $6.54 billion in 2013).[124] By some accounts Israel is the world's fourth largest arms exporter,[125] or the sixth,[126] or the tenth.[127]

Israel itself claims to vie with Britain, Russia, China and France, if upgrades in military equipment and other forms of servicing are taken into account.[128] Thus its 400-plus public and private defense firms sold $10.8 billion of arms during 2000–07, on a par with China. Ministry of Defense figures, however, estimate Israel's total exports in this period as nearer to $29.7 billion, since they include upgrades and other services in its calculations.[129] That would place Israel third among arms-exporting countries, well behind the US and Russia, but tied with France.

An economics of scale requires Israel to export between 70–85 percent of its military products.[130] Ranked by SIPRI tenth among the largest arms exporters between 2009 and 2013, its largest target markets are in North America, Europe, Latin America and Asia, fully a third of its major conventional arms going to India.[131] Four Israeli companies, the state-owned Israel Aircraft Industries (IAI), Israel's biggest employer outside government, Israel Military Industries (IMI) and Rafael, plus the publicly traded Elbit Systems, are among the world's hundred largest arms-producing companies.[132] The Tadiran-Elisra Group is another major private-sector Israel arms manufacturer.

Military sales are but a part of arms industry, however, which also includes homeland security, surveillance and policing. In the realm of domestic security, the Israeli government and private companies work with security agencies the world over on issues of counter-terrorism, crime, border controls, prison management and disaster control. Israel's experience in controlling the Occupied Territories and its population, as well as insulating its own population from resistance and terrorism, has become a major selling point. Israel has moved aggressively in turning homeland security into one of its biggest exports. More than 350 Israeli companies export about $1.5 billion annually in domestic security goods and technology. Israel's share of the $175 billion global domestic security market is less than 1 percent, but growing rapidly.[133] Just as the military shades into homeland security, so does homeland security shade into policing—yet another branch of the Israeli arms industry exported throughout the world.[134]

Israel's security politics, I have suggested, entail serving hegemons big and small while nonetheless pursuing its own strategic agenda. But what is it exactly that Israel provides those hegemons? We now turn to a more detailed consideration of what technologies, weapons and security systems, tactics and models of control it "contributes" to the global pacification system, locating Israel as a "pivotal" player able to skillfully "niche-fill." We will explore in particular three macro-niches of pacification that Israel has carved out for itself:

- Niche 1: developing weapons of hybrid warfare and securocratic control;
- Niche 2: constructing a comprehensive model of securitization, a Global Matrix of Control, and
- Niche 3: framing and "lawfare" (although, for reasons of space and focus, we will just touch upon this but briefly).

3

Niche Filling in a Global Matrix of Control

As a country embroiled in a potentially debilitating, endemic, resource-draining and alienating conflict, Israel has managed, as Klieman shows, to parlay its disadvantages into potent assets. Not only does Israel possess broad military and securocratic experience, but its global reach—if expressed in depth of involvement with regimes and non-state actors throughout the world—rivals, perhaps surpasses, that of the US. The American military presence is a relatively straightforward one of bases, soldiers, weapons and surveillance, with some covert and Special Ops activity.[1] The Israeli presence, lacking bases and the weaponry of the US, is no less extensive in range: it does a *formal, reported* arms business with 130 countries. It surpasses the US in depth, however. In addition to ingratiating itself into the military-industrial complex of the core, its presence in "Third World" countries, including many Arab and Muslim ones, runs far deeper. Israelis can be found training army units, elite Presidential Guards and security agencies, national and local police, as well as providing protection and services to private companies in "markets difficult to penetrate."

Other core armies provide training for foreign forces, of course, but for the IDF, technical training is merely an ingredient of security politics. Foreign military units are brought through its International Training Branch. According to the IDF website:

> ... the main aim of the Branch is true ground diplomacy. These training situations bring about meetings, without mediators, between soldiers and officers from the armies of the world and those of the IDF—and there is no better way to have soldiers bond than to have them eat from shared field rations. Maj. Limor Leon, head of the Marketing and Sales Department within the Branch, says that the foreign trainees in Israel

and the coordination delegations for each training exercise in Israel are invited to a day of touring and familiarization with the country. "Whether we are talking about a visit in the Yad Vashem Holocaust Memorial, or a tour of Sderot, we try to bring to them the story of Israel in the shortest amount of time and on the most personal level. When they return to their countries, they definitely feel closer to us and understand the complex daily reality of our lives in Israel and the threats against us ... ."[2]

A Pivotal Israel

What can explain this breadth and depth of Israel's security politics? Israel, after all, numbers among the second tier of arms industries allied with those of the core: the Czech Republic, Australia, Canada, Norway, Japan and Sweden, the BRICS/MINT nations and newly industrialized countries with modest military-industrial complexes (Argentina, Indonesia, Iran, Singapore, South Korea, Taiwan and Turkey). These are the "Adapters & Modifiers," that is, integrated but subordinate parts of a globalized, interdependent arms industry ruled by the major "critical innovators" which produce 85 percent of the world's arms and dominate weapons development.[3]

One explanation has to do with its "niche-filling" strategy. In addition to being broadly competent, Israel specialized in producing high-tech components of weapons systems, middle-range and smaller platforms (from UAVs, APCs and missiles to rifles, micro-UAVs and nanoweapons), surveillance technologies and tactics of counter-insurgency and counter-terrorism. Its technological capabilities rises above those of other middle-level competitors in large part because of its embeddedness in a chronic, ongoing conflict that both drives its need to produce advanced weaponry and offers unique opportunities to do so, as well as to test and perfect them on an actual population. Add to that privileged access to American and European military technology and a readiness of core governments and corporations to involve Israeli scientists, engineers and IT specialists in joint military projects, all supported by massive funding from major governments and corporations alike, and one begins to comprehend how Israel has forged for itself a uniquely pivotal position (Figure 3.1).

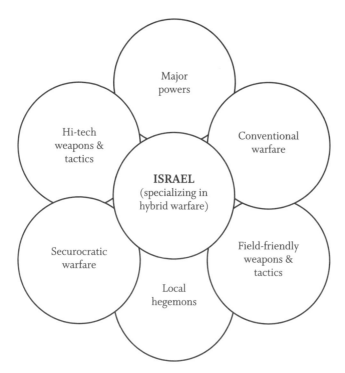

Figure 3.1   A pivotal Israel

Israel Between Conventional and Securocratic Warfare

Israel tops the list of countries most involved in intense international conflicts of the last two hundred years.[4] Besides being embroiled in an intense civil conflict during the half-century before the establishment of the state in 1948, it has fought four conventional wars (1948, 1956, 1967, 1973, plus the 1967–70 War of Attrition), at least seven hybrid or asymmetric ones (First Lebanon War 1982, with an occupation lasting until 2000; First Intifada 1987–93, Second Intifada 2000–05, Second Lebanon War 2006, and three assaults on Gaza 2008/9, 2012, 2014), plus mounting or participating in innumerable operations and engagements inside Israel, in the Occupied Territory, throughout the Middle East and well beyond. It continues to be engaged in one of the longest securocratic wars of modern times: its occupation of the West Bank, East Jerusalem, Gaza and the Golan Heights over the past nearly five decades. Throughout, it has honed its military skills and arsenal to meet the challenges of cutting-edge forms of warfare, including urban warfare, that have emerged since 9/11, defined by the Pentagon as "non-traditional challenges" to US hegemony. It has done all this while also securing—even insulating—its own population against terrorist attacks and other forms of armed resistance, creating models and systems of securitization and policing sought after the world over.

Israel Between the Major Powers and Lower-Level Hegemons

Israel's long involvement in both conventional wars and local-level, low-intensity conflict gives it operational experience and an arsenal in many ways superior to those of more powerful core countries, an edge that carries over into counter-terrorism, urban warfare, internal security, policing and securitization as well. Not only do major hegemonic powers find this range of securocratic prowess valuable, but so do lower-level governments, warlords and armed forces ever vigilant over any signs of rebellion, dissent, or challenge to the vital resources they control. And, again, Israel's security politics operates with no strings attached, political ideology and human rights swept aside.

Israel Between High-Tech Weapons and Tactics and Field-Friendly Weapons and Tactics

Israel develops its weapons and security systems "in action." They are the products of continuous engagement in the real-life, on-the-ground laboratory of the Occupied Palestinian Territory, augmented occasionally by periodic "operations." Indeed, combat soldiers play a key role in suggesting new military applications, testing new weapons and instruments during development and providing valuable feedback to the manufacturers, most of whom are military men themselves. Israeli arms are both effective and user-friendly. Thus the IDF keeps a skeptical distance from such "fancy" security doctrines as RMA (the vaunted Revolution in Military Affairs, which the Americans also call "network-centric warfare"), preferring instead to rely on operational flexibility in finding an effective mix of military technologies and operational needs. "In Israeli eyes, sophisticated conventional warfare responds only to a narrow range of threats," write military analysts Eliot, Eisenstadt and Bacevich, who themselves question whether RMA is genuinely a "revolution" or merely a culmination of developing technologies and tactics, and are critical of its top-down nature as well. The Israeli military, they report approvingly, prefers the concept of "the future battlefield," which more closely weds technology to actual operational needs.[5]

This is not to exaggerate Israel's military prowess or over-inflate its political clout. It is still "only" a middle-tiered country whose various areas of expertise are shared with other "Adapters & Modifiers." Yet the range of its security politics, its need to act on the global stage if only to protect its occupation policies, the scope and scale of the hostilities in which it is engaged and the array of services, products and tactics it offers lends it a more strategically pivotal position than most other nations, large or small. Among its offerings is yet another "service" unique among the nations: a model of control and pacification applicable to conflict situations the world over, a global Matrix of Control arising from its occupation.

The Global Matrix of Control

Sandwiched between the 9/11 attacks and the American assault on Iraq in 2003, Israel's own war on Palestinian "terror" suddenly acquired a larger, more immediate relevance. The rise of the Global War on Terror placed a premium on Phase 4 skills, tactics and weaponry, precisely put forward as Israel's specialty. Subsequent military campaigns have failed to effectively counter terror or insurgency, both growing in proportions. This in turn has sown fear and insecurity in the core countries themselves, which have devoted vast resources to "homeland security" and the militarization of their police. Israel's success in setting itself up as the "go-to" country in the war against terrorism and insurgency only endeared it more to another key market: the leaders of authoritarian human-security states in the semi-periphery and peripheries of the world-system.

If pacification represents a fundamental element by which hegemons maintain their domination over the world-system, how is it operationalized? Two countries, I would argue, disseminate globalized doctrines of militarized securitization: the United States, which as the "world's policeman" has taken upon itself the task of protecting the capitalist world-system and which is actively engaged in producing the military and securocratic means of doing so, and Israel, the predominant authority on securitization and prolonged pacification. Among the major military powers—China, France, the UK, Russia, India and Israel—the US's political and military agenda is the only one that is truly global. To be sure, the French and the British also deploy troops abroad, and their military organizations and weaponry resemble those of the Americans, yet both play merely a supporting role limited to participation in coalition operations—the French in West Africa, or when deploying missions to train, advise and assist weaker militaries; the British mounting specific Special Forces operations, as in Iraq or Afghanistan. China and India focus mainly on immediate external as well as internal threats. They participate in few deployments abroad, and then almost exclusively in non-combat "peace-keeping" operations conducted under the auspices of the UN. Russia seeks to hold sway predominantly in its broader region of influence.[6]

Israel's armed forces share operational demands similar to those of other major militaries. The IDF is trained, organized and equipped for high- and low-intensity operations, conventional warfare, focused "operations" bordering on brief wars and counter-insurgency (COIN) alike. It is organized primarily around general-purpose forces deployed in conventional combat operations, yet like France and India it is able to quickly "devolve" into focused operational, Special Forces, or COIN missions, abroad or at home. The UK, France and Israel are each prepared for limited military actions abroad—Israel takes pride in its "long-reach" capacity to attack supplies of arms to Hamas passing through Sudan or nuclear facilities in Iran—but no military other than the US sees itself as a truly global force engaged in sustained and simultaneous operations spread throughout the world.[7]

That being said, the dictates of Israeli security politics mandate that it make itself as useful to the US as possible, aiding it in its efforts at global pacification, thus advancing its own interests as well. The two countries' military-industrial-security complexes are integrated to a degree "that it might now be reasonable to consider them as a single diversified, transnational entity ... [f]ueled by the two states' similar ideologies of permanent war."[8] Indeed, the "Americanization" of Israel's arms industry is traceable to the two countries' close technological and financial cooperation in developing major weapons systems, the Lavi jet fighter and the Arrow missile defense system in particular.[9] Britain and France may provide supporting forces and equipment in US-led campaigns, but they are far less embedded in weapons development and deployment with the Americans than are the Israelis.

The United States has defined what I call the Global Matrix of Control in the lexicon of its own military; Israel has provided many of the operational strategies, tactics and weaponry from which pacification flow. Figure 3.2 sets out the overall concept and structure of the global Matrix of Control, a necessary framework for assessing both the nature of global pacification and the role Israel plays in enforcing it.

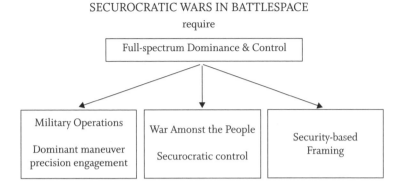

Figure 3.2   The global Matrix of Control

The United States and its core allies have articulated their intent to impose "full-spectrum dominance and control" over an unruly global battlespace. This fluid form of domination and control ranges across the civilian-military divide and spans conventional warfare, counterinsurgency, surveillance, policing and pacification—essentially "doing what has to be done," especially as warfare moves increasingly to the world's cities. Operationally, it is divided into three spheres, overlapping yet kept conceptually separate for different legal and public relations reasons: (1) military operations; (2) war against the people, or counter-insurgency operations, shading into securocratic control (surveillance and policing), and (3) a security-based framing necessary to "sell" pacification to the public, accompanied by "suitable" alterations in international law that strengthen the hand of states over non-state actors.

Military Operations

Traditionally, outright war has been the most overt, if often passing, form of "dominance and control." Modern technology, however, holds out a possibility long dreamed of but never remotely possible of totalized, unassailable, "full spectrum" domination and control of the world system. This is the potential of the Revolution in Military Affairs (RMA) of the 1990s. RMA conceived of battlespace as encompassing not only the traditional spectrum of the battlefield—land, sea, air—but new dimensions as well: space and the "human terrain" beyond military formations. And not only the physical battlespace but also the electromagnetic spectrum, cyber-space and information space. The effect and purpose of full spectrum dominance, in the Pentagon's view, is that it "permits the conduct of joint operations without effective opposition or prohibitive interference"—the ability to rapidly translate global power projection into decisive force in any circumstance and environment.[10]

Operationally, full spectrum dominance hinges on two key elements: dominant maneuver and precision engagement. The Pentagon defines *dominant maneuver* as the gaining of decisive advantage by controlling the breadth, depth and height of the battlespace through the integrated application of information, engagement and mobility capabilities. It reflects three global developments that impact in fundamental ways on American armed forces:

> First, the United States will continue to have global interests and be engaged with a variety of regional actors … Our security and economic interests, as well as our political values, will provide the impetus for engagement with international partners. The joint force of 2020 must be prepared to win across the full range of military operations in any part of the world … Second, potential adversaries will have access to the global commercial industrial base and much of the same technology as the U.S. military … Increased availability of commercial satellites, digital communications, and the public Internet all give adversaries new capabilities at a relatively low cost … Third, we should expect potential adversaries to adapt as our capabilities evolve … In the face of such strong capabilities, the appeal of asymmetric approaches and the focus on the development of niche capabilities will increase …
>
> To meet the challenges of the strategic environment in 2020, the joint force must be able to achieve full spectrum dominance.[11]

With the advent of RMA, computer-based Intelligence, Surveillance and Reconnaissance (ISR) systems have greatly enhanced "total battlespace awareness," dependent in turn on establishing early dominance over the electromagnetic spectrum, the "information environment" upon which ISR depends. When combined with other technological systems—C^4 (command, control, communications, computers) and high-tech target acquisition (TA) abilities—C^{4}ISTAR forms the basic architecture of "network-centric" warfare. It is this what enables precision engagement with minimum casualties on "our" side. ISTAR data permits the attacking forces to make "kinetic" adjustments during an operation, to conduct sustained and synchronized operations from dispersed locations across the entire range of military operations (air and/or ground to sea, space and/or ground to air, etc.), and to carry out ongoing assessments of the situation on the ground in the aftermath. Overall, full-spectrum dominance aims to completely control a battlespace for as long as it takes to defeat or pacify the enemy and "stabilize" the situation.[12]

"Over the past 30 years," observes Yiftah Shapir, an Israeli military analyst,

> ... it has become increasingly clear that the nature of warfare is undergoing a radical change. Enormous battles between two regular, mechanized, and well-equipped armed forces of the industrial age have become a thing of the past. In fact, the Yom Kippur War in 1973 was the last time classic battles of this kind were fought, either in this region or beyond. Other types of warfare, of an absolutely different kind, have taken their place.
>
> One type, commonly called the Revolution in Military Affairs (RMA), rests on three main components: the use of precision guided, long range weapons; absolute intelligence superiority throughout the battle arena; and systems of Command, Control, Communications, Computers, and Intelligence (C⁴I) that allow for integration of all the other elements. The war in Iraq in 2003 proved the absolute superiority of a military that adopted this approach over a traditional mechanized military.[13]

Two other systems support dominant maneuver, each an important Israeli "niche." "Focused logistics" fuses information, logistics and transportation technologies, enabling a rapid and coordinated response to crisis. Focused logistics keeps track of shifting "assets" (weapons, materiel and personnel) while en route and delivers tailored logistics "packages" directly to the appropriate level and site of operations. It is crucial for "rapid power projection," a key US strategy in which Special Operations Forces (SOF), based in the United States, can be deployed anywhere in the world at short notice. The Air Force's version, a Prompt Global Strike (PGS) Mission capacity, means

> ... the United States should be able to strike globally and rapidly with joint conventional forces against high-payoff targets; that the United States should be able to plan and execute these attacks in a matter of minutes or hours—as opposed to the days or weeks needed for planning

and execution with existing forces—and that it should be able to execute these attacks even when it had no permanent military presence in the region where the conflict would occur.[14]

Information technologies, the essence of RMA, lighten deployment loads, extend logistical reach and pinpoint logistics delivery systems, resulting in a smaller but more capable force with a smaller logistics footprint, thereby decreasing the vulnerability of lines of communication.

"Full dimensional force protection," another Israeli "niche," offers the protection necessary for the unencumbered deployment, maneuver and engagement of forces as they take control of the battlespace—while precision engagement denies the adversary similar capabilities. Force protection extends from overall, multi-dimensional battlespace awareness to enhanced deception and camouflage measures, plus the ability to withstand and recover from WMD attacks. In essence, admits the Pentagon, "We must protect our own forces from the very technologies that we are exploiting."

Dominant maneuver, whether in battle or in COIN, militarized counterdrug operations, counter-terrorism, peace-keeping, or "stability operations," depends on *precision engagement*. An RMA "system of systems" enables joint forces to locate a target, provide an appropriate command-and-control response, generate the "desired effect" (i.e., destroying or disabling the target), assess the level of success and, if necessary, retain the flexibility to re-engage with precision. Precision-guided weapons for the most part are ballistic missiles. Be they surface-to-air, air-to-air, or anti-tank missiles, their explosive "payloads" are guided to their targets by homing sensors and GPS. They play an increasingly central role in modern warfare due to their accuracy and power. Able to traverse great distances rapidly carrying a wide range of payloads, including weapons of mass destruction—a long-range ballistic missile can travel to the other side of the world in 30 minutes—precision missiles can destroy a target in a single shot, rather than with dozens or even thousands as in carpet bombing. They supposedly reduce the danger of collateral damage—and are more affordable than large-numbers of conventional "dumb" bombs.[15] Ballistic weapons are highly destructive and difficult to defend against because they give so little advance warning—although anti-missile defense systems also employ them. Even from extended ranges, then, precision engagement, supported by information superiority related to dominant maneuver, enables commanders to "shape" the battlespace.[16]

Armed forces organized by these doctrines and technologies are very different from traditional armies, and have far greater pacification power. They are able to:

- Engage in both regular and irregular warfare, and crucially with low rates of casualties ("zero-casualty warfare");
- Control territory and the people inhabiting it;
- Deploy smaller units equipped more lightly for agility (since expeditionary forces will need to intervene over great distances), supported by lighter classes of armored fighting vehicles, on-call (as opposed to organic) firepower and a reduced logistic trail ("demassification");
- Coordinate forces using C^{4}ISTAR network-centricity, so that all units wage war from a genuinely common script and the "OODA loop" (observation, orientation, decision and action) can be sequenced almost instantaneously;
- Control space, vital for the operation of C^{4}ISTAR systems;
- Control global airspace, necessary for the increasing use of unmanned aerial vehicles (UAVs), including unmanned aerial combat vehicles (UACVs);
- Be able to deploy precision missiles, ballistic and cruise;
- Be able to deploy a globally dominant navy for both attack and securing access to distant landmasses often inaccessible by land or air because of "sovereignty issues"; and
- Be able to deploy special operations (SO) units as supplements to, at times even replacements of, regular troops.[17]

"War Amongst the People"

Conventional wars attempted to achieve decisive conclusions—victory— over major rivals to hegemony, regional or global. Their successors, securocratic wars, aspire to "securitize everything." They are by definition open-ended and totalized, striving for a greater degree of long-term control, stabilization, or pacification than do conventional wars. Since securocratic wars span a continuum from "hybrid" conflicts against objectively weaker state or non-state actors of the Global South to police actions against perceived domestic threats, all but the formal distinctions between external militaries and internal policing disappear, subsumed under such rubrics as "homeland security."

While guerrilla warfare has long been a feature of war in general, British General Rupert Smith contends that a fundamental paradigm shift has occurred in recent decades as "wars amongst the people," as he calls them, have replaced conventional interstate, "industrial" wars. He defines wars amongst the people, or securocratic wars, by six dominant trends:

- The ends for which we fight are changing from the hard absolute objectives of interstate industrial war to more malleable objectives to do with the individual and societies that are not states.
- We fight amongst the people, a fact amplified literally and figuratively by the central role of the media: we fight in every living room in the world as well as on the streets and fields of a conflict zone.
- Our conflicts tend to be timeless, since we are seeking a condition, which then must be maintained until an agreement on a definitive outcome, which may take years or decades.
- We fight so as not to lose the force ["achieving dominance" or "projecting power"], rather than fighting by using the force at any cost to achieve the aim [of "winning"].
- On each occasion new uses are found for old weapons ... since the tools of industrial war are often irrelevant to war amongst the people.
- The sides are mostly non-state ... .[18]

The change in paradigm, Smith argues, reflects the fact that the goals of post-interstate warfare have changed fundamentally. Rather than engaging with "official" state enemies whose militaries pose clear threats and can be defeated in a trial of strength after a definable period of "warfare," after which a political outcome is generally dictated by the victor, the best a commander can hope for today is to achieve "a condition."

"The condition" of which Smith speaks, a kind of steady-state situation "which then must be maintained until an agreement on a definitive outcome, which may take years or decades," I would argue can never be attained. Perhaps the steady-state situation can be maintained for a period, but it can never become an "outcome" since it does not, cannot, address the systemic conflicts underlying the conflict without fundamentally altering the hegemonic relationships, which is unacceptable to the capitalist ruling classes of the Global North. Indeed, the only "condition" that might be attained through military force is the relatively smooth flow of resources to the core.

In war against the people, the securocratic part of warfare, i.e., Phase IV operations, eclipses actual combat or police actions. Even the Pentagon seems to recognize this since 2001. The Pentagon's Quadrennial Defense Review of 2006, entitled *The Long War*, states:

> ... the U.S. military has been continuously at war, but fighting a conflict that is markedly different from wars of the past. The enemies we face are not nation-states but rather dispersed non-state networks. In many cases, actions must occur on many continents in countries with which the United States is not at war. Unlike the image many have of war, this struggle cannot be won by military force alone, or even principally. And it is a struggle that may last for some years to come.[19]

As conflicts with non-state actors and "rogue states" extend into global battlespace, including cities, "victory" is replaced by prolonged, low-intensity military engagement accompanied by permanent, repressive securitization. The new paradigm of war amongst the people, explains Smith

> ... is based on a concept of a continuous crisscrossing between confrontation and conflict ... Rather than war and peace, there is no predefined sequence, nor is peace necessarily either the starting or the end point ... war amongst the people is mostly a tactical event, with occasional forays into the theatre level.[20]

And just as the aftermath of "asymmetrical warfare" is policing, "peacekeeping" and militarized humanitarian intervention—what Graham calls the "policizing" of the military—so, too, in core societies brought to the brink of paranoia by endemic insecurity, are the traditional lines between police and the military blurred, as police forces become increasingly militarized.[21] What stands at the heart of war amongst the people, whether Phase IV operations or domestic policing, is the integrated MISSILE Complex: Military, Internal Security, Surveillance, Intelligence-gathering and Law Enforcement. Seen in its securocratic form, war amongst the people is in fact war *against* the people.

Thus homeland security becomes an integral part of the Global War on Terror. In the United States and other core countries, the "wall" erected over the centuries between foreign intelligence and domestic surveillance, military campaigns "outside" and policing within, has now been breached. North America has been placed under a Northern Command, the first time the US government established a military command over the homeland itself. Dozens of federal agencies belonging to the Departments of Defense, Homeland Security, Justice, Treasury and Transportation engage in domestic data-mining operations, all connected by Total Information Awareness (TIA), designed to link all government and commercial databases worldwide—with all the threats to civil liberties highlighted in the Edward Snowden case and by Wikileaks.[22] Just as the US leads (by far) the military fight against global counterhegemons, so, too, does it "lead" in the fight against counterhegemons and other sources of "security threats" domestically. Besides Britain, whose Prevention of Terrorism Act of 2005 has been amended several times, European countries have generally avoided the excesses of the Orwellian-named US PATRIOT Act.

Yet another indication of the interconnection between securocratic war and domestic law enforcement are the common weapons deployed. Although major weapons systems are identifiably military, under the 1033 Program the Pentagon is authorized to transfer excess military equipment to law enforcement agencies. As of 2014, 8,000 local American police forces have received $5.1 billion in military hardware from the Department of Defense, including surplus aircraft, tactical armored vehicles, weapons and watercraft.[23]

More common around the world is the military/police convergence of "small arms" and "light" weaponry (SALW), together with surveillance and crowd-control equipment. Electronically equipped patrol and crowd-control vehicles, chemicals and light machine guns for crowd control; souped-up assault rifles with thermal sights, sensor-activated alarms, lethal "smart fences" monitored from far-away command posts or biometric controls on movement, night-vision equipment, network and data mining systems, UAVs, body armor—all these and more integrate military, security, police and civilian applications.[24] "There is now a dominant military culture within modern police agencies," writes Radley Balko in *Rise of the Warrior Cop: The Militarization of America's Police Forces*. In 1982, only 59 percent of US cities with populations of over 50,000 has a SWAT team; by 1995, that number had risen to 89 percent—and that was before homeland security grants of $34 billion were made available to local police forces in the wake of 9/11.[25] The combination of militarized police and the enhanced powers given to law enforcement by the PATRIOT Act has invariably led to an all-out attack on civil liberties, most of them having nothing to do with terrorism. In 2002 alone, the New York Police Department conducted over

450 drug raids per month, the vast majority under "no-knock" warrants; in 2005, between 50–60,000 SWAT raids were conducted.[26]

Security-Based Framing and Laws

Bertram Gross, in his book *Friendly Fascism*, wrote:

> Anyone looking for black shirts, mass parties, or men on horseback will miss the telltale clues of creeping fascism … In America, it would be supermodern and multi-ethnic—as American as Madison Avenue, executive luncheons, credit cards, and apple pie. It would be fascism with a smile.[27]

Framing has to do with creating a security issue by labeling it as such:

> A securitizing actor, by stating that a particular *referent object* is threatening to its existence, claims a right to extraordinary measures to ensure the referent object's survival. The issue is then moved out of the sphere of normal politics into the realm of emergency politics, where it can be dealt with swiftly and without the normal (democratic) rules and regulations of policy making. For the content of security this means that it has no longer any given meaning but that it can be anything a securitizing actor says it is. Security—understood in this way—is a social construction with the meaning of security dependent on what is done with it.[28]

By claiming the need to securitize against a threat, the securitizing agent also creates an inherent justification of its actions. An "enemy" is identified and demonized, or a "threat" is identified and an "emergency"—often a permanent emergency—is declared, all of which casts the securitizer as the victim, the one acting in self-defense. This, of course, obfuscates the self-serving aspects of conflict and framing. Warfare is often less about defeating genuine enemies or making the world a safer place than it is about profiteering and power.[29]

Monitoring uncomfortable laws and enforcing them in tendentious ways is another understated element of securitization. One can regard the emergence of international humanitarian law (IHL) and human rights covenants as an example of how non-hegemonic actors arising out of civil society have acted through the UN system to institute laws and articulate norms that constrain the actions of hegemonic powers. One can argue, as do Dillon and Reid, that the "universal" values they promote are themselves a mechanism of capitalist hegemony hiding behind liberal forms of govern-mentality, capable of imposing core discipline over the entire world-system if applied in self-serving ways. The fact that IHL is implemented mainly by the stronger on the weaker; the trial by the International Criminal Court only of people from Third World countries, and then primarily Africans, is a case in point, as well as the fact that the US has refused to join it. And, of course, as with the rulings of the International Court of Justice and even UN resolutions, the hegemonic elites can simply ignore them. All this reinforces the impression that IHL is wielded more as a weapon of the core against the unruly peripheries than as an instrument of the weak to redress structural inequities.

The most graphic example of this is the "lawfare" campaign, being led globally by Israel and its supporters, which actually accuses those resisting the core hegemons (framed invariably as "terrorists") of "exploiting" IHL to defeat "democracies." Thus:

> The enemies of the West and liberal democracies are pursuing a campaign of lawfare that complements terrorism and asymmetric warfare. Terrorists and their sympathizers understand that where they cannot win by advocating and exercising violence, they can attempt to undermine the willingness and capacity to fight them using legal means. Moreover, serious legal questions remain unanswered which must be resolved in the best interests of democracies, such as: *What legal limits should be placed on those who fight the war against terrorism and what rights should be granted to the terrorists we are fighting? Should a U.N. voting bloc comprised largely of non-democratic member states have the power to dictate international human rights norms?* The precedents set by lawfare actions threaten all liberal democracies.[30]

Military operations based on dominant maneuver and precision engagement, securocratic "war amongst/against the people," framing and the manipulation of human rights and IHL—these, then, are the main components of "full-spectrum domination and control," the operational element of enforcing hegemony, of imposing a Global Matrix of Control. It works from the top (the core) down, but also from the bottom (human-security states) up. Like Neocleous and Graham, Whitehead sees the Global

Matrix of Control from the microcosm of his own society. "A police state," he writes,

> ... is characterized by bureaucracy, secrecy, perpetual wars, a nation of suspects, militarization, surveillance, widespread police presence, and a citizenry with little recourse against police actions ... By "police" I am referring to the entire spectrum of law enforcement and surveillance personnel from the local police and state troopers to federal agents (the FBI and intelligence police that work locally through "fusion centers"), as well as the military and agents employed by private corporations who work in tandem with government-funded police.[31]

Conceptualizing a Global Matrix of Control in this truly global way suggests key niches in the promotion of pacification that a country like Israel can fill. In so doing, it helps us understand Israel's "contribution" to that core enterprise.

Israel's Three Macro-niches of Pacification

Few countries span the spectrum from conventional inter-state war to domestic securitization and policing like Israel. Being embroiled in a prolonged securocratic struggle with the Palestinians, punctuated by occasional "hybrid" operations, means that Israel has more to offer in terms of security-state structures, tactics and weaponry than the weak Phase IV activities of the major powers, which they have trouble applying to either post-war situations or their own domestic scenes. War amongst the people constitutes, perhaps, Israel's most sought-after "niche."

Over time, sensitive to their country's security politics, Israeli government officials, military officers, members of the defense industry and business people have carved out several "macro-niches" in the Global Matrix of Control.

Niche 1: Weapons of Hybrid Warfare, Including Securocratic Control

Israel's experience in conventional warfare with Arab countries (plus exercises with NATO, the US and other countries and tangential involvement in other conflicts such as Iraq and Afghanistan) has given it military capacities at the level of the strongest European countries.

Irregular warfare during its ongoing century-long war with the Palestinians, and its attempts at permanently pacifying the population of the Occupied Palestinian Territory, together with its success in securing its own population, have all given it skills, tactics and instruments of control that make it a leading practitioner of securocratic war. Taken together, this adds up to an Israeli specialization in hybrid warfare, the cutting edge of modern-day securitization.

A key part of this niche is the development and export of several major weapons systems, high-tech components of weapons systems and securocratic weapons for Phase IV or domestic control, plus such accessories as force protection equipment, logistical support services and upgrades for aircraft and other weapons systems. This niche places Israel at the table with the major weapons producers and militaries, crucial for its security politics.

Niche 2: The Securocratic Dimension of Warfare Amongst the People

Addressing what happens after combat, from Phase IV stability operations through policing, Israel offers a model of sufficient pacification, its own Matrix of Control developed and imposed by Israel on the Palestinians since 1948.

Niche 3: Framing and "Lawfare"

Framing and lawfare comprise a third macro-niche of pacification. The ability of Israel to cast itself simultaneously as the aggrieved party defending itself against threats to its security, yet also a proactive securocratic power capable of empowering hegemons to take effective steps in enforcing their rule, is crucial to its security politics. Its ability to cast itself as "the only democracy in the Middle East" despite decades of occupation in violation of IHL, particularly the Fourth Geneva Convention, is the product of a carefully constructed campaign of image control studied by other countries embroiled in disputes of their own. In fact, so effective is Israeli PR that the Hebrew term for it, *hasbara*, has virtually entered the popular vocabulary. With a workforce of some 70 officers and two thousand soldiers, the IDF Spokesperson's unit is the largest PR office in the country, and one of the largest in the world.[32]

Related to framing is "lawfare." The former Military Advocate General of the IDF, Avihai Mandelblit identifies "four fronts" of modern war, and in particular in asymmetrical war. Besides the military and political ones, there is a "media/consciousness front" ("we fight in every living room"), served by framing, and a "legal front." The latter is the focus of Israel's campaign of "lawfare." In order to grant itself the freedom to pursue its own war against the Palestinian people, framed as "terrorists" by Israel as it does all non-state actors resisting state hegemony, it pursues a global campaign to address the limitations imposed by IHL in general on state actors fighting wars against the people.[33] Claiming that "terrorists" exploit IHL as a weapon to constrain the power of state militaries—waging "lawfare against democracies"—Israel seeks to change the rules of the game. In particular, it advocates the nullifying of two fundamental principles of IHL: the prohibitions against attacking civilians (the Principle of Distinction) and employing disproportionate force (the Principle of Proportionality).

Framing and lawfare represent two key ingredients of Israel's security politics, a niche designed to strengthen hegemons' ability to sell and pursue their various securocratic wars. Since I have written about them elsewhere,[34] I reference them here but will focus instead in this book on Niches 1 and 2.

Israeli security politics provide the context for examining its niche filling, which in turn provides the rationale and logic for the types of weapons Israel develops and sells as part of its "contribution" to global pacification. I do not mean to imply that Israel merely niche fills. As the stress on security politics emphasizes, the country possesses political agency beyond purely market calculations. In the next five chapters we will examine these "niches" in greater detail.

Part III

Weaponry of Hybrid Warfare and Securocratic Control (Niche 1)

4

The Israeli Arms and Security Industry

The shift to niche filling proved a smart decision. In the post-Cold War period, as the battlefield/battlespace became ever more technologically complex but sending large armies abroad less popular, the importance of force multipliers grew. This was indeed a key niche in an increasingly globalized and competitive arms market. Israel's ability to supply unobtainable technological components and systems to the international market would give it qualitative advantages and the ability to surprise its enemies.[1] Israel's high-tech security industry, today one of its main military-civilian niches, grew out of this change in strategy.[2]

Ze'ev Bonen, former director general of the Israeli arms manufacturer Rafael, describes the process of determining strategic "niches":

> Each niche is subdivided by weapon/platform range and payload characteristics. The law of niche-filling may be stated as follows: The technological arms race drives in the direction of filling ever more existing niches and in the direction of opening up new niches … Thus in the past we had a major investment in an air force plus a minor one in anti-aircraft defense. Now [with the improved capabilities of anti-aircraft systems and the subsequent development of anti-anti-aircraft systems] we have three major battlefield systems devoted to fighting each other, with none of them defeating the other completely. This is the situation in most cases: the various niches are filled with ever more systems, counter-systems and counter-counter systems.[3]

Even if Israel lacked the productive and financial capability to produce major platforms, the fact that it possessed the technological know-how to do so stood it in good stead. It might not have the capacity to export entire platforms such as the Lavi or the Merkava tank (which is today being exported in small numbers), but their very production—together with that of satellites, launch rockets, missile and other systems—contributed in a major way to the acquisition of the necessary technological prowess. The primary achievements of the Israeli defense industry, reports Shapir,

> ... lie mainly in missiles, electronics, and optronics. Israel produces surface-to-air, air-to-air, and anti-tank missiles, guided bombs, and anti-missile defense systems: the Arrow ballistic missile defense system against mid-range missiles is already operational, and two anti-rocket systems against short-range rockets, David's Sling and Iron Dome, are under development. Israel also has a sophisticated aerospace industry and produces both satellite launchers (the Shavit) and satellites of various kinds—the Amos communications satellites, and the Ofek, Eros, and TecSAR lines of surveillance satellites. Israel produces guidance and target acquisitions systems for fighter planes and ground and airborne radar systems, including airborne early warning (AEW) and surveillance planes ... for use by the American forces in Iraq. These forces use, among other items, made-in-Israel unmanned aerial vehicles (UAVs) and modular armor for vehicles.[4]

To Shapir's list, Eisenstadt and Pollock add "important niche suppliers of innovative high-tech items and systems that fill US capabilities gaps" that include robotics, mini-satellites, passive and active defenses for armored vehicles, conventional and smart munitions, and cyberwarfare.[5] In Table 4.1, Sadeh provides a more detailed if similar list of core Israeli military export technologies.[6]

By producing high-tech systems and components, Israeli technology carries the advantage of not being "black boxed," meaning that it is more freely circulated and applied than other European and American technologies, with their constraints.[7] Israeli arms and component exports are coordinated by SIBAT, the marketing arm of the Israel Ministry of Defense. Combining, as its website says, "in-depth and up-to-date knowledge of the defense world's relevant concepts" and

> ... a close, ongoing relationship with Israel's defense and homeland security industries, SIBAT identifies cooperation opportunities with the Israeli defense industry, pinpoints relevant technological solutions for specific requirements, establishes joint ventures, manages the marketing and sale of IDF inventory and organizes the Israeli national pavilions at international defense exhibitions, among other services.[8]

Table 4.1   Core Israeli military export technologies

Field	Subject/System
Navigation and ranging	Range finders
Energy and laser	Non-lethal weapons; laser designators; range finders
Aeronautics	Structure and aerodynamics
Battle protection	Survival suits; reactive armors
Electronics	Radar; pulse output modules
Ergonomics	Cockpits
Communications	Encoding systems and techniques
Electro-optics	Image processing; display and surveillance systems
Control	Gimbals control
Micro-electronics	Sensors and signal processing; superconductivity
Computing	Software
Structure and materials	Low radar cross-section; low infrared signature materials
Platforms	UAV and aircraft; ballistic missiles; launchers; tanks
Electronic warfare	Passive and active electronic countermeasures
Propulsion	Engines for space, land, airborne and naval uses
Simulation	Flight, missile and naval simulators

As I've mentioned, over 95 percent of the arms produced in Israel are manufactured by five companies—state-owned ELTA, IAI, IMI and RAFAEL, which sell about 75 percent of the country's arms sales, while Elbit systems and its subsidiaries, a mix of private/government ownership, make up the rest.[9]

Tables 4.2 and 4.3 present a brief overview of Israel's arms and security industry.

Already in the early 1990s, at the advent of network-centered RMA warfare, Klieman and others (Dvir and Tishler,[10] Lewis,[11] Reiser[12]) were urging the Israeli military industry to "prepare itself for the future by specializing in optimal areas of comparative advantage, [namely] the development of quality weapons systems [in which] Israeli firms have a relative advantage over western military industries in selected categories of smart weaponry."[13] They foresaw a competitive advantage in nurturing Israeli-specific weapons systems that would simultaneously address Israel's own security needs but, rooted in the nitty-gritty of actual conflict, would then find ready markets abroad—plus "Israelizing" major platforms other countries already possessed through upgrading and retrofitting, be they

Table 4.2   The Israeli arms and security industry at a glance

---

- Israeli arms exports: $7 billion (2012). Ranked sixth by Janes, tenth by SIPRI.
- Israel exports 75% of the arms it produces. In 2013, it produced 18,000 defense commodities and issued 30,000 marketing licenses to 190 countries and end-users.
- 25% of Israel's arms exports are aerial defense systems/missiles; 14% radar systems; 10% naval systems; 3% UAVs (IDECA).
- 20% of Israel's military export is to the US ($1.5 billion in 2012). Focus also on India, China, Poland, South Korea, Australia, Thailand, Colombia, Brazil and Chile; Azerbaijan and Vietnamese markets growing.
- Israel is ranked the world's eleventh strongest military power (not including nuclear capability) (Global Firepower Index 2015). Declared "the most militarized nation in the world" for the sixth year running by Global Military Index (2012).
- Israel's military budget was $16.6 billion for 2015 (without the $2.5 billion price of Operation Protective edge in Gaza). Percentage of Israeli GDP spent on the military: 5.8% in 2014. (The US by contrast spent 4.4%.) Military was 15.1% of overall budget in 2013 (SIPRI, Hamushim).
- Israel has received some $121 billion in aid (overwhelmingly military) from the US since 1949.
- Israel was the tenth largest supplier of major conventional weapons in 2013: 23% to South Asia; 19% to Middle East; 18% to Europe; 18% to Latin America; 9% to SE Asia; 4% to Africa (SIPRI, 2013).
- Israel is one of only about a dozen countries that export $100 million or more in such weapons (Small Arms Survey 2011).
- There are more than a thousand arms companies in Israel, and 312 homeland security companies. 6,784 people deal in arms (*Ha'aretz*, July 15, 2013).
- Three Israeli arms companies are listed in the SIPRI Top 100: Elbit, with sales of $2.68 billion in 2011 (#34); IAI, with sales of $2.5 billion (#41); and Rafael, with $1.9 billion in sales (#51) (SIPRI 2013: 233–7).
- Israel has become the world's No. 2 exporter of cyber products and services, after the US. 200 homegrown cybersecurity companies exported $3 billion in 2012, about 5% of the $60 billion global market (*Washington Post*, October 8, 2014).

---

either of NATO or Warsaw Pact origin. All this, again, would be crucial to Israeli security politics.

The "unique high-tech weapons systems" identified in the mid-1980s still largely define Israel's defense industry today. Placing the specifics into a broader "macro" framework, Israel's key weapons niches may be summarized as follows (following Lewis[14] and Sherman[15]):

- Tactical and strategic intelligence systems and C⁴ISTAR systems, based on information sharing. In order to carry out a military action,

Table 4.3   The structure and finances of the five largest Israeli arms companies

Israel Aerospace Industries (IAI)
Main areas of activity: Satellites and space systems, defense systems, missiles and loitering weapons, special mission and early warning aircrafts, unmanned aerial systems (UAS), radar and electronic intelligence, passenger to freighter aircraft conversions, command and control strategic systems, cyber solutions, robotics.

Sales: $3.6 billion (75% for export in 2013); 17,000 employees

Key Israeli Subsidiaries: Bedek Aviation, Elta Systems

Elbit Systems
Main areas of activity: military aircraft and helicopter systems, helmet mounted systems, commercial aviation systems and aero structures, unmanned aircraft systems, naval systems, land vehicle systems, command/control/communication/ computer/ intelligence (C⁴I) systems, electro-optic and countermeasures systems, homeland security systems, electronic warfare (EW) and signal intelligence (SIGINT) systems, various commercial activities.

Sales: $2.3 billion (76% for export in 2013); 11,200 employees

Key Israeli Subsidiaries: Elop Electro-Optics, Elbit Land and C⁴I, Elisra EW & SIGINT

Rafael Advanced Defense Systems
Main areas of activity: Rafael develops and manufactures advanced defense systems for the Israeli Defense Forces and the defense establishment, as well as for foreign customers around the world. The company provides innovative solutions from underwater, naval, land, and air and space systems, focusing on EW, C⁴I, training and simulators, armor, precision-guided weapon systems and anti-missile defense systems.

Sales: $2 billion (70% export in 2013); 7000 employees

Key Israeli Subsidiaries: CONTROP Precision Technologies, Rafael Development Corporation (RDC)

Israel Military Industries (IMI)
Main areas of activity: IMI is a defense systems house specializing in the development, integration, manufacturing and life cycle support of modern land, air and naval combat systems. It focuses on armor protection and survivability; weapons ranging from rockets and guided missiles, heavy aerial weapons, tank, artillery and infantry ammunition, advanced guided mortar and artillery rounds, to less-than-lethal and small caliber ammunition; integrated weapon systems including rockets and defensive suites for aircraft and armored vehicles; anti-terror doctrine and training capabilities; and weapons upgrading.

Sales: $1.9 billion (70% export in 2013); 3,200 employees; state-owned

Key Israeli Subsidiaries: Ashot Ashkelon, IMI Academy for Advanced Security & Anti-terror Training

Israel Weapon Industries (IWI)
Main areas of activity: Production and marketing of small arms in close collaboration with the IDF: Uzi and Negev sub-machine gun, Galil sniper and assault rifles, Tavor and X95 assault rifles and Jericho pistols.

Sales: 90% export in 2013; 500 employees

Member of the SK Group

the required information about what is transpiring must be passed on to the military decision makers as well as to those executing the action, who must be able to respond in the quickest and most effective way. The rise of Network-Centric Warfare within RMA requires interlinking systems of ISR (intelligence, surveillance and reconnaissance), information gathering from vehicles ranging from spy satellites and UAVs to ground-based communications and intelligence passed between people (COMINT). This information is useful only if passed quickly to units who integrate it into their command mode and are able to act on it, a C^4 (Command, Control, Communications and Computers) system that then feeds into target acquisition (TA).

- Air-defense suppression systems such as the HARPY RPV already deployed by Israel to attack radar systems and presaging such projects as Iron Dome and David's Sling.

- Anti-ballistic defense systems like the Arrow ABMs, being developed jointly by Israel and the US.

- Deep-strike air-attack systems such as the Popeye air-to-surface missile, which led into the development of precise targeting using weaponry of multiplied force in which Israel was later to specialize: missiles (surface-to-air, air-to-air, and anti-tank missiles, guided bombs and anti-missile defense systems, including the Delilah missile and the Arrow ballistic missile defense system).

- Electronic warfare systems, anticipating RMA, which came to include airborne early warning (AEW), electronic intelligence and electronic support measures (ELINT/ESM), signals intelligence (SIGINT), smart weapons, navigation systems and Intelligence Preparation of the Battlefield (IPB), along with robotics, a major Israeli military/security product.

- Space systems: Israel, together with Britain and Germany, had already emerged as a major participant in Reagan's Strategic Defense Initiative (Star Wars) and had already launched two Ofek spy satellites. It was later to begin development of directed-energy weapons (lasers), kinetic-energy weapons (ABM missiles) and other weapons to be deployed from space, as well as producing satellite launchers (the Shavit) and a range of surveillance and communications satellites.

- Systems for verifying and supervising demilitarized zones, which would develop into perimeter security.

- UAVs, now a major Israeli military/security product.

- The development of other high-tech specialty systems—notably in optronics/electro-optronics, avionics, navigation, surveillance and sighting systems (optronic and optical sensors, thermal imaging devices, laser rangefinders, cameras, night-vision and infrared devices) and guidance and target acquisitions systems for fighter planes and ground and airborne radar systems, plus
- Upgrading and retrofitting weapons platforms, particular key to servicing militaries of the semi-periphery and periphery, a mainstay of Israel's military industry.

To this list we may add:

- Medium-sized versions of what Klieman refers to as "the four chief types of weapons systems": aircraft, small naval vessels, armored fighting vehicles and missiles, together with satellites and launchers, ballistic and cruise missiles and anti-missile defense systems;[16]
- Cutting-edge military technologies of cyber-warfare, surveillance, nano-weaponry, biometrics, robotics, reactive body armoring and others that have emerged in the past two decades;
- A wide variety of homeland security, perimeter security and police products, including high-tech small arms and force protection gear; and finally
- Technologies of future warfare: weapons based on combinations of genetics, nanotechnology and robotics (GNR), stealth material, the application of artificial intelligence to weaponry and more.

Israel, argues Ettinger:

… constitutes a bonanza for the US defense industries, advancing US national security, employment, research & development and exports. In addition, Israel is a battle-proven laboratory, which has upgraded and refurbished hundreds of US military systems and technologies. It shares with the US most of these improvements, enhancing the competitive edge of the US defense industries, thus saving many US lives and mega billions of dollars in terms of new jobs, research and development. For instance, the current generation of the F-16 includes over 600 modifications introduced by Israel.[17]

In order to understand the political as well as operational significance of Israeli weapons development and deployment, we have to examine three interrelated dimensions: how they are used in war, how they are used for securocratic control, and what role they play in Israeli security politics. Since a key aim of Israel's security politics has to do with integrating Israel into the world's arms and security industries—and that of the US first and foremost—it must strive to address the industries' preoccupation with conventional interstate warfare. Thus, Israel is active in developing weapons for full-spectrum dominance and control. But as the major powers come to the realization that Phase 4 stability operations are crucial for creating that strategic "situation" over which operations were commenced in the first place, and as securocratic control becomes a preoccupation domestically, Israel finds a significant niche in applying the weaponry and tactics arising from its own prolonged COIN conflict with the Palestinians to wider global conflicts. Let's approach Israel's niche filling, then, through the two main elements of full-spectrum superiority set out by the Pentagon: dominant maneuver and its subsets, force protection and focused logistics (Chapter 5), and precise engagement (Chapter 6). Following that we will examine the application of niche filling to securitization-as-pacification.

5

Dominant Maneuver

Dominant maneuver is the first component of gaining full-spectrum dominance over all the dimensions of battlespace: land, sea, air, the subterranean and terrestrial, cyberspace, the biological and the psychological. Dominant maneuver works in tandem with precision engagement; neither can be effective without the other, and finding the right balance is essential. "Maneuver and fires have always been primary elements of combat power," writes General Dennis J. Reimer, former US Army Chief of Staff:

> Dominant maneuver allows forces to move into positional advantage to deliver direct or indirect fires to control or destroy an enemy's will to fight. Fires provide the destructive force and facilitate maneuver. Precision engagement significantly contributes to successful operations. However, it cannot fully dominate battlespace across the conflict spectrum by itself. While precision engagement can shape the battlespace, it cannot accomplish all operational tasks. In practical terms there are never enough fires, and many of them can be countered. Following the first strikes, the track record of precision engagement in recent operations indicates that no matter how effective a weapon system may be at first, the surviving enemy soon adapts psychologically and technologically … Thus it is even more important to balance dominant maneuver, particularly on the ground, with precision engagement. Ground forces employing dominant maneuver in a show of force may resolve many issues without using lethal means.[1]

My apologies if the discussion of weapons systems in the next two chapters is overly technical. Its aim is to begin to acquaint us with weapons systems, military technologies and the uses to which such equipment is applied, as well as with military terminology and jargon. For people like me (and probably you) who know little if anything about this domain, this is crucial. We cannot effectively resist militarism and attempts to securitize and pacify us if we don't know what we're up against. Hence the "lifting" of terms and phrases from the marketing and professional literature. This does not mean we must take the military-industrial complex's hype about its weapons systems at face value; there is obviously a huge gap between the descriptions of defeating adversaries in a neat and overpowering RMA battlespace and the realities we all see. But neither must we underestimate the totalizing and growing power of these systems, especially given the intrusion of militarized battlespace into our domestic lives.

It is impossible to catalogue all the available weapons and their assorted support systems, not to mention ISR technologies. Since I am taking Israel as our guide into global securitization, I have focused mainly on weapons and technologies it produces. Although this represents only a fraction of the available systems—in fact, something like 95 percent of Israel's weaponry comes from the US—the fact that Israel must scramble to stay on the cutting-edge of military technology if it is to effectively "niche-fill" means that it offers us a revealing window into that ever-emerging pacification industry. Israel's focus on developing technologies that span conventional warfare and domestic policing, its century-long experience (and counting) in war amongst the people and its global reach deep into the internal security of core countries and those of the peripheries alike, lend it a special relevance to our exploration of the MISSILE Complex. Ready? Let's dive in.

Space-Based ISTAR Systems

If the entire planet ultimately consists of a single battlespace, surveillance from space offers the ultimate in what military strategists call "situational awareness." This is an area on which Israel has focused starting as far back as 1973, when its military elite came to believe that the US had withheld crucial satellite information regarding Egyptian and Syrian military build-ups, information that might have prevented the surprise attack that almost overwhelmed the IDF. The US, however, continued to restrict access to its satellite imagery, especially after it discovered that Israel had used the information to strike Iraq's nuclear facility in 1981. Indeed, many in the US government feared that access to American satellite intelligence would only spur additional Israeli attacks.[2]

The subsequent decision to develop independent space reconnaissance capacity over the entire Middle East and beyond illustrates the double-edged thrust of Israeli security politics: pander to the world's superpower—or, better, to a number of powers like the members of NATO—but, disabused of the illusion that friendships trump broader national interests, acquire the skills and equipment to pursue one's own interests. In 1982, Israel inaugurated a space agency, primarily under the pretense of pursuing commercial and scientific goals, but based on a partnership of the Ministry of Defense and Israel Aircraft Industries. Unsurprisingly, the first satellite launched, in 1988, was the first in the Ofeq ("horizon") series of spy satellites focused on patrolling the Middle East. Israel became only the eighth country to achieve an indigenous launch capability, and the smallest to do so. Ofeq 9 upgraded Israel's intelligence gathering and enabled it to monitor sensitive areas like the Iranian nuclear sites and facilities.[3] The latest spy satellite, Ofeq 10, launched in 2014, focuses on the Middle East and the southern half of the globe. It is able to detect objects being carried by people on the ground.

The Ofeq satellite series was developed for the Ministry of Defense by Elop, a subsidiary of Elbit Systems, Israel's leading electro-optics (EO) company specializing in "cutting-edge space projects," together with IAI, which manufactured both the satellite and its launcher, the Shavit rocket. At the heart of the Ofeq satellites are a series of progressively more sophisticated cameras developed by Elop: the Neptune, Uranus and Jupiter models. Ofeq makes a half-dozen or so daylight passes per day over Israel and the surrounding countries, versus only one or two by US and Russian spy satellites. "With Ofek 9, Israel now has about 10 satellites working in a joint system—a commercial amount," says Israel Space Agency Chairman Isaac Ben-Israel:

> One of them completes a round every 90 minutes, then the second one comes along, then the third one, and so on. At a given moment, there is not one place which interests us in the Middle East and is not being shot. In fact, a country will not be able to conduct any secret operations in the Middle East without the area being covered by one of our satellites.

"There are seven independent countries in space," he added, "and in terms of quality and technology only the United States comes before Israel."[4] According to reports, Ofeq 9 has a resolution of "less than half a meter."[5]

IAI and Elbit/Elop have launched other "families" of spy satellites, many through Elbit's ImageSat subsidiary. Registered in the Dutch Antilles, ImageSat's principal business, according to its website, is "operating high-resolution satellites and providing exclusive, autonomous high-resolution satellite imaging services to Governments and their Defense Forces for National Security and Intelligence applications"[6]—in short, launching and operating spy satellites. ImageSat claims to be only the second company in the world to deploy a non-governmentally owned high-resolution imaging satellite, a perfect example of government-corporate—or, more menacingly, corporate-corporate—cooperation on worldwide surveillance.

Notable among the IAI/Elbit/Elop/ImageSat products is the EROS family of satellites (EROS stands for Earth Remote Observation Satellite): eight light, low-earth-orbiting, high-resolution satellites designed to view virtually any site on earth as often as two to three times per week. Based on the Ofeq satellites, EROS A was launched in 2000 from Siberia, as was EROS B, launched in 2006, whose primary task has been monitoring Iran's nuclear program. The rest in the series will eventually give Israel and its partners full global surveillance coverage. From being dependent on the US for surveillance images from space, Israel has turned into a premier supplier of such images to governments and corporate clients alike. India recently launched an IAI-built RISAT-2 all-weather spy satellite from the Sriharikota launch site in southern Andhra Pradesh state, thus forging strategic cooperation in space projects between the two counties.[7]

TecSAR is yet another Israeli reconnaissance satellite. Built by IAI and its subsidiary, Elta Systems, which specializes in ISTAR capabilities, early warning, electronic warfare and homeland security, it is the first Israeli satellite to employ the German-developed Synthetic Aperture Radar (SAR) system which produces extremely high-resolution images day or night regardless of weather conditions. Described by IAI as a Low Earth Orbiting (LEO) Satellite designed for strategic Image Intelligence (IMINT), TecSAR is ranked among the world's most advanced space systems.[8] One TecSAR satellite, the Polaris, developed with Northrop Grumman and launched in 2008, provides a graphic example of Israeli security politics. Launched from India on an Indian missile, it not only considerably enhances Israel's intelligence-gathering capability—in particular Israeli monitoring of Iran and Syria—but also provides a platform from which India can closely monitor.[9]

Israel has launched other spy satellites as well, in particular the miniature early-warning Techsat 2 in 1998 (built primarily by students at the Technion, Israel's technical university). Other satellites—OPSAT, an optical observation satellite, the series of five Amos communication satellites, ShloshSat, INSAT-1/INSAT-2 nano-satellites and TAUVEX (also launched with India)—are classified as scientific and communications platforms. They are based largely on Ofeq designs, however, and carry out military applications; in general, they illustrate well the dual-use military/civilian blend. The Israeli Space Agency, as well Israeli military and commercial firms, have signed cooperation agreements with the space agencies of the US (NASA), Canada (CSA), India (ISRO), Germany (DLR), Ukraine (NSAU), Russia (RKA), the Netherlands (NIVR), Brazil (AEB) and France (CNES).[10]

Overall, Israel has contributed vital targeting information for the air campaign against ISIS in Iraq and Syria, since its spy satellites are dedicated to covering the Middle East more thoroughly than those of the US and other countries. That data is "scrubbed" to remove any evidence that it came from Israel, but we should note that none of the Arab nations contributing warplanes to the operation have complained—an example of the subtle workings of security politics.[11]

Air-Defense Systems

Not all warfare is offensive, of course, and dominant maneuver has its defensive side as well. Beginning in the 2006 Lebanon war when some 4,000 missiles (mainly Katyushas) were fired into Israel by Hezbollah and continuing through the firing of another 8,000 Palestinian-made Qassam rockets, Russian Grads and mortar shells into southern Israel from Gaza in the period preceding the 2008 assault on Gaza, Israel faced an urgent need to be able to intercept and destroy short-range rockets and artillery shells fired from distances of 4–70 kilometers, whose trajectory would take them into populated areas. For this Rafael adapted its Spyder system into the Iron Dome anti-missile defense system, declared operational in 2011. It uses a radar system supplied by the Israeli defense company Elta to detect a launch and track its trajectory. If it is determined that it will land in a populated area, two Tamir interceptor missiles, equipped with electro-optic sensors and several steering fins for high maneuverability, are fired to detonate the rocket before it impacts (at a cost of $35–50,000 per missile, versus $800 for each Qassam). The system, which has a success rate of about 90 percent, will eventually be housed in 10–15 batteries throughout the country, each battery consisting of three launchers with 20 missiles each.[12]

Iron Dome is the bottom tier of a planned four-level Israeli air defense shield. A second layer consists of Rafael's David's Sling, under joint development with Raytheon and the Pentagon. This system will intercept medium- to long-range rockets and cruise missiles such as those possessed by Hezbollah, which are fired at ranges from 40 km to 300 km.[13] A third layer, Arrow 2 missiles produced by IAI and Boeing, will deal with the ballistic missile threats from Iran and Syria, while Arrow 3 provides an upper-tier exo-atmospheric intercept. Arrow 2 is able to intercept its targets above the stratosphere, high enough so that any nuclear, chemical, or biological weapons do not scatter over Israel. Arrow 3, which could conceivably be used against satellites, can be launched into an area of space before it is known where the target missile is going. It will be able to intercept salvos of more than five ballistic missiles within 30 seconds.[14]

When it was declared operational in 2000, the Arrow 2 ABM became the first theater missile defense system in the world to be deployed, and it is still the only operational system that has consistently proven that one missile can shoot down another at high altitudes and speeds.[15] "We are the first to succeed in developing, building and operating a defense system against ballistic missiles," crowed the IAF Commander Eitan Ben Eliyahu.[16]

Unmanned Aerial Surveillance Vehicles (UAVs) or "Drones"

Unmanned Aerial Vehicles, UAVs or drones, play a key role in establishing dominant maneuver. Israel, the first country to appreciate the combat value of UAVs, began developing drones in the early 1970s during the War of Attrition waged by Egypt against Israeli military positions in Sinai. In 1971, the IAF established its first UAV squadron, the "200"; already in the 1973 war it reduced its manned aircraft losses by using inexpensive Chukar decoys to deceive and saturate Egyptian surface-to-air missile battles.[17] In the occupied Golan Heights as well, UAVs were deployed to "fool the Syrians into thinking that a massive combat plane strike had begun against their [anti-aircraft] positions."[18]

Israel's first deployed real-time video capable surveillance UAVs in combat during the Operation Peace in the Galilee invasion of Lebanon in 1982, where images and radar decoy provided by the Scout drone helped Israeli jets destroy some 30 anti-aircraft missile batteries and more than 80 MIGs; not a single Israeli jet was downed.[19] During the first Gulf War, US Navy battleships used the IAI's Pioneer UAVs to locate Iraqi targets, the first time the US used drones for real-time surveillance in combat.[20] In another watershed moment, "a group of Iraqi soldiers saw a Pioneer flying overhead and, rather than wait to be blown up by a 2,000-pound cannon shell, waved white bedsheets and undershirts at the drone—the first time in history that human soldiers surrendered to an unmanned system."[21]

UAVs contribute to situational awareness by providing ISTAR information: intelligence, surveillance and reconnaissance (ISR), together with target acquisition (TA). When deployed as part of an integrated strategy of war, counter-insurgency, control and pacification, UAVs can map the physical landscape of the battleground in real time, guide the attacks of approaching ground forces and identify targets for air and artillery strikes. Increasingly, they are being weaponized, transforming them into UACVs— Unmanned Aerial *Combat* Vehicles.

In 2003, the IAF established a second UAV squadron, the "166," charged with operating Elbit's Hermes drone systems.[22] The speed of Israeli technological advancement in the field reflects an important aspect of its pacification laboratory. During wartime, research and development in industrial nations operates at an accelerated pace. After more than four decades of consistent conflict in the Occupied Territories and nearly two decades in Lebanon, Israel has benefited immensely from a permanent wartime level of militarized technological investment, not to mention the laboratory for battlespace deployment the Occupation affords. Indeed, it was in Gaza during Operation Cast Lead (2008/9) and Operation Protective Edge (2014) that Israeli drones really had a chance to strut their stuff.

The IDF's own drone of choice is Elbit's Hermes 450. Comparable in size to IAI's Eitan or the Predator and capable of staying aloft for about 20 hours, it is designed principally to perform ISTAR operations, providing real-time intelligence data to ground forces. Yet it is also a UACV. The Israeli Air Force, which operates a squadron of Hermes 450s out of Palmachim Airbase south of Tel Aviv, has adapted the aircraft for use as an assault UAV, reportedly equipping it with two Hellfire missiles or, according to various sources, two Rafael-made missiles. According to Israeli, Palestinian and independent reports, the Israeli assault UAV has seen extensive service in the Gaza Strip. About 20 of the aircraft served the IDF in the 2006 Lebanon war. The Hermes 450 has been deployed in Afghanistan by Britain since 2007 and has been incorporated into the Singaporean Air Force, among others.[23]

During the 2014 assault on Gaza, Elbit's Hermes 900 became operational, one of the weapons systems whose deployment was rushed so as to take advantage both of its capabilities and the marketing opportunities that the label "combat-tested" would accrue. The Hermes 900 is a long-endurance tactical UAV capable of performing ISTAR missions (for area dominance, persistent intelligence, surveillance, target acquisition and reconnaissance). Designed for medium-altitude long-endurance (MALE) tactical missions, it can fly for over 30 hours, giving the IAF the ability to conduct surveillance flights over hostile territory as distant as Iran, some 950 miles away. Flying at a maximum altitude of 30,000 feet, the 900 can be fitted with a variety of payloads such as electro-optical and infra-red sensors, thermal surveillance equipment, laser designator and electronic intelligence sensors—all of which enable the aircraft to convert electromagnetic waves into electronic signals for capturing high-resolution images, real-time data and videos at night, even in clouds, rain, smoke, fog and smog, and targeting enemy battlefields. The 900 is also equipped with synthetic aperture radar, a ground moving target indicator, electronic warfare capabilities, signal intelligence (SIGINT) and communication intelligence (COMINT), allowing it to detect "over the horizon" ground or maritime targets over a wide spectral range. In addition, it carries the SkyJam airborne communications jamming suite.[24] The Hermes 900 recently beat out IAI's newest drone, the Super Heron, as the Swiss Air Force's new UAV.[25]

IAI's Heron UAV, with a range of 300 km, is able to stay aloft for 45 hours and to carry a payload of 250 kg, is designed for "deep penetration, wide-area, multi-role surveillance, reconnaissance, target-acquisition and fire adjustment missions." The Australian army deploys them in Afghanistan.[26] The Searcher family of MK I, II and III UAVs began operational duties with the IAF in 1992 over Lebanon and since then has served to "locate terrorist targets" and aid "IAF planes while they carry out their attacks."[27] They are IAI's latest versions of the Scout and Pioneer UAVs and are related to the Heron. The Searcher is a multi-mission tactical Unmanned Air System used for surveillance, reconnaissance, target acquisition, artillery adjustment and damage assessment.

Ground-Based Intelligence Gathering and Cyberwar

Complementing wide-ranging surveillance systems in space are ground-based intelligence-gathering sites. The IDF's Urim facility in the northern Negev is part of the network of Echelon satellite interception ground stations initially set up in the early 1960s by the US, Britain, Canada, Australia and New Zealand ("Five Eyes") to monitor the military and diplomatic communications of the Soviet Union and its Eastern Bloc allies during the Cold War—although its controversial spying on private individuals on the context of the War on Terror has led Edward Snowden to characterize the program as a "supra-national intelligence organization that doesn't answer to the laws of its own countries."[28] As such, it monitors the communications of governments, international organizations, foreign companies, political organizations and individuals. Urim itself is considered "among the most important and powerful intelligence gathering sites in the world."[29]

At the Urim SIGINT (signal intelligence) base, super-computers garner words and phone numbers "of interest" from intercepted phone calls, e-mails and the mass media as they travel via communications satellites, undersea cables, radio transmissions, or other sources; indeed, at a time when non-state actors, from protesters in Egypt to ISIS supporters at home, to local cells, or even individuals capable of mounting an attack, have become actors, monitoring the social media has become a central focus. SIGINT emanating from anywhere in the Middle East, Europe, Africa and Asia, as well as from ships, is transferred to Unit 8200, the Central Collection Unit of the Intelligence Corps, and the largest corps in the IDF. Its headquarters are located at the Glilot Junction just north of Tel Aviv, where information is collected, translated and passed on to other agencies, including the army and Mossad. Unit 8200 and its counterparts—the British Government Communications Headquarters (GCHQ) and the American National Security Agency (NSA)—are less well-known than other foreign intelligence and special operations agencies (MI6, the CIA and Mossad), yet they are far bigger.[30] Israel also runs programs of data mining cyberspace.[31]

Unit 8200 engages in field operations as well. Beginning in Lebanon in the 1990s and extending throughout the Second Intifada and into the assaults on Gaza, it has provided tactical information for IDF combat units on the ground—although its failure to provide useful information to the troops in the 2006 war in Lebanon led to considerable reorganization. In 2011, 8200 even established a combat unit of its own, whose members are embedded with other field units. The new unit utilizes intelligence technology to thwart enemy plans in real time (by breaking into Palestinian computers, for instance) or gather immediately relevant tactical intelligence. In 2011, it carried out some three hundred missions on the ground, mainly in the West Bank. In Gaza, 8200 operatives gathered information relating to movements of Hamas fighters or wanted individuals, even listening in to

Hamas's plan to boobytrap particular buildings. The field unit has one other function: to attract new recruits who seek out combat action. "We want to reach young people [through] a place that also offers a lot of challenging, combat-related things," a commander is quoted as saying. "[A soldier's] mother can tell her friends that he's in 8200, and his father can tell people that he's a combat soldier."[32]

Unit 8200 has expanded its activities into cyberspace as well. In fact, it has been implicated in initiating the first act of cyberwar, infesting Iranian computers with the Stuxnet worm. Electronic warfare extends into cyberspace, the "fifth domain of warfare," defined as "actions by a nation-state to penetrate another nation's computers or networks for the purposes of causing damage or disruption."[33] In 2007, it was estimated that at least 120 countries were actively developing cyberwarfare capabilities.[34] Cyberwar can take many forms. It can disseminate propaganda or disinformation to a population via the Internet, vandalize or take down websites, embed malicious software in computer systems, spy, disrupt military computer and satellite systems (thus countering full-spectrum dominance) and mount full-scale cyber-attacks on critical infrastructure.

Some cyber-attacks are minor, expressions of psychological warfare. During Operation Cast Lead in late December 2008, for example, the IDF hacked into Hamas's television station, broadcasting an animated cartoon showing the deaths of Hamas's leadership with the tag line: "Time is running out."[35] Others constitute full-scale acts of war. Thus, on September 6, 2007, Unit 8200 launched a combined electronic/cyber/conventional attack on a site in Syria thought to be a nascent nuclear facility. Israeli aircraft, including intelligence-gathering aircraft, not only penetrated Syrian air space in order to bomb the facility, they succeeded in doing so using normal non-stealthy aircraft without being engaged or even detected, although Syria at that time had one of the largest air defense systems in the world. What enabled that was an assault on a Syrian radar site with a combination of electronic/cyber-attack and precision bombs, thus knocking it out, accompanied by networked penetrations—hacking—of the Syrian command-and-control capability. *Pravda* called the operation "the first live example of the military application of network warfare ... heralding a frightening new era."[36]

Then, in 2010, Iran became the first country attacked by an official act of cyberwar when the Stuxnet worm, developed and launched jointly by Israel and the US, targeted the Siemens industrial software and equipment upon which Iran's uranium enrichment infrastructure depends. That represented the first time an army attacked using malware, which spies on and subverts industrial systems. It was also the first attack to utilize a programmable logic controller rootkit, and the first in which a cyber-attack was used to effect physical destruction, damaging the Natanz nuclear facility.[37] Since then, it should be noted, at least five high-ranking Iranian nuclear scientists have been killed in targeted assassinations, another signature of the American and Israeli militaries, ironically aided by the MEK, the People's Mujahedin of Iran, long designated a terrorist group by the United States.[38]

The next year yet another new cyber malware was found, Duqu, thought to be related to Stuxnet, and in April 2012, Iran's oil ministry, its national oil company and a number of other companies affiliated with the ministry were also hit by a cyberattack. Then came what has been called "the most sophisticated cyber-weapon yet unleashed": Flame, a state-sponsored cyber espionage malware that circumvented anti-virus programs and remained undetected between two and five years. Aimed to map Iran's computer networks and monitor computers of Iranian officials, it was designed to provide intelligence to help in a cyber campaign against Iran's nuclear program. It also infected computers in the West Bank, Sudan, Syria, Lebanon, Saudi Arabia and Egypt.

Flame was capable of stealing data from infected computers, logging keystrokes, activating computer microphones to record conversations, and taking screen shots. What made it so effective was its ability to constantly evolve in order to send home intelligence to an unknown spy-master controlling servers around the world. Then, once it needed to be extracted, the virus could clean out the insides of a computer where it had been hiding, leaving behind no evidence that it had ever been activated. The data-mining operation involved the National Security Agency, the CIA and Israel's military.[39]

Ironically (or not), the Israeli company that pioneered the development of Internet firewalls, Check Point, was founded by Gil Shwed, a graduate of Unit 8200 and Israel's youngest billionaire, a graphic example of how military technology enters directly into the Israeli economy.[40]

Early Warning Systems

IAI and its Elta Systems subsidiary produce the Phalcon Airborne Early Warning system. Phalcon helps establish aerial dominance through early warning, tactical surveillance of airborne and surface targets and the gathering of signal intelligence. Suitable to a wide variety of aircraft, the Phalcon system is based on four interacting sensors and is the first to use an Active Electronically Scanned Array rather than a slowly rotating dome for better coverage, whether of a particular point in a battle zone or wider battlespace.[41] After the US pressured Israel to back out of a $1 billion agreement to sell China four Phalcon phased-array radar systems, Russia and Israel signed a tripartite $1.1 billion agreement in 2004 to facilitate the equipping of the Indian Air Force with the more advanced EL/W-2090 Phalcon airborne warning and control systems.[42]

"Enhancing" Soldiers: HPE Accessories and Equipment

In the end, actual soldiers are needed to direct, conduct and conclude a military operation. Considered a "system" amongst other systems, soldiers must become virtual cyborgs integrated seamlessly with their machines, weapons and C⁴ISTAR interfaces if they are to fully perform effectively in battlespace and carry their weight with other weapons systems.[43] C⁴ISTAR and strike capabilities will be steadily built into human warfighters through bionics, implanting brain/computer interactive applications, genetic engineering and the drugs that "enhance" and fundamentally alter human perceptions—all products of a branch of science known as HPE, Human Performance Enhancement, lavishly supported by the Pentagon's Defense Advanced Projects Agency (DARPA). MIT's Institute for Soldier Nanotechnologies is a leader in this field.[44] In the other direction, robotsoldiers will be endowed with "strong" artificial intelligence that matches or exceeds that of humans.[45]

The "soldier-as-system" is not merely a medium for precise engagement, but is seen as essential to dominant maneuver itself. It provides a proactive presence on the ground, one whose broad situational awareness of the battlespace enables effective engagement with adversaries while holding or expanding positions in coordination with other combat units. "Future Infantry Ensembles" enable infantry to perform as integral elements of "soldier-centric combat systems" seamlessly coordinating with tanks, artillery, missiles, and unmanned air and ground systems."[46]

A wide range of Israeli companies specialize in particular pieces of the ensemble, but major companies such as Elbit offer a complete package. DOMINATOR (in capital letters) is advertised as "an Integrated Infantry Combat System that equips warfighters with advanced, miniaturized hi-tech tools empowering them with never-before capabilities." Sold under the slogan, "Every Soldier is a Sensor, Every Soldier is a Platform," DOMINATOR enables infantry units and individual warfighters to dominate the field by presenting them an up-to-the-minute Common Operational Picture on personal displays, combined with the ability to send and receive information. DOMINATOR also links to Elbit's silent mini-UAV, Skylark, empowering special operations teams with constant reconnaissance. DOMINATOR ensures simple, swift planning, targeting and coordination with armored units, artillery and close air support in the most intense combat situations.[47] The Australian Army recently awarded Elbit a $298 million contract to integrate the DOMINATOR system into its ground forces.[48]

A more modest yet extremely useful piece of the soldier's "ensemble" is the Xaver 800 and 400 Ultra-Wide Band radar systems (including a hand-held version). This small device allows soldiers to literally "see" through walls, thus providing situational awareness in otherwise unknowable surroundings. Developed for military and law enforcement agencies during urban operations in Jenin and other Palestinian cities by the Israeli company Camero, the portable, high-performance sensor presents 3D images of people and other objects otherwise hidden behind solid barriers and allows them to be watched from multiple angles.[49]

The Military Applications of NBIC/GNR/BANG

Miniaturization takes various forms, but some of the most insidious have to do with the fusion into weapons of such emerging technologies as NBIC (nanotechnology, biotechnology, information technology and cognitive science), GNR (genetics, nanotechnology and robotics) and BANG (bits, atoms, neurons and genes)—of which Israel is a leader.[50] Future weaponry is taking the form of inner drones, whether nanoweapons through which intelligence can be gathered, surveillance drone and targeted killing carried out in undetectable forms, or nanobots implanted into humans that can cause fundamental physical or psychic distortions. But these are not mere applications. When endowed with artificial intelligence and given the ability to replicate themselves, nanoweapons become autonomous weapons systems (AWS), capable of deciding on their own when and whom to strike.[51] Future war will indeed be waged amongst and against the people, with self-directed nanoarmies battling each other and, likely, bypassing each other and attacking humans and their societies directly.

The Technion, Israel's main technical university, is also the IDF's largest laboratory, a key source of the military applications of GNR. Described as "an incubator for the Israeli military-industrial complex," it operates three research centers that focus on the development of autonomous systems, one focusing on UAVs, another on "autonomous agent networks."[52] According to its website:

Autonomous systems represent the next great step forward in the fusion of machines with sensors, computers, and communication capabilities. The objective is to develop intelligent systems that can interact dynamically with the complexities of the real world. These systems make their own decisions independently about how to act, even in groups, especially in unplanned, changing, or unexpected conditions. Autonomous systems applications include performance-enhanced unmanned aerial vehicles (UAVs); swimming medical micro-robots that can travel through the human body; unmanned vehicles for under-water, land-based, and space exploration; environmental disaster cleanup operations; rescue operations; detection, identification, and neutralization of chemical or biological weapons and explosives; transportation and traffic control systems; communication networks; and a wealth of other implementations that will drive progress in defense, medicine, and industry. Developments in micro- and nanotechnology are critical to the development and practical application of such autonomous systems.[53]

Israeli commercial companies as well as the military benefit from these technologies. For example, an Israeli company, Nanoflight, has developed a special paint that makes drones, missiles, or warplanes "disappear" or, more accurately, difficult to detect by covering them in a nano layer that absorbs radio waves emitted by the radar and then releases them as heat energy scattered in space. In this way the material disguises the object, making it difficult to identify by radar.[54]

"Enhanced" soldiers will internalize weapons capabilities, not simply wear or use them. They will become "transhuman platforms." GPS technology implanted in the brain, augmented reality and *in vivo* health monitoring nanoplatforms are just a few of the physical engineering "enhancements" soldiers will endure.[55] Israel's scientific/military know-how plus the demands of security politics has propelled it into the forefront of implanted enhancements, just as it has with other weapons systems.

Personal Protective Gear

As Israel learned when it attempted to defeat Hezbollah in Lebanon and Hamas in Gaza exclusively through air operations, close combat involving ground troops, special operations forces if not entire infantry units, remains an integral part of warfare and counter-terrorism. Israeli-produced force protection of ground troops takes the form of external systems: body armor that protects against ballistic and blast injuries or against chemical and biological weapons; uniforms and backpacks made of specially treated materials (infrared-, fire and water-resistant), with built-in hydration systems; thermal-control systems and physiological sensors integrated into personal gear to monitor individual health and performance capability; ballistic-shock resistant helmets; high-tech tents; varieties of combat boots and shoes and combat goggles; ammunition links, lightweight battery packs and more.[56]

Focused Logistics

Full-spectrum superiority relies on focused logistics, the fusion of information, logistics, and transportation technologies, to provide rapid crisis response, to track and shift assets even while en route, and to deliver tailored logistics packages and sustainment directly at the strategic, operational and tactical levels of operations. The Israeli defense industry has not ignored the less glamorous but critical field of logistics, particularly by computer coordinating all IDF systems related to inventories, personnel, procurements, storage, production and budgets. Space prevents us from entering into this realm in depth, but it is worth noting Israeli contributions, especially in robotics. IAI, for instance, has developed REX, a relatively small robotic platform designed to accompany ground forces. A battery-powered robotic beast of burden, Rex can carry up to 550 pounds/200 kilograms, run three days without a recharge, and follow and respond to the voice commands of its master utilizing IAI-developed technology.

Putting It All Together: Battle Management Systems

Battle management systems are designed to cut through the "fog of war" by enabling accurate tactical coordination between battalion, company and platoon mounted forces and systems. A harmonized network of computers and sensors linking the battalion HQ with field units and a wide array of field units with each other, Elbit Systems' WINBMS (Weapon-Integrated Battle Management System) accelerates and clarifies mission planning, improves force efficacy, and raises mission survivability by establishing a common and clear language across all combat elements. WINBMS thus enhances the common operation picture from the earliest stages of pre-planning and intelligence collection, through maneuvering and actual combat operations, where it steps up the pace of battle and target destruction. In the field, on-board networked BMS computers support the operational needs of tactical units by facilitating direct fire engagement and maneuver, indirect fire support, intelligence and logistics, universal situational awareness, in-depth collaborative mission planning and management, and a continually updated common operation picture. At the headquarters level, WINBMS facilitates rapid definition and enforcement of areas of responsibility, clear line of separation and safety margin delineation, automatic distribution of intelligence updates, target information and alerts throughout the battle group. Added on to virtually any combat vehicle, the mounted sensor or weapon system creates highly coordinated joint battalion combat teams comprised of battle tanks, armored fighting vehicles, armored personnel carriers, and other combat and combat support vehicles.

Elbit Systems' BMS systems are in use today by over 20 militaries worldwide, with the Netherlands and Australia being among the latest to sign up.[57]

6

Precision Engagement

Dominant maneuver prepares the battlespace for precision engagement—the ability of joint forces to locate, destroy, or disable a target, as well as to revisit the target, deploying accurate weaponry based on C⁴ISTAR capabilities—even as precision engagement creates the conditions for dominant maneuver.

Precision-Guided Ballistic and Cruise Weapons

Ballistic missiles are guided during powered flight and unguided during free flight, when the trajectory that it follows is subject only to the external influences of gravity and atmospheric drag. Cruise missiles, by contrast, are long-range, low-flying guided missiles that can be launched from air, sea and land (and which can shade into a UAV). Unlike a ballistic missile, a cruise missile, designed to deliver a large warhead over long distances with high accuracy, is propelled towards its target, usually by a jet engine. Traveling at supersonic or high subsonic speeds, it can fly on a non-ballistic, extremely low-altitude trajectory and is self-navigating.

The most formidable and secret of Israel's ballistic missile programs is that of the Jericho I, II and III long-range surface-to-surface missiles, all produced by IAI and nuclear capable. *Jane's Defense Weekly* and the International Institute for Strategic Studies estimate that Israel currently possesses between 100 and 300 nuclear warheads, making it the world's sixth nuclear power, alongside Britain, with warheads deployable by land, air or sea.[1] The key delivery force is the Jericho series of missiles: Jericho II has a range of up to 4,500 kilometers (2,800 miles) and Jericho III up to 7,800 kilometers. Nuclear warheads could also be delivered by American-supplied F-16 fighter jets, or by sea on Israeli-modified American Harpoon missiles—or on Israeli Popeye Turbo missiles—deployed on at least four *Dolphin*-class submarines supplied by Germany, which the German government has admitted have nuclear capabilities.[2] Israel, it should be noted, has refused to sign on to the Missile Technology Control Regime (MTCR).

Jericho II, developed with South Africa and still in service, is a solid-fuel, two-stage medium-range ballistic missile system that can be launched from a silo, a railroad flatcar, or a truck, enabling it to be hidden, moved and deployed quickly, or kept in a hardened silo to ensure survival against attack. Jericho II is reported to have a range of about 1,300 km carrying a 1,000-kg payload, whether a considerable amount of high explosives or a one megaton (MT)-yield nuclear warhead.[3]

The Jericho III intercontinental ballistic missile (ICBM), which entered into active service prior to 2008, is capable of carrying a payload of 1,000–1,300 kg—two or three low-yield MIRVs (multiple independently targetable reentry vehicles), warheads that can be dispersed against multiple targets across a broad area, for example—or a single 750-kg nuclear warhead. A three-stage solid propellant missile, Jericho III has an estimated range of 4,800–7,800 km (2,982–4,800 miles); the range is significantly greater if fitted with a smaller payload (like one of Israel's smaller nuclear warheads). That gives Israel a nuclear strike capability covering the entire Middle East, Africa, Europe, Asia and almost all parts of North America, as well as large parts of South America and Oceania.[4] Jericho III's extremely high-impact speed enables it to avoid ballistic missile defenses.[5] Jericho III ICBMs could be used in an attack on Iran.[6]

Beginning in the early 1970s, IAI developed the Gabriel series of sea-skimming anti-ship missiles. Development of the Gabriel was a model of niche-filling, in this case Israel's own urgent need for an independent navy in the wake of the French embargo of 1969 and the offensive capability of Arab navies equipped with Soviet missile systems, culminating in the sinking of the destroyer *Eilat* in October 1967.[7] The latest version, Gabriel-V, is a naval attack missile equipped with an advanced active radar seeker, sophisticated electronic counter-countermeasures and weapon controls for operational effectiveness in "target congested littoral environments"—the naval equivalent of urban warfare. Gabriel missiles are sold to Chile, Ecuador, India, Kenya, Mexico, South Africa and Sri Lanka.[8]

IAI's Missiles and Space Division has also developed other ship-based missiles, part of an integrated offensive and defensive "suite" of systems. Most prominent is the Barak-8 long-range air defense missile, a project undertaken jointly with the Indian Navy, though it can be used by land forces as well. Barak-8 offers effective protection from multiple aerial threats, manned or unmanned, as well as from guided weapons, and it covers both low and high altitudes. The missile is equipped with a two-way datalink, supporting mid-course updating and terminal updating and validation, and is able to integrate surface-based radars and communications elements with airborne manned and unmanned elements.

Barak-8 functions within a sophisticated "phased array" shipborne radar developed by Elta, a subsidiary of IAI which specializes in electronic warfare. Phased array radars allow a warship to use one radar system for surface detection and tracking (finding ships), air detection and tracking (finding aircraft and missiles) and missile uplink capabilities. Phased array systems can be used to control missiles during the mid-course phase of the flight. During the terminal portion of the flight, continuous-wave fire control directors provide the final guidance to the target. As the ship's primary sensor, the radar system also provides 3D long-range air surveillance.[9]

Rafael has also developed a number of specialized missile systems. The Python family of dogfight air-to-air missiles is a "beyond-visual-range missile" capable of locking on to a target either before or after launch and regardless of the target's location relative to the direction of the launching aircraft (including rearward attack ability). The Python features an advanced electro-optical imaging infrared seeker which scans the target area for hostile aircraft, then locks on for terminal chase, as well as effective countermeasure capabilities. Like previous models, the Python-5 is integrated with the Elbit Systems' display and sight helmet-mounted (DASH) system. It was first deployed in combat during the 2006 Lebanon War.[10]

The beyond-visual-range Derby air-to-air missile is essentially a Python-4 missile deployed as an interceptor; it is designed to destroy a wide spectrum of threats, from attack aircraft, bombers and drones to cruise missiles, precision-guided munitions and stand-off weapons. Both Python and Derby missiles adapted for surface-to-air anti-missile defenses are incorporated into the advanced ground-based SPYDER (Surface-to-air PYthon and DERby) systems whose command-and-control units can be loaded on trucks or used as fixed assets. The system is capable of multi-target simultaneous engagement and also single, multiple and ripple firing, by day and night and in all weathers.[11] In 2009, Rafael contracted to sell 18 Spyder surface-to-air missile systems to India for $1 billion,[12] and has sold them to the Philippines,[13] Peru,[14] Singapore,[15] Poland[16] and perhaps Georgia, among others.

High-Tech Components for Weapons Systems: C⁴ISTAR, Avionics, Optronics and Electro-Optics (EO)

At the heart of modern net-centric warfare is the electronic battlespace, where a wide range of electronic systems and devices are deployed to deal with a complicated electromagnetic, or information, environment. Dominant maneuver depends upon the degree to which forces have unimpeded access to and use of that environment in order to control it, which C⁴ISTAR addresses. And in a contested electromagnetic environment, forces must have the ability to destroy counter-capabilities, including altering or channeling forces of the global environment for its purposes.

Electronic warfare is a cutting-edge niche into which Israel has stepped with both feet. The Israel Export Institute lists 14 companies specializing in the key field of avionics—the design and manufacture of all of the electronic systems used on aircraft, satellites and spacecraft—although many are subsidiaries of larger Israel conglomerates.[17] Aeromaoz, for example, specializes in basic, though sophisticated, illuminated display and control systems for manned aircraft (fighter jets, attack helicopters, reconnaissance or transport). Elbit's Helmet Mounted Display (HMD) system places vital flight information directly into the pilot's line of sight through a built-in yet unobtrusive helmet display. Another Israeli-developed device, a Tactical Air Launched Decoy, protects US warplanes from enemy fire.

Israel allegedly possesses several one-megaton bombs, which give it significant EMP (electromagnetic pulse) strike capability. If such a weapon were to be detonated 400 kilometers over Iran, there would be no blast or radiation effects on the ground. Instead, if the bomb were coupled with cyber-attacks, the electric power grid, communications and oil refineries would all shut down, transportation would gridlock, food supplies would run out and Iran would face economic collapse. No less significant, the uranium enrichment centrifuges in Fordo, Natanz and widely scattered elsewhere, would freeze for decades. Serious damage would also occur to all of the electrical systems in the Middle East, and much of Europe.[18]

Electronics built into navigation systems is also an Israeli specialty. Elbit's HMD system integrates the information formerly on the pilot's dashboard into the helmet itself, bringing vital and fast-changing information into the pilot's sight and "enslaving" the aircraft's sensors, avionics and weapons to the target. Simply by moving the angle of his head, a pilot can direct air-to-air and air-to-ground weapons seekers or other sensors to a target, then shoot. The pilot and the pilot's aircrew, sharing the same pilot-acquired information, can attack and destroy nearly any target seen by the pilot with no verbal communication among them, minimal aircraft maneuvering, minimum time spent in the threat environment, greater lethality, greater survivability and far greater situational awareness. Elbit has HMD systems for both combat airplanes and helicopters, and also has adapted them for tank and infantry commanders.

The US Marine Corps awarded Elbit a $11.6 million contract to provide helmet display tracker system (HDTS) kits on their Bell AH-1W attack helicopter fleet. Using 3D symbology and geological digital terrain information, HDTS provides pilots with visual approach and drift cues so they know where they are in relation to the ground and obstacles.[19] Although Israel is not one of the nine formal partners in the project, it is also participating in the production of the F-35. Elbit Systems has been selected to join the production of the F-35's helmet-mounted display systems together with Rockwell Collins from the US (de Vries 2015).

Electro-optically (EO) guided weapons, yet another Israeli micro-niche, joins dominant maneuver with precise engagement. Rafael's LITENING pod offers all-weather, day and night precision strike capability to a wide variety of aircraft, significantly increasing their combat effectiveness. Its sophistication and capabilities comes through in this concise description:

> LITENING is an integrated targeting pod that mounts externally to the aircraft. The targeting pod contains a high-resolution, forward-looking infrared (FLIR) sensor that displays an infrared image of the target to the aircrew; it has a wide field of view search capability and a narrow field of view acquisition/targeting capability of battlefield-sized targets. The pod also contains a CCD [charged coupled device digital] camera used to obtain target imagery in the visible portion of the electromagnetic spectrum. An on-gimbal inertial navigation sensor establishes line-of-sight and automatic boresighting capability.
>
> The pod is equipped with a laser designator for precise delivery of laser-guided munitions. A rangefinder provides information for various avionics systems, for example, navigation updates, weapon deliveries and target updates. The targeting pod includes an automatic target tracker to provide fully automatic stabilized target tracking at altitudes, airspeeds and slant ranges consistent with tactical weapon delivery maneuvers. These features simplify the functions of target detection and recognition, and permit attack of targets with precision-guided weapons on a single pass.[20]

Electro-opticals applied to guided missiles represent yet another micro-niche. Rafael's family of electro-optically guided Spike missiles are designed primarily to penetrate, disable, or destroy armored vehicles, be they tanks, armored personnel carriers, other types of armored combat vehicles, or ships. They come in a variety of sizes, from the Mini-Spike and Spike-MR that can be carried and launched by a single infantryman to the long-range Spike-ER or Spike NLOS (Tamuz) that can be mounted on helicopters, naval vessels, or combat vehicles. In 2012, Rafael unveiled its Mini-Spike electro-optic guided missile, marketed as the world's smallest military missile and the first to implement an anti-personnel precision attack missile. The Mini-Spike is small enough, weighing only 4.4 kilos (8.8 pounds), that one soldier can carry four of them. Using wireless communications to view and guide the missile to its target, it has a range of 1.5 km (three-quarters of a mile) and is intended for deployment against enemy forces in shelters or trenches.[21]

The Delilah cruise missile, developed by IMI, is another EO precision-guided weapon that combines the capabilities of an unmanned aerial vehicle and guided missile. Fitted with a variety of warheads, Delilah can be fired from most combat aircraft, from ships, or from ground launchers. With a range of 250 km, it can "loiter" over the target area for extended periods of time in order to hit well-hidden threats, as well as attack moving targets on sea and on land. The weapon can be commanded to "go around," wait for better conditions, or strike the target from a different angle. The "flagship" of IAF weapons, Delilah is used mainly for hunting such targets as surface missiles and launchers, rocket launching sites, surface-to-air weapons, as well as supply vehicles and urban targets.[22]

Rafael's basic Popeye is an air-to-surface standoff cruise missile deployed in particular against such "high-value" targets as power plants, bridges, bunkers and missile sites, but it has more deadly members in the "family," such as the Popeye Turbo mounted on the German submarines capable of reaching Iran.[23] Rafael's SPICE (Smart, Precise Impact and Cost-Effective) "Guidance Kit," a derivative of Popeye, converts a standard bomb into an EO-guided air-to-surface missile. An ingenious device, SPICE is loaded with an array of sophisticated but lightweight systems—satellite guidance so as to engage camouflaged and hidden targets; a "drop-and-forget" option good for several simultaneous targets, the ability to operate in all weather and lighting conditions, electro-optical guidance for high precision, the ability to engage relocatable targets and more—all fitted onto one conventional bomb. Aircraft carrying reduced loads of munitions gain increased combat range and maneuverability. SPICE can be programmed to hit up to a hundred targets.[24]

IMI's MPR-500 Deep Penetration Bomb represents a somewhat more conventional air-to-ground munition, optimized for operation against "challenging targets," such as reinforced concrete structures. Capable of penetrating more than a meter of reinforced concrete or four floors of a building, the MPR-500 is especially suited to attacking urban targets.[25] Among other members of IMI's "family" of bombs are the IFB-500 anti-materiel/anti-personnel Improved Fragmentation Bomb, which spews 12,000 steel balls over a wide area, and utilizes a proximity electronic fuse for optimized lethality, and MIMS, IMI's Miniature Intelligent Multipurpose Submunition for area denial. When fired from a warplane or from artillery rockets, the miniature munitions is a pod, uses sensors to detect tanks, armored personnel carriers and other combat vehicles and then attacks their most vulnerable parts.[26]

IAI has also developed the Fireball, a laser-homing 120/121-mm mortar shell launched from rifled or smooth-bore tubes designed for single-shot kill. Reaching almost twice the range of conventional mortar bombs (up to 15 km), Fireball uses fragmentation warheads for soft targets, percussion for armor and penetration for bunkers, and is optimized for urban environments.

Electro-optical and optronic sensors represent an important sub-niche of EO. Whether embedded in satellites, reconnaissance pods of fighter aircraft, UAV payloads, observation posts, or other platforms, these devices enable surveillance and sighting systems to "see" through total darkness, haze, smoke, or fog. Such sensors utilize a wide range of technologies, including laser rangefinders embedded in artillery, mortar and other precision munitions, thermal imaging devices and EO jammers against incoming infra-red missile threats, plus cameras, night-vision and infrared (IR) devices. According to SIBAT:

> Israel offers a wide range of systems, from basic components such as optical and IR lenses, coatings and filters, through detectors, signal processors and subsystems, to complete multi-sensor systems and sensor-to-shooter systems. Israel is among the exclusive producers of advanced thermal imager technology (Forward-Looking Infra-Red— FLIR) employing different bands of the IR spectrum … used for a wide range of applications, including observation, reconnaissance, targeting and force protection.[27]

Directed-Energy Weapons: Lasers, High-powered Microwaves, Particle Beams and Advanced Optics

Directed-energy Weapons—the "death ray" of science fiction—have the potential capability of shooting down incoming missiles and of attacking pinpoint targets at the speed of light; they will eventually replace current chemical-powered guns.[28] "My idea" says Oded Amichai, an Israeli expert on laser weapons, "is to build a defense wall based on lasers which will prevent any missile from leaving Gaza. The laser is fast, low cost and it will destroy the enemy's missile by melting it."[29] Rafael might be close to doing that. At the 2014 Singapore Air Show it unveiled its laser-based, mobile Iron Beam system, whose High-Energy Laser Weapon System (HELWS) is designed to counter short-range rockets, artillery and mortars too small for the Iron Dome system to intercept effectively, as well as UAVs.[30]

UACVs

UAVs have such obvious attack potentials that it didn't take long for unmanned aerial *combat* vehicles (UACVs) to enter battlespace. The IAI's Harpy, developed in the 1990s, is a "lethal UAV," a kind of guided bomb with loitering capabilities, tipped with a high-explosive warhead. In 2009, IAI unveiled the Harop UAV (or Harpy 2), a remotely piloted suicide drone which can extend its operations to hunting elusive ground targets, such as anti-aircraft systems and mobile or concealed ballistic missile launchers.[31]

The IAI's *Eitan*, although designated as a reconnaissance craft, can also be weaponized and deployed in armed roles including missile defence and long-range strategic strike, and it has been reported to have been deployed in a 2009 airstrike against a Gaza-bound Iranian arms convoy traveling through Sudan.[32] Regardless, Israel has developed a number of assault UACV models adapted for targeting and firing Hellfire or higher-precision Israeli-made Spike missiles. IAI's Heron, of which Eitan is a late variation, is deployed in Afghanistan by Australian, Canadian, French and German forces. The Hermes 450 has also been modified by Israel to carry up to two Hellfire or Spike missiles.[33]

Another Israeli firm, UVision, offers the Hero-400, a medium-size (40-kg) "loitering munition." A hunter-killer sensor/weapon equipped with advanced electro-optical day/night imaging sensors, it is able to loiter for four hours at ranges of up to 150 km searching for targets and relaying their location back to the command center, which can decide best how to attack them. Toward the end of its mission, or when a priority target appears, the Hero-400 itself can be directed to attack fixed or moving targets with an 8-kg warhead.[34]

From here to killing people is a small step. Needless to say, Israel was one of the first to use UACVs for extrajudicial executions, beginning in Lebanon and the Occupied Territory in the early 1990s. Since then their use in "targeted killings" has become commonplace, although "hits" are not as precise as advertised and many innocent bystanders have been killed.[35]

Tanks and Armored Combat Vehicles

The Merkava ("Chariot") tank is one of the few major weapons platforms produced by Israel. Its development goes back to the mid-1960s when Israel and Britain joined in the development of the Chieftain tank. By 1977, under the direction of General Israel Tal, an all-Israeli tank, the Merkava Mark I, was introduced into the IDF, where it saw combat in the 1982 Lebanon War. Since then, several models of the versatile and innovative Merkava have been introduced. As of mid-2012, Israel's arsenal included 1,140 Mk-3 and Mk-4-model tanks, with more Mk-4s to be delivered. Another 1,970 older models are in operational storage.[36]

The following description of the latest Mk-4 tank is useful in that it illustrates in detail both the sophistication of the platform itself—lest anyone think it is just a clunky machine too heavy and awkward to be a "precise" weapon—and the degree to which systems from different Israeli companies have been integrated into it (SIBAT's sales directory lists 50):

> The Mk-4 is equipped with a 120 mm gun ... [and] a modern fire control and sighting system ... with an improved tracking system which enables tracking of moving targets, such as tanks, helicopters, vehicles or soldiers. It also enables locking the sight and gun on targets when the tank is on the move, utilizing the ultra-fast gun stabilization and electrical turret drive system ... The tank also utilizes the Battle Management System (BMS) designed by Elbit Systems' Elop ...
>
> The Merkava Mk-4 is equipped with the new VDS-60 digital data recorder produced by Vectop; it records and restores the sight images and observation data collected during the mission. The capture of such images can also be shared by other elements, which are networked with

Elbit's Weapon-Integrated Battle Management System (WINBMS), to enable reporting of enemy targets. This concept is rapidly becoming an essential part of the "digitized land forces" integrated battlefield concept, combining tanks, anti-tank and combat helicopters in a combined task force at various levels ... Merkava Mk-4 uses four cameras installed in hardened cases embedded outside the tank. These cameras are providing full peripheral view displayed on high resolution monitors ...

Unique among the main battle tanks of the world, the Merkava design features a front-mounted power pack, which presents a heavy mass in the forward area, which protects the crew from enemy attack. This configuration also cleared room at the rear section for a safe exit and enough space to carry a few fully armed infantrymen, in addition to the crew ... Special modifications installed on Merkava Mk-4 are preparing the tank to operate in the urban environment of Low Intensity Conflict.[37]

"The [Merkava] tank is one of the most technologically advanced platforms around," contends Col. Yigal Slovik, commander of the IDF's 401st Armored Brigade. "It is like flying an airplane, only on the ground."[38] Until recently, however, it has never sold the tank as an entire system out of fear that its secretive domestic technologies might be exposed, and because of the American components built into it.[39] In order to offset costs, the Ministry of Defense recently authorized for the first time sales of the Merkava Mk-4 tank and its derivative, the Namer APC—though only to "friendly countries." Colombia has shown an interest in purchasing between 25 and 40 Merkavas at about $6 million each.[40]

The need to deploy in Palestinian cities or the confined battlespaces of southern Lebanon pointed to a need to either develop new weaponry for urban terrain, or to modify existing weapons into more agile ones suited for close quarter combat. Out of that shift came the Merkava LIC (LIC standing for "low-intensity conflict"). Rather than using a cumbersome and heavy gun which anyway is ineffective against individual enemy combatants and causes tremendous "collateral damage," the Merkava LIC employs a smaller, more maneuverable turret carrying a 12.7-mm caliber coaxial machine gun, enabling the crew to lay down heavy but more accurate cover fire from inside the tank, without exposing the crew to small-arms fire and snipers.[41] The Merkava LIC saw extensive combat in Gaza.

The Namer ("Tiger"), a middle-level Armored Infantry Fighting Vehicle (AIFV) falling between a tank and an armored personnel carrier (APC), represents the joining of precision engagement with force protection in close battlespace quarters. An offshoot of the Merkava and Soviet BMPs, it received its baptism by fire during Operation Cast Lead in Gaza. The Namer, the IDF's next-generation armored personnel carrier, can carry twelve people, including a commander, gunner and driver. But the Namer, seamlessly combining defensive and offensive capabilities, blurs the distinction between an APC and an AIFV. It is a completely armored vehicle equipped with special folding seats that reduce the possibility of injury by anti-personnel mines, with the engine installed in front as in the Merkava tank as additional protection against antitank weapons, yet it can also carry a 12.7-mm machine gun, a 7.62-mm machine gun, or 40-mm MK19 automatic grenade launcher. A control and inspection system, 360-degree cameras and computerized weapon systems will enable the soldiers to destroy a threat while remaining in the APC, yet maintaining direct contact with the Division Commander.[42] The IDF has ordered about 130 such vehicles, at a cost of $3 million each, and there are plans to acquire as many as 800. Israel and Azerbaijan are negotiating on the production of BMP. The cost of a fully equipped modern BMP "Namer" is estimated at $2 million.[43]

The idea of converting tanks into combinations of armored fighting vehicles and APCs preceded the Namer by many years. The Nagmachon, based on the body of British Centurion tanks, and the Achzarit ("Cruelty"), converted Soviet T-54 and T-55 tanks that were captured in the hundreds during the Arab–Israeli wars, are still in service with the IDF. Protected by reactive armor, both are used in patrolling and security missions in hazardous areas—meaning the Occupied Territories, where they have been deployed especially during the Intifadas and the attacks on Gaza. They are described as being ideal for urban warfare, where they carry Israeli troops into Palestinian cities. A distinctive feature of the Nagmachon is its elevated superstructure with rings of machine guns enabling the troops inside to shoot soft targets (i.e., targeted people) without being exposed to enemy fire. Fitted with heavy armor plate and anti-mine systems, the Nagmachon also breaches routes through minefields and booby-trapped areas, therefore being classified as yet another type of fighting vehicle, a combat engineering vehicle (CEV). As such, they supervised and secured armored Caterpillar D9 bulldozers in dangerous combat zones.[44]

The Achzarit APC is the best-protected infantry carrier in IDF service and can withstand both HEAT (high-explosive anti-tank) and kinetic energy missiles which would destroy conventional IFVs. It is fitted with either Rafael's Overhead Weapon Station or the more advanced Samson

Remote Controlled Weapon Station, also known as Katlanit ("lethal"), which remotely fires machine guns, grenade launchers, anti-tank missiles, or observation pods. During fighting within Palestinian cities in the summer of 2002, many Israeli casualties were caused by snipers firing downwards from surrounding buildings. Machine gunners firing from the hull tops of Ml 13s and other AFVs were particularly at risk. The Achzarit, equipped with its own weapons station, could fire at Palestinian positions whilst the gunner remained safe under armor. The most "celebrated" use of the Achzarit's abilities came during the Second Intifada, when in March 2002 the APCs destroyed the Muqata, Palestinian President Yasser Arafat's HQ in Ramallah.[45]

Force Protection

The key element of deployment is full-dimensional protection for armed forces as they maneuver and gain control of the battlespace—keeping in mind that only about 10 percent of an army's equipment is weapons.[46] Freedom of action during deployment and the ability to effectively engage and prevail will continue to depend upon such traditional tactics as deception and camouflage, but as information systems provide greater multi-dimensional awareness, the ability to assess and identify all forces in the battlespace will also grow, together with the ability to avoid, withstand, or counter threats without compromising effective levels of precise engagement—capabilities rendered all the more complicated by the close quarters in which counter-insurgency and urban warfare are increasingly fought.

Israel has long used the Merkava as a kind of laboratory for developing military subsystems; anti-tank force defense systems is one of them. In the 2006 Lebanon war, the IDF discovered that non-state actors such as Hezbollah could disable or destroy the vaunted Merkava tanks; of several hundred tanks fielded, 52 were damaged and five totally destroyed, 45 of them by anti-tank guided missiles.[47]

Israel offers two active defense systems: Iron Fist, developed by IMI, and Trophy, a system developed jointly by Rafael and IAI. Both intercept and destroy incoming anti-tank missiles and rockets. Iron Fist employs radar to detect threats, and as a missile approaches, it either jams its guidance system or launches an explosive projectile interceptor towards it, destroying, deflecting, or destabilizing it without detonating the missile's warhead. Iron Fist may also be used to protect sensitive installations or patrol boats, or to protect from RPG attacks frequently encountered in counter-insurgency operations. Besides intercepting, Iron Fist can also fire non-lethal, anti-personnel, smoke, or illumination projectiles.[48]

Trophy employs a threat detection and warning subsystem consisting of several sensors placed at strategic locations around the vehicle that surrounds it with a hemispheric protected zone where incoming threats are intercepted and defeated. Once an incoming threat is detected, a countermeasure device is positioned so as to effectively intercept it and is launched automatically into a ballistic trajectory. The system has an automatic reload mechanism to handle multiple attacks, and can simultaneously engage several threats, arriving from different directions. It also locates and eliminates the source of the threat.[49]

Both Iron Fist and Trophy are designed to effectively operate in dense urban environments where armored vehicles operate closely with integrated infantry forces. The countermeasures taken against incoming missiles are designed to ensure effective target kill, but with low collateral damage and low risk to nearby troops. Trophy-Light is a variant made to protect lighter armored vehicles, and permits the removal of some of their permanent armor, thus increasing both their mobility and transport. Rafael has signed a marketing agreement with General Dynamics, offering the Trophy system to US and other armies worldwide.[50]

Israeli companies produce other force protectors as well: automatic threat-detection systems; advanced countermeasures, hybrid passive, reactive, active (hard-kill) and soft-kill countermeasures; gunshot detection and location systems; and camouflage and signature reduction.[51]

The Lebanon experience also spurred the development of new types of armor protection—though Israel pioneered the concept of reactive armor from the early 1970s and has fitted it to US tanks for years.[52] Rafael specializes in both passive armor (the kind of nuts-and-bolts armor we are most familiar with) and reactive armor that reacts in some way to the impact of a weapon to reduce the damage.[53]

Conventional Naval Vessels

Israel is also upgrading its navy with precision targeting capabilities. New air defense systems derived from the joint Israeli-Indian Barak-8 missile program have been incorporated into its Littoral Combat Ships. Its navy is also acquiring fast patrol boats for operating in shallow waters close to shore. Funded by the US, IAI will supply four Super Dvora Mk-IIIs and Israel Shipyards will supply another three Shaldag boats.[54]

Most dramatically, the German subs have been described as part attack submarine, part strike ship and part commando taxi. More than 225 feet long, the diesel-electric Dolphin II class subs' armaments include non-nuclear anti-ship Harpoon and anti-helicopter Triton missiles, plus sophisticated German- and Israeli-made radar systems. The latest submarines—the *Tannin* (which was delivered in early 2015), the *Rahav* and a third unnamed submarine—each contain ten torpedo tubes capable of launching fiber-optic cable-guided DM-2A4 torpedoes. Four of these tubes are larger 26-inch tubes capable of launching small commando teams or firing larger cruise missiles. Although not admitted by the Israeli government, it is widely believed that the Dolphin II will soon possess nuclear-tipped Popeye Turbo cruise missiles.[55]

These subs are capable of traveling 9,200 miles without refueling, putting them in range of Iran and far beyond. Indeed, one of the Dolphins' main tasks is deterrence. In 2009, Israel sent a "message" to Iran by sending one of its nuclear-capable subs through the Suez Canal into the Persian Gulf. As part of Israel's undeclared nuclear strike force, they contribute measurably to its "second strike" capability, and constitute a deterrent to any threat to its homeland. Obviously meant for regional deployment, they extend Israel's reach from Sudan over much of Europe and beyond Iran to the broader Middle East, making it able to defend its own interests as well as those of its patrons as well.[56] On a more mundane level, the submarines are also designed for littoral operations off Lebanon, potentially Syria and including commando operations both into Gaza itself but, no less crucial, to protect Israel's massive deposits of natural gas.[57]

USVs—Unmanned Surface (Naval) Vehicles

Another area in which Israel is taking a lead is in the development of USVs, Unmanned Surface Vehicles. Over the years, the Israeli Navy has had to cope with increasingly more complex challenges, from "normal" patrolling of its sea-lanes (99 percent of Israeli imports arrive by sea) and enforcing the sea blockade of Gaza (which includes intercepting flotillas of peace activists like me, as well as attempts to bring arms—and fish—into Gaza) to engaging in occasional sea battles off the coast of Lebanon and, in general, monitoring the region by sea. In Operation Cast Lead, the navy coordinated closely with the land forces for the first time, leading to a decision to bolster the capability of landing ground forces amphibiously in places like Lebanon and Gaza. Again, the need has arisen to protect the natural gas rigs off the coast, particularly given disputes with Palestinians, Lebanese and Turks alike, regarding drilling rights.[58]

Now Israel cannot afford a major navy—although it is debating whether to invest $100 billion in two major warships. But niche-filling, applying its technologies to the development and manufacture of specialized unmanned naval vessels, provides an affordable avenue for merging its own needs with the demands of the marketplace. Rafael has produced the Protector SV, heralded as the first unmanned stealth patrol vehicle on the seas. Based on its own Mini-Typhoon system—a remote-controlled, stabilized weapon station capable of operating a heavy MK-49 machine gun with laser accuracy up to a range of 50 kilometers, sticking to its target whether on land, air, or sea even if bouncing on waves—and a Close-in Weapon System that detects and destroys incoming anti-ship missiles and enemy aircraft at short range, it fills a niche in anti-terrorist/anti-pirate operations, the guarding of merchant shipping, naval vessels, oil and gas rigs and coastal power plants, naval force protection, early warning, sea-to-sea and anti-submarine warfare, mine detection, and on to homeland security tasks like patrolling ports.

Called a "naval combat system" by Rafael, a "wonder boat" by several military analysts, but popularly known by the nickname "Death Shark," the crewless 9-meter-long speedboat-drone is fitted with sophisticated subsystems, including a 360-degree panoramic camera capable of reading a license plate from a distance of 26 kilometers. The Protector is operated by remote control from a shore base, though it is capable of interfacing with aerial and other naval platforms.[59] After its successful performance with the Singapore Navy, India and South Korea have ordered the Protector. Western naval experts rate it one of the most effective military and intelligence craft afloat, able to take over tasks of high-cost warships with large crews. It can easily cruise off the shores of Lebanon, Syria and Iran undetected for long periods due to its tested stealth design.[60]

Similar to the Protector in concept and capability is Elbit's Silver Martin USV, a robo-boat designed for force protection/anti-terror missions, mine warfare and search and rescue, as well as a smaller version, Stingray.[61]

In 2014, IAI unveiled its own combat marine system, the Katana, which detects and tracks ships and boats, protects exclusive economic zones, harbors and offshore platforms, patrols shallow coastal and territorial waters, and contributes to surface and electronic warfare by providing long-range surveillance.[62]

Unmanned Ground Vehicles (UGVs)

While unmanned ground vehicles (UGVs) have obvious offensive roles and capabilities, they are used mainly for reconnaissance, perimeter security, force protection, combat support, combat logistics support and convoy security, and thus relate to two additional principles of full-spectrum dominance: force protection and focused logistics.

IAI and Zoko Enterprises are developing an unmanned D-9 Caterpillar bulldozer, one of the prime weaponized machines of the IDF Engineering Corps, used among other things to demolish Palestinian homes, apartment buildings and urban infrastructure. G-NIUS, a joint subsidiary of IAI and Elbit Systems that specializes in developing and manufacturing autonomous unmanned ground systems, produces the Guardium, a UGV deployed along the Gaza and Lebanese borders to patrol for, or ambush, infiltrators. Marketed as "the world's first robot soldier," the Guardium is a small, armored, high-speed, off-road car, based on the Tomcar chassis, an all-terrain vehicle developed in Israel, equipped with a suite of optical sensors, C^4I command and surveillance gear, including fancy cameras. Operating in the perimeter fence area, the Guardium, carrying both lethal and non-lethal weapons, continuously patrols, surveys and reports on the status of the perimeter area, and reacts immediately to intruders, containing and even communicating with them until backup arrives.[63]

Avitar-2004, developed by Elbit, and ROEE of the Israeli Technion Land Systems Division are two other lightweight, tele-operated UGVs being developed as patrol systems.

Fighting Robots

Israel is one of the world's leading innovators of military robotics, of which drones and Iron Dome are only part. Although over 40 countries have military-robotics programs, Israel moves more quickly to develop and deploy new devices to meet battlefield needs; in 10–15 years, one-third of Israel's military machines will be unmanned.[64] "We can be a world superpower in robotics," crows Prof. Zvi Shiller, the chairman of the Israeli Robotics Conference and a faculty member of the Ariel University Center of Samaria, located in the West Bank settlement of Ariel.

Adapted to the needs of combat soldiers "on the ground," robots add considerably to their ability to execute precision engagement, especially in enhancing their accuracy and force.[65] The IDF-developed VIPeR (Versatile, Intelligent, Portable Robot), for instance, is a remote-controlled "force multiplier" robot designed to accompany dismounted troops in urban environments. Just nine inches tall and weighing 11 kilos (25 pounds, light enough to be carried by one soldier), the VIPeR uses various sensors to map buildings, or scout out caves or trenches for IEDs. Guided by an operator wearing a helmet-mounted display, it moves on a "Galileo Wheel" system, a patented Israeli innovation whereby the robot's treads change shape to adapt to any terrain, be it stairs, rubble, dark alleys, or narrow tunnels. Equipped with an explosives sniffer and a device that shoots jets of water to disarm bombs, it can also be weaponized, equipped with a mini-Uzi submachine gun or with grenades that it releases from a 4-ft-long robotic arm.[66]

Another type of versatile robot, the Eyeball, is a spherical camera used by IDF troops for the first time during Operation Cast Lead to survey homes and suspicious areas before entering them. Developed by the Tel Aviv-based company ODF Optronics, the Eyeball is an advanced, audio-visual surveillance sensor, only slightly larger than a baseball, that can be thrown into an area that needs to be surveilled, or mounted on a pole, or lowered on a cable into a tunnel. The same company also produces the Eyedrive, a lightweight, four-wheel, remote-controlled, observation and surveillance mini-robot. Durable enough to be thrown on the ground, go down stairs, flip over and keep on going, it provides continuous, real-time 360-degree audio and video surveillance.[67]

The robotics department at the IDF's Ordnance Corps has developed a prototype robot that can spray tear gas and allow troops to "paralyze" suspects during raids. The innovation is meant to improve the forces' ability to operate in populated areas.[68]

Miniature UAVs and UACVs—MAVs or Micro-Drones

Miniaturization makes it harder for "targets" to detect an impending attack and is especially useful in crowded urban areas where attacks by larger

UAVs or other major weapons systems is impractical. Micro-air vehicles or MAVS are bug-sized devices that fly and are also called "entomopters." Guided by sensors, a military force is able to carry out precise, deadly strikes without sending its own soldiers into danger.

Elbit and other Israel companies produce cutting-edge mini-UAV systems (MAVs) designed for squad-level combat, battle damage assessment, air or artillery spotting, sensor dispersal, communications relay, detection of mines and hazardous substances, and jamming radar or communications equipment at short range. Since they are capable of hovering and vertical flight, they are also useful in scouting out buildings for urban combat and counter-terrorist operations, and for use in complex topographies such as mountainous terrain with caves, heavily forested areas with dense foliage and triple canopy jungle and high concentrations of civilians.[69] Elbit's Skylark family of electrically powered, human-portable, hand-launched, "counter-terror oriented" mini-UAVs send real-time video to a portable ground station over a range of 10 km. The armies of Australia, Canada, Croatia, the Czech Republic, France, Hungary, Israel, Macedonia, Netherlands, Poland, Slovakia and Sweden all deploy Skylarks, which have seen considerable action in Afghanistan and Iraq.[70]

IAI's mini-UAV, the BirdEye, comes as either a 7-kilo or a half-kilo kit, and performs "Over the Hill" reconnaissance and surveillance for small unit infantry.[71] Rafael produces SkyLite, which can be fired from a vehicle mount or shoulder-launched and has an hour's endurance. SkyLite B performs ISR missions in adverse weather conditions, navigates autonomously up to an altitude of 11,000 m and detects armed persons on the ground day or night.[72]

The Malat Division of IAI produces no less than ten types of UAVs. On the other end of IAI's UAV offerings is the Mosquito, a half-kilo flying video camera that can be launched by hand and can survey urban areas for up to an hour. In October 2010, IAI unveiled two more state-of-the-art mini-UAVs, the Panther and Mini-Panther, both for use by infantry unit and special forces, which combine the flight capabilities of an airplane with helicopter-like hovering. The Panther, weighing only 65 kg, is capable of loitering for six hours at altitudes of up to 3,050 m, with an operation radius of over 60 km. It is equipped with IAI's Mini-POP (Plug-in Optronic Payload), a day/night stabilized camera with a laser range finder, pointer and laser designator. The UAV control station—which is compact enough to be transported on a mid-size vehicle—stores up to three aircraft, a ground data link, support equipment and spare parts.[73]

Again ahead of the curve, IAI, which has a department of mini-robotics, has developed two mini-drones: Ghost, a silent, miniature, electrically powered, 4-kilo spy helicopter that can be carried in a backpack by a single soldier, and Bat, both of which are intended for day or night surveillance missions in urban settings, which could include tracking suspects marked for assassination by armed UAVs, helicopter gunships, or F-16 strike jets using precision-guided munitions.[74]

Already in 2003, however, IAI introduced a much smaller micro-drone, the Mosquito, weighing only 450 grams (about a pound). Launched by hand, even from within moving vehicles, the Mosquito has an endurance of an hour, carries a miniature video camera and can range up to two kilometers even in stiff winds. Once it locates a target, it activates a "hive" of three JUMPER canisters, each containing eight missiles, linked via an integrated command-and-control unit. Requiring no crew to operate it, the Jumper precision strike munitions missile system, guided by a GPS/INS system, delivers weapons carrying several possible warhead options with pinpoint accuracy up to a range of 50 km. By providing ground forces with autonomous fire support, especially in constricted urban areas where, it is claimed, its accuracy reduces "collateral damage," the Mosquito/JUMPER system leverages the combined capabilities of missiles, C^4 systems and miniaturization. Major General (Ret.) Eyal Ben-Reuven, the Deputy Commander of Israel's Northern Command during the second Lebanon War, says: "The JUMPER's unique mode of operation is very relevant to the asymmetric warfare characteristics of the complex battlefield under which the IDF and other modern armies have to operate."[75]

In 2012, IAI unveiled a butterfly-shaped drone weighing just 20 grams, the smallest in its Miniature Autonomous Robotic Vehicle (MARV) range so far, for gathering intelligence inside buildings. The miniscule surveillance device can take color pictures and is capable of a vertical take-off and hover flight, like a helicopter. "The butterfly's advantage is its ability to fly in an enclosed environment. There is no other aerial vehicle that can do that today," said Dubi Binyamini, head of IAI's mini-robotics department. In ground clashes, especially in cramped urban environments, a soldier could merely take it out of a pocket and send the butterfly behind the enemy's line. The virtually noiseless "butterfly" flaps its four wings 14 times per second. Almost translucent, it looks like an overgrown moth, but is still smaller than some natural butterflies. A soldier, putting on the helmet, finds himself in the "butterfly's cockpit" and virtually sees what the butterfly sees utilizing Israeli avionics. The butterfly-MARV can be deployed to observe in buildings, offices, or other sensitive sites, to survey battlefields and even forests like those in southern Lebanon where Hezbollah hides its ambush squads.[76]

MAVs, basically miniature spy planes, are rapidly evolving into MARVS. "The war in Lebanon proved that we need smaller weaponry," then-Deputy Prime Minister Shimon Peres was quoted in a newspaper article. "It's illogical to send a plane worth $100 million against a suicidal terrorist. So we are building futuristic weapons." One weapon is a "bionic hornet" that could track, chase, photograph, record and ultimately kill a "terrorist." Peres envisions bionic hornets hovering over the heads of terrorists as they record them and transmit their images back to an IDF Control Room: "The hornet comes within touching distance of the terrorists—and then the 'sting': a huge explosion is heard and the members of the cell are killed on the spot." According to the reporter, Peres "speaks at almost every opportunity of the hidden potential of nanotechnology."[77]

Moving quickly from idea to application, Peres, the father of Israel's nuclear bomb industry, selected 15 experts, "the best brains of the military and high-tech industries plus academic researchers," divided them into working groups, gave them budgets and the best research facilities, and set them to work on "futuristic applications of nanotechnology that will serve the security of Israel." The Israeli government planned to invest $230 million in nanotechnology research and development over the first five years of the project, beginning in 2006, which would make nanoscience one of Israel's most heavily-invested R&D fields. (Recall the establishment of a joint nanotech laboratory between the Weizmann Institute of Science and the LENS Institute for Atomic Physics in Florence with its initial €250 million endowment.) Prototypes for these futuristic weapons, including bionic gloves that give soldiers superhuman strength, new light-weight, super-strong armor for tanks based on NOLES (Nanotubes Optimized for Lightweight Exceptional Strength) and "smart dust" sensors to detect suicide bombers, could, says Peres, be ready within three years.[78]

One innovative research project is "Lessons from Insects for the Design of Nano Unmanned Aerial Vehicles" of the Technion's Faculty of Aerospace Engineering, whose students have developed the "Dragonfly" drone. Its 9-inch (23-cm) wing span makes it small enough to "easily enter rooms through small windows and to send back photos from a miniature camera."[79] Snake robots, also developed by the Technion, represent sophisticated biorobotics in which snake-like machines of varying sizes (including micro), equipped with cameras and occasionally explosives, are deployed for surveillance in open terrain, in contested buildings in urban battlespaces or, potentially, to implant poisons or debilitating devices in targeted individuals.[80]

Rather than rely only on biomimicry, MARVs also harness real insects for military purposes. The creation of cybernetic insects by placing micro-mechanical systems inside insects during the early stages of metamorphosis and thus transforming them into tools of surveillance, has been pioneered by the Pentagon's DARPA in its Hybrid Insect Micro-Electro-Mechanical Systems project. Funded by that program, Israeli scientists at Technion's aeronautics laboratory in Haifa, one of five laboratories around the world conducting similar research, are conducting experiments that would allow them to control the flight of insects from afar, as if they were mechanical flight vehicles. "The important thing is not just to control the insect from afar," explains Dr. Gal Ribak, an expert in animal biomechanics. "The challenge is to prod an insect to fly, to have it do what it already knows how to do, and to intervene only when we want to intervene"[81]

In another project funded by DARPA, Prof. Joseph Terkel of the Center for Applied Animal Behavior for Security Purposes at Tel Aviv University is focusing on the natural advantage of birds: flying, communicating, having superb eyesight, yet being unobtrusive. He is training birds to respond to visual stimuli for surveillance missions. In the project, birds are being trained to cover a large area or to remain within a particular site; when the "target" they have been taught to locate appears in their vision, they respond as trained.[82] Yet another DARPA program in Israel focuses on developing NAVs, extremely small (less than 15 cm), ultra-lightweight (less than 20 g) air-vehicle-systems that can perform indoor and outdoor military missions within an operating range less than 1 km and endurance of less than one hour—such as the "smart dust" Peres alluded to. Such research is progressing at the Satellite and Wireless Communication Laboratory at Ben Gurion University, where "smart dust" is more formally known as "optical wireless communication in distributed sensor networks."[83]

In another, though related, direction, Yoram Shapira, a Tel Aviv University professor specializing in microelectronics, has developed "smart dew," sensors the size of dewdrops that can be scattered across an enclosed space or around the perimeter of an area to detect any intrusion within a range of 5–50 m. Each "droplet" in this early warning system is sensitive to a single parameter, such as noise, magnetic fields produced by metal in cars or tanks, vibrations, carbon monoxide emissions, or light. Issuing a signal every few seconds, it instantly identifies an intruder, be it mechanical, human, or simply a bird flying by. And each droplet, equipped with its own micro-battery and able to operate for several months, communicates via radio frequency to a base station that analyzes the data and issues an alarm if warranted. "Smart dew" drops are about one-tenth of an inch (2.5 mm) and are sturdy enough to be dropped from an airplane.[84]

Artillery and Mortars

Soltam Systems specializes in artillery: towed and self-propelled howitzers, mortars of various kinds, mortar ammunition and their delivery systems. A subsidiary of Elbit since 2010, Soltam serves customers in more than 60 countries, including the US Army and NATO. Among its "family" of artillery systems is the Atmos Autonomous Truck Mounted Howitzer System, mountable on a variety of military vehicles, whose shells are aimed by computerized navigation systems and whose potential range is more than 50 km. The Slammer can be mounted on tank chassis and is capable of firing nine rounds per minute. The ATHOS 2025 Autonomous Towed Howitzer receives digital radio target data directly from a forward observer or a remote target acquisition system and prepares itself for firing, able to move its carriage and position itself. The Rascal is a self-propelled 155 mm howitzer so compact and light that it can be deployed in narrow urban streets or narrow mountain roads.[85]

IAI's LORA long-range surface attack missile is an artillery weapon designed to engage strategic targets—infrastructure assets (communications, power stations), surface-to-air missile batteries and the like—deep in the enemy's territory, from mobile or maritime platforms, and with an accuracy of less than 10 m, equal or better to that of an aerial guided weapon. LORA can be launched within a few minutes from unprepared positions and hit any target within its range in less than ten minutes. The missile can be equipped with a 400-kg high-explosive warhead, or with a 600-kg penetration warhead, to hit hardened targets; like smaller artillery pieces, it can hit a target at high angle of attack. LORA can perform pre-programmed maneuvers after launch and after re-entry, to conceal its launch point and intended target, thus preventing the enemy from taking defensive measures or attempting to intercept the missile or launcher.[86]

Elbit Systems has unveiled a mortar-firing system called Spear, which has entered service in the IDF and other militaries. The system can be installed on light combat vehicles, including Humvees and jeeps, due to its lightweight gun barrel firing recoil loads that weigh less than 10 tons. Firing 120-mm mortars, the system—described by Elbit as a fully autonomous soft-recoil mortar system—"significantly improves the maneuverability and operational performance of infantry forces, as it delivers immediate indirect artillery support for effectively engaging a wide range of targets."[87]

Senior IDF sources said 40 percent of artillery shells are being converted into precision shells that can accurately strike specific buildings from 40 kilometers away—a 150 percent increase in range from the older shells. The upgrades will mean that a battalion commander on the ground who identifies threats in a Lebanese village dozens of kilometers away does not need to call in the air force and wait. He will be able to immediately direct precision artillery fire at a building of his choice.[88]

Small Arms/Light Weapons (SALW)

No matter how sophisticated the technology of "engagement at a distance" might become, armies will still need ground forces, even if Special Operations Forces (SOFs) replace larger units in urban warfare and pinpoint engagements. Small arms and light weapons (SALW) at the service of individual soldiers are no less a key to precision engagement than larger weapons systems. Indeed, versatile small arms are often more appropriate for close quarter combat in urban environments than cumbersome infantry weapons such as assault rifles, machine guns, mortars and grenades.

Since the early 2000s, for example, the IDF has been transitioning from the American M-16 and the M-4—and even from its own lightweight Galil— to the Micro-Tavor. Known officially as the MTAR-21, the Micro-Tavor can easily be converted from an assault rifle to a sub-machine gun (with a silencer), and is also fitted with an integral, advanced and accurate sighting system attached directly to the barrel. Developed by the Israeli company ITL Optronics—optronics being another key Israeli industry—the sighting system consists of a multi-purpose aiming reflex sight (MARS), combining a reflex sight that aims a red dot constantly on the target with a laser sight that renders the dot either visible or seen only by soldiers equipped with special night-vision infrared devices. The Micro-Tavor, which also carries a traditional iron sight, can be mounted with an array of other scopes.

A product of Israel Weapon Industries (IWI), the Tavor line of assault rifles was developed in close cooperation with the IDF and underwent extensive field-testing in the Palestinian laboratory. The Tavor and

Micro-Tavor employ a bullpup configuration, meaning it can use either a very short barrel for urban warfare, thereby minimizing the silhouette of the soldier, especially when coming around corners, or a very long and easily attached one for more open terrain. Variations of the Micro-Tavor include the CTAR-21, a compact assault rifle for commandos and Special Forces, the STAR-21 designed for snipers and the G-Tar 21, equipped with a grenade launcher.[89]

All together, the various components and capabilities of the Micro-Tavor line conform to the type of "modular" weapon needed to extend the precise, lethal firepower of the infantry: one that lends itself to the "arms room concept," under which each soldier would have multiple options available in a single weapon, supported by magnified optics for mid-range engagements or non-magnified optics for close range or urban engagements.[90] The Tavor line spans the MISSILE Complex of war amongst the people, homeland security and policing, where it has become a favorite among special operations units and SWAT teams. Indeed, IWI's TAR Msw and five variations of its X95 assault rifles are designed particularly for law enforcement.[91] Not surprisingly, it has also become popular among drug dealers, arms dealers, the mafia and common criminals, just as its cousin the Uzi was and still is.

IWI's Negev Light Machine Gun, also standard equipment in the IDF, is highly versatile, suitable for infantry, vehicle-mounted operations, or mounted on helicopters or naval craft. The Negev SF and the latest Negev NG7, designed for special forces, can switch from automatic to semi-automatic fire in urban combat where precision shooting is essential.[92] (*Defense Review* is less concerned about "collateral damage." "Assuming the IWI NEGEV NG7 works as advertised, it will be a welcome infantry warfare tool for the Israel Defense Forces (IDF)," it enthuses, "especially if/when they end up having to fend off the enemy Arab and Iranian/Persian/Aryan hordes in a World War III (WWIII)/Armageddon-style war).")[93]

Yet another Israeli company, Silver Shadow Advanced Security Systems, describes itself as "specializing in military firearm design and customized solutions for special operations units … [and] led by a former senior officer of the Israel Defense Forces and Israel Police, who holds a remarkable operational track record." The company produces various models of its Gilboa assault rifle. Its compact APR (assault pistol rifle) is designed specifically for close quarter combat, VIP protection and special forces, while snipers have the Silenced Timna high-precision rifle, among other specialized firearms.[94]

IMI's multi-purpose rifle system (MPRS) promises nothing less than to "completely change the way infantry soldiers engage targets and hit them." IMI uses the same technology found in fire control systems of advanced tanks like the Merkava to develop sensors that transform any assault rifle into a precision grenade-launcher. The rifle's sight displays the ubiquitous red dot aiming point at just the right elevation necessary for an accurate shot, then automatically sets the time-delay fuse in the grenade to activate it just before impact at a preset altitude over the target. A 40-mm grenade can also be set to explode at a preset delay after impact, to enable penetration of a relatively "soft target," such as a window.[95]

CornerShot is another innovative weapon of urban warfare, special ops and law enforcement. Composed of a forward swiveled pistol mount attached to a specially designed gun frame equipped with a video display, it is capable of shooting around corners, thus protecting the shooter. The brain child of Lt. Col. Amos Golan who "was frustrated by the mounting [Israeli] casualties in the West Bank," CornerShot, a product emerging directly out of the Palestinian lab, can fire bullets or tasers, although its heavier models can launch grenades and even anti-tank rockets.[96]

For all this, as with other weapons systems, Israel adapts foreign weaponry to its own uses or enters into joint development projects, making its valuable "lab" available to others. During Operation Protective Edge, for example, the IDF tested the HTR 2000, a new sniper rifle distributed to all infantry battalions, made by H-S Precision in the United States, but called the "Barak" locally because of various Israeli improvements—likewise with the IDF's standard sniper rifle, the Remington M24.[97]

Munitions

IMI produces munitions for weapons ranging from air-to-ground systems, artillery and tanks down to rifles and pistols—explosive rounds and rockets, general purpose and "smart" ammunition, urban bombs, deep penetration bombs, runway penetrators and small caliber ammunition. Indeed, IMI is a leading supplier of munitions to the US Army and NATO members (IMI Munitions; IMI/Small Calibre). Here, too, innovation is constant. One new anti-personnel/anti-material (APAM) tank cartridge, the HE-MP-T, has become standard IDF ammunition. It is equipped with a high-explosive fragmentation warhead that "enhances lethality" *in the anti-personnel role* (i.e., against people) by using tungsten fragments to envelop "targets" such as "dug-in personnel" in an intensely hot airburst over an area. So intense is the tungsten-based burst—it is hot enough to melt glass—that it penetrates walls, thin armor, or fortification.[98]

This munition, known as a Focused-Lethality Munition, was initially developed by the US Air Force but was used for the first time in 2005 in the Gaza lab. Dropped on groups of people, a DIME bomblet of "dense inert metal explosives" is nonetheless considered a "low collateral damage" weapon because, though reliably killing every human within the blast zone, it does so within a blast zone that is small and concentrated, "only" a 50–100-foot circle. As the former chief of the IDF's weapons development program, General Yitzhak Ben-Israel, explains it, "one of the ideas is to allow those targeted to be hit without causing damage to bystanders or other persons." It is therefore presented as a "humane" weapon.[99]

DIME bombs, which are chemically toxic, carcinogenic, damaging to the immune system and, in that they attack DNA, genotoxic, explode just above the heads of the targeted persons and the unfortunate others standing nearby, releasing a powerful blast that sprays a superheated, powdered heavy metal tungsten alloy.[100] "When the shrapnel hits the body," reported Dr. Joma Al-Saqqa, chief of the emergency unit at Gaza's largest hospital, Al-Shifa

... it causes very strong burns that destroy the tissues around the bones ... it burns and destroys internal organs, like the liver, kidneys, and the spleen and other organs and makes saving the wounded almost impossible ... There were usually entry and exit wounds. When the wounds were explored no foreign material was found. There was tissue death, the extent of which was difficult to determine ... A higher deep infection rate resulted with subsequent amputation. In spite of amputation there was a higher mortality. The effects of the weapon seemed "radioactive." As a surgeon, I have seen thousands of wounds during the Intifada, but nothing was like this weapon.[101]

The opposite of focused-lethality munitions are cluster bombs, bomblets dropped in their millions that spew submunitions when set off, killing indiscriminately, often for years after a conflict has ended. Israel is a major producer and exporter of cluster bombs and landmines; it has not joined either the Landmine Ban Treaty or the Convention on Cluster Munitions, both of which it in fact actively opposes. IMI produces the MI-85 air-dropped cluster bomb, used by British forces in Basra. For its part, Rafael produces the ATAP-300, ATAP-500, ATAP-1000 RAM, TAL-1, and TAL-2 cluster bombs, as well as the BARAD Helicopter Submunition Dispenser. Israel is also reported to have laid approximately 1 million operational and non-operational landmines in the Golan Heights and the Occupied Palestinian Territories.[102]

Hype or Reality?

In the last two chapters, I've tried to convey the range and power of modern weaponry as reflected in the Israeli arsenal. We have entered into new realms of killing ability and control. There are no grounds to doubt that the capabilities built into the systems just reviewed can perform as advertised, but that does not mean their ability to impose totalized securitization is a given, or that resistance is futile. There still exists a significant gap between technological power and precision—and the death, destruction and suffering it can certainly cause—and the ability to actually enforce hegemony or achieve pacification. Nowhere is this more evident than in tiny, exposed Gaza. There, for all Israel's vaunted strength, technological sophistication and long experience in counter-insurgency, it has not succeeded in "defeating" the Palestinians. In fact, as the French learned in the Battle of Algiers, the rate of attrition in the ability of an strong oppressor to withstand the loss of moral legitimacy that comes with massive violations of human rights, IHL and simple justice is often greater than that of the oppressed with little to lose. Again, this is not to minimize the totalizing power arrayed against us, but rather to urge us to look for and exploit the vulnerabilities that such systems must invariably contain.

We'll now move from weaponry to the Matrix of Control, Israel's model of securocratic control, of a globalized Palestine, being marketed abroad.

Part IV

The Securocratic Dimension—A Model of "Sufficient Pacification" (Niche 2)

7

Israel's Matrix of Control

If the development of high-tech weaponry and components for weapons systems constitutes the first Israeli macro-niche in the global pacification system, then providing a model of securocratic control, what I call Israel's Matrix of Control, embodies the second. The Occupied Palestinian Territory has been transformed into probably the most monitored, controlled and militarized place on earth. It epitomizes the dream of every general, security expert and police officer to be able to exercise total biopolitical control. In a situation where the local population enjoys no effective legal protections or privacy, they and their lands become a laboratory where the latest technologies of surveillance, control and suppression are perfected and showcased, giving Israel an edge in the highly competitive global market. Labels such as "Combat Proven," "Tested in Gaza" and "Approved by the IDF" on Israeli or foreign products greatly improves their marketability.

As much as Israel has refined its Matrix over the years, it did not invent it whole cloth. Much of it reflects, in fact, British colonial practices. Laleh Khalili points out that

> ... a large number of legal apparatuses that [the Israeli military] use as part of their counterinsurgency, including their emergency regulation, comes from the British. Many of their administrative procedures come from the British military experience, and finally a lot of the punitive forms that they use in their counterinsurgency including closures and curfews, house demolitions, and the uses of walls and other security apparatuses are all borrowed from the British. The first set of walls that were built as a kind of an offensive counterinsurgency measure was by the British in the 1930s.[1]

What's more, the Matrix emerged (and continues to emerge) out of field-based necessity. Boaz Ganor, a leading Israeli authority on counter-terrorism and the author of *The Counter-Terrorism Puzzle*, contends that "Israel does not have—nor did it ever have—a written, structured and unambiguous counter-terrorism policy." Instead its approach is based on "several underlying principles" and an "operational policy," an approach far removed from a formal strategy. In fact, the IDF's goal regarding terrorism has been limited to minimizing the scope and damage of attacks, not to eliminating them.[2]

Ganor's reservations about the existence of an Israeli doctrine of counter-terrorism notwithstanding, surveying Israeli policies and practices over seven decades, including almost fifty years of occupation, reveals a coherent approach that, while constantly adapting to new situations and actors, does constitute a "model" that can be taught, followed and described. What I present here may not be accepted by Ganor and the military establishment—starting with my framing of the Matrix's overall conception as "warehousing"—but it rests on a thorough search for the myriad pieces of the "puzzle" that, when fit together, do indeed present an intelligible picture.

Between Phase 4 and "Sufficient Pacification": Israel's Approach to Warfare, Conventional and Securocratic

As warfare moves from its conventional interstate forms to hybrid wars, war amongst the people, securitization at home and abroad, counter-terrorism and militarized domestic policing, Israel is able to parlay its interminable struggle against the Palestinians (and Hezbollah) into an exportable commodity. The fact that Israel has failed miserably in both combating terror and resolving its conflicts doesn't seem to tarnish its reputation as a leading authority on the War on Terror, as military commentators such as Gazit, Maoz and Peri sardonically note. In fact, Israel has turned its inability to resolve its conflict with the Palestinians into a marketing advantage, for the failure to come to terms with the Palestinians is not presented as a failure at all, but as a successful case of pacification—or at least "sufficient," ongoing pacification.

Indeed, Israel's focus on pacification departs fundamentally from Western counter-insurgency doctrine which holds, with Clausewitz, that the ultimate aim of war is to achieve the strategic goals for which the war was fought in the first place or at least to "create a condition in which a strategic result is achieved," as General Smith says. "Winning hearts and minds," striving "less to kill insurgents than to protect the civilian population" and, eventually, returning political control (if not overall hegemony) to the local population lie at the heart of the American approach.[3] "In a COIN environment," says the US Army's Counterinsurgency Manual

> ... it is vital for commanders to adopt appropriate and measured levels of force and apply that force precisely so that it accomplishes the mission without causing unnecessary loss of life or suffering ... An operation that kills five insurgents is counterproductive if collateral damage leads to the recruitment of 50 more insurgents.[4]

Israel is incapable of adopting a "hearts and minds" approach because it cannot give the Palestinians precisely what would end the conflict: either political independence or equal civil rights. It thus seeks neither to end the conflict (so no Phase IV) nor turn over political control to the local population in any hypothetical resolution of the conflict. The only alternative is therefore pacification with all that entails: intimidation, isolation, confrontation and the use of disproportionate force, all intended to induce despair over attaining national rights and breaking the Palestinians' resistance. Overt repression replaces counter-insurgency—and hence the lack of a counter-terror doctrine, which Ganor himself says is dependent upon a political solution.[5] Nonetheless, because repression achieves more rapid and dramatic results in the short term than does genuine counter-insurgency or counter-terrorism, Israeli tactics are lauded and copied. In the long term, however, the Israeli approach is indeed limited and likely even counter-productive for countries seeking political solutions, or at least more sustainable forms of hegemony.

Khalili[6] doubts that defeating revolutionaries/insurgents in order to create political conditions in which popular government could be restored has ever been the genuine agenda of counter-insurgency practitioners from Galuta to Petraeus. If, in fact, a neo-imperial agenda most obvious in the "resource wars" waged by the core capitalist states and their local allies against the peoples of the periphery pits them uncompromisingly against each other, then the Israeli "zero-tolerance" approach of permanent repression makes sense. So, too, does the aspiration to core pacification as expressed in the "clash of civilizations" and the Global War on Terror. If securitization, control and pacification are the true goals, as they are in Israel's policies toward the Palestinians, the aim of Israeli counter-insurgency, "undermining the adversary's determination and to lead to the adversary's abandoning his objectives, through a cumulative process of inflicting physical, economic and psychological damage, [and] to lead the adversary to realize that his own armed engagement is hopeless,"[7] has much to commend it on the global stage.

"Sufficient victory over terrorism"—that is how Major-General Ya'akov Amidror, formerly Netanyahu's National Security Adviser, president of Israel's National Defense College and currently a fellow at the Begin-Sadat Center for Strategic Studies, describes Israel's goals. In "a protracted intractable conflict," he contends, "sufficient victory" can be attained through continuous counter-terrorist measures, what the IDF refers to as "mowing the grass."[8] Following a strategy of attrition, the IDF

> ... just "mows the grass" of the enemy capabilities, with no ambition to solve the conflict. It also attempts to achieve some deterrence to extend the time between the rounds of violence. Periods of tranquility are important for Israel because its mere existence is a success over its radical non-state enemies and sends them a constant reminder that their destructive goals are not within reach. The longer the absence of violence along its borders, the lower the price Israel pays for being engaged in such a protracted conflict. [Nonetheless, mowing the grass] contains traditional elements of Israel's military modus operandi, such as retaliatory raids and preemptive strikes.[9]

The IDF measures its progress, according to Amidror, not only by the usual military standards of casualties inflicted, enemy equipment destroyed, or battles won, but by the degree of security and tranquility it engenders (among the population being defended, in this case the Israelis) and by indices of economic growth attained even in the course of the conflict. Counter-insurgency/counter-terrorism, war amongst the people, is for Israel much more securocratic war than it is for the Americans in Iraq or Afghanistan, in which the counter-insurgents leave. Instead, it is more akin to the Russian suppression of Chechnya or the Chinese in Tibet: intimate, close-quartered and permanent. This may give Israeli tactics special appeal to militarized security and police forces—the Brazilian Pacification Police in the Rio *favelas* or US police in the inner cities— but it carries severe implications, as warfare or pacification move into domestic securitization.

A Warehouse Within a Fortress

It is impossible to avoid the image of a prison when describing Israeli control of the Occupied Territory. But prison captures only part of Palestinian reality. More than 1.5 million Palestinians live as citizens of Israel within Israel "proper," but are confined by zoning and restrictions on land-use by non-Jews to just 3.5 percent of their own country's land, 94 percent of the land of the state being reserved for Jews. Of the 4.5 million Palestinians living in the Occupied Territory conquered in 1967, an area representing but 22 percent of historic Palestine, 96 percent are confined to dozens of enclaves on small bits of their country: some 70 cells on only 38 percent of the West Bank; isolated pockets of "east" Jerusalem comprising just 11 percent of the urban area, and the cage of tiny Gaza, besieged and closed from all directions, including Egypt and the sea. Naomi Klein calls these enclaves "holding pens," different from prison cells only in that their inmates have not been convicted and can leave by permanently exiting the country altogether—holding pens until people leave. "What Israel has constructed," she writes

> … is a system … a network of open holding pens for millions of people who have been categorized as surplus humanity … Palestinians are not the only people in the world who have been so categorized … In South Africa, Russia and New Orleans the rich build walls around themselves. Israel has taken this disposal process a step further: it has built walls around the dangerous poor.[10]

These holding pens are scattered throughout the country, and since all Palestinians live within a *de facto* or *de jure* "Jewish" state extending from the Mediterranean to the Jordan River, it is often difficult to distinguish between life for Palestinians within Israel or in the Occupied Territory. If they reside in slightly more porous "holding pens" rather than cells, "warehousing" might better describe their situation better than imprisonment. The concept of warehousing emerges from the American prison system, where "surplus populations" are locked up.[11] Their situation is static: Palestinians can neither negotiate it collectively nor have the right to change it. Unless they emigrate as individuals, they exist as permanent inmates, their confinement de-politicized and even normalized. Being parts of a "terrorist collective"—Israel has never recognized them as a people with national rights of self-determination—their warehousing has been emptied of all political content and possibility of resolution. In Israeli terms, warehousing is cast as "autonomy." According to the former IDF Chief-of-Staff and Minister of Defense Moshe Ya'alon:

> Israeli policy immediately following the Six Day War in 1967, and up to the Oslo Accords in 1993, centered on finding a formula that would enable Israel to avoid ruling over the Palestinians, without returning to the unstable pre-war '67 lines. It was on this basis that Israel did not annex Judea, Samaria and Gaza, yet at the same time did not speak of a Palestinian state within those territories. In fact, nothing that Israel did or said in those years—including at the 1978 Camp David Accords between Israeli Prime Minister Menachem Begin and Egyptian President Anwar Sadat, which called for "autonomy for the Palestinian people," and later, in 1993, when Prime Minister Yitzhak Rabin entered into the Oslo Accords—constituted intent or consent to establish a Palestinian state within the pre-war '67 lines. Those Israeli leaders understood that these lines were indefensible ... Rabin was very clear on the need to provide Palestinian autonomy, yet maintain defensible borders for Israel.[12]

If Palestinians are warehoused in discrete holding pens, Israeli Jews live freely on the entire Land of Israel, more than half a million of them residing in the Occupied Territory. Their expansive and contiguous national space is also circumscribed however: the entire Land of Israel under Israeli control taking on the form of a fortress encircled by highly militarized borders—or in the strange but more felicitous image offered to Israelis by Ehud Barak, a "villa in the jungle." Indeed, it was Barak, a former prime minister and minister of defense, who first gave a name to Israel's concept of co-existence with the Palestinians: *hafrada*, meaning "separation," or "apartheid" in Hebrew. As in South Africa where "separate development" concealed a system in which one population separated itself from the others, then created a permanent and institutional regime of domination, *hafrada* does the same. Thus the official name of the barrier that snakes through the West Bank, the "Separation Barrier," hides under the rubric of security the incorporation of half of the West Bank into Israel and the truncation of the Palestinian areas into small, impoverished "cantons."

Israel's warehouse within a fortress constitutes a model society congruent with the needs of emerging human-security states of the core. Guided by a set of operational doctrines, its structure, what I call a Matrix of Control, consists of four main elements that can be exported, either singly or as an overall system of securocratic control: (1) a strategic matrix of "facts on the ground," (2) a legal and administrative regime, (3) effective tactics and weaponry of control, all within (4) a regime of economic control and dependence (see Table 7.1).

Table 7.1   Israel's Matrix of Control over the Occupied Palestinian Territory

Framing: A Tendentious Definition of "Terrorism"

Strategic "facts on the ground"
- Borders and Walls
- The Iron Wall
- Kitur/Encirclement, isolation and layered defense systems
- Monitoring movement/Surveillance

An expedient legal and administrative regime
- Military government/"Civil" administration
- Planning and zoning regulations
- Mass detentions and limitations on civil liberties
- Creating categories of people with differential rights and life-spaces
- Blurring civil/military lines in the enforcement of internal security

Operational doctrines and tactics
- Interactive intelligence gathering
- Limited use of unlimited force, disproportionate force, cumulative deterrence and escalation domination
- Aerial occupation
- Targeted assassinations
- Urban warfare
- Weapons of suppression

A regime of economic control and dependence

Framing: A Tendentious Definition of "Terrorism"

If warehousing has a chance of succeeding, of becoming somehow sustainable over time, it requires a compelling "framing" that turns the oppressed into the threat and the oppressors into the victims merely defending themselves. Appeals to the need for security to protect the "innocents" and the casting of those resisting colonization or suppression as "terrorists" has long served the various powers-that-be.[13] Israel possesses yet another powerful resource: the widespread perception that the Jews are history's ultimate victims, a view it encourages and cynically exploits even as it claims that Zionism has normalized Jewish/Israeli life—and even as its security politics compels it to project an image of a major military power.

A key to Israel's framing and central to its "lawfare" campaign is a tendentious definition of "terrorism" which lets it off the hook as an Occupying Power and places the onus squarely in the Palestinians living under its control. The definition, put forward by none other than Benjamin Netanyahu in his book *Terrorism: How the West Can Win*,[14] has been endorsed by Israel's military/academic establishment. As articulated by Ganor, who heads the International Policy Institute for Counter-Terrorism known as the Interdisciplinary Center, a right-wing Israeli think-tank/college, terrorism "is a form of violent struggle in which violence is deliberately used against civilians in order to achieve political goals."[15]

On the surface, this definition would seem to apply to Israel's own policies towards the Palestinians, beginning with the expulsion of half the Palestinian people from their country, the systematic destruction of 536 villages, towns and urban neighborhoods and the expropriation of their lands, and up to today where a military occupation of five decades has resulted in the deaths and injury of tens of thousands of civilians, massive arrests and torture, the demolition of some 60,000 homes, impoverishment, further displacement and expulsion—and open "punishment" for the crime of turning to the ICC for protection.

But here is the catch in the Netanyahu/Ganor definition. It is based not on the human rights/IHL approach by which all attacks on civilians (or non-combatants) is prohibited by all sides, state or non-state, but rather "intention," giving states in particular the ability to ascribe to the non-state adversaries and themselves motives that serve their ends. Thus, says Ganor, "terrorism is not the result of random damage inflicted on civilians who happened to find themselves in an area of violent political activity"—"collateral damage" in military terms—"rather it is directed a priori at harming civilians."[16] In other words, the 2,200 people killed in Israel's 2014 assault on Gaza, two-thirds of whom were civilians, cannot be counted as victims of terrorism because the Israeli government did not *intend* to kill them (though who could ever prove that remains to be seen, especially in light of such IDF procedures as the Dahiya Doctrine). By contrast, the five Israeli civilians killed by rockets from Gaza *were* victims of terror because Hamas "intended" to kill them, despite the fact that their missiles cannot be effectively aimed—unlike the "precision" missiles of the IDF, which could not have killed civilians unless they were intentionally targeted. The four boys playing on a beach near Gaza City who were killed in a "precision" strike were, in the words of the IDF, "a tragic outcome," while it blamed Hamas for its "cynical exploitation of a population held hostage."[17]

"Selling" its occupation and periodic mauling of the Palestinians as justifiable self-defense against terrorism is key to perpetuating the Matrix of Control and legitimizing its methods and practices. (A spokesman for the Chinese Army traveled to Israel after Operation Cast Lead to learn from his counterparts just how the IDF framed its attack. The IDF for its part reported, "The Chinese delegation will be presented with the public-relations lessons learnt during … Operation Cast Lead."[18]) Given that protective covering, the Israeli government and army are at liberty to formulate, execute and proudly export their model of securitization and pacification. Let's look now at how its done.

Creating Strategic "Facts on the Ground"

Borders and Walls (The "Iron Wall")

The primary goal of the Matrix is to create a sanitized and secure space for Israelis that is both expandable (allowing Palestine to be "Judaized") and separated from the (ever-shrinking) Palestinian holding pens (de-Arabization and *hafrada*), yet secured by highly militarized borders and internal divisions. The use of walls not as borders but as kinetic internal instruments for controlling territory and populations has a distinguished history in Zionist thought. As far back as 1923, Ze'ev Jabotinsky, the political mentor of Begin, Netanyahu and the Likud Party, formulated his doctrine of the Iron Wall. Recognizing that, as he put it, "Every indigenous people will resist alien settlers as long as they see any hope of ridding themselves of the danger of foreign settlement," he proposed that the Zionist settlement of Palestine develop "under the protection of a force that is not dependent on the local population, behind an iron wall which they will be powerless to break down."[19]

Israeli military doctrine has always emphasized "secure defensible borders" augmented by deterrence and a culture of initiated offensive strikes.[20] In the early 1990s, however, the IDF reassessed Israel's "threat environment," leading to a reordering of its military's priorities. WMD and long-range delivery systems in the hands of distant states were designated primary threats, with terrorism and counter-insurgency "promoted" to second place. The threat of conventional warfare with neighboring states, long the first priority, was demoted to third place.[21]

Writ large, "secure defensible borders," then, refers to control of space, airspace and all the potential battlespace that separates Israel from adversaries who can reach it in any way, a conception that feeds into Niche 1. In regards to Niche 2, more immediate securitization "on the ground," it refers to borders over which non-state insurgents ("terrorists") might surge or take control—or even which fail to protect the state from threats to its integrity. Until recently, for example, the border with Egypt was merely a rusty, semi-dilapidated fence. As African asylum seekers (called "infiltrators" or "illegal aliens" by Israeli officials) began reaching Israel through the Sinai, it has been up-graded to a hi-tech 245-mile (395-km) barrier complete with advanced surveillance equipment so as to "secure Israel's Jewish and democratic character."[22] The barrier on the Egyptian border is an extension of that constructed around Gaza, completed in 1996; as in Gaza, it also protects against attacks by Hamas fighters and their allies. As the Syrian civil war gained strength, fears that jihadist terrorists or Lebanese Hezbollah fighters might spill into Israel prompted the construction of an additional 44-mile (70-km) "smart fence" on the occupied Golan Heights, together with a 50-mile (80-km) barrier on the Lebanese border, armed with concertina and razor wire, touch sensors, motion detectors, infrared cameras and ground radar. The final section of barrier around Fortress Israel will be constructed along a 250-mile (400-km) route extending the length of the border with Jordan, again, more against the infiltration of asylum seekers than "terrorists."

The "border" of greatest concern to Israel, however, is its "demographic border" with the Palestinians, now guarded by the "Separation Barrier." This internal border expands Israeli-controlled territory and settlements over half the West Bank while separating the Jewish population of East Jerusalem and the settlement "blocs" from the Palestinians locked into their disconnected "cantons" (all while securing it from Palestinian attacks). The border between the West Bank and Jordan is a more conventional "security border" defending the Fortress from the east. Both borders carry out political decisions by effectively eliminating the two-state solution.

Construction of the "Separation Barrier" (*mikhshol ha-hafrada*) commenced in mid-2002. Although sold to the Israeli and international publics alike as an installation to prevent terrorism, its very name denotes its basic purpose of demarcating Israel's demographic border. "There is no doubt that the most important and dramatic step we face is the determination of permanent borders of the State of Israel, to ensure the Jewish majority in the country," Acting Prime Minister Ehud Olmert told the Herzliya Conference in January 2006. "We must create a clear boundary as soon as possible, one which will reflect the demographic reality on the ground. Israel will maintain control over the security zones [and] the Jewish settlement blocs ... ."[23]

The Separation Barrier extends along a tortuous route of about 420 miles (680 km), even though the "Green Line" itself is only 217 miles (320 km) long. (As prime minister, Ariel Sharon insisted that it not follow the 1967 border so as not to signify space in which a Palestinian state might emerge.) For most of its length, in the rural areas, the Barrier consists of electronic fences fortified by watchtowers, sniper posts, mine fields, ditches 13 ft (4 m) deep, barbed wire, security perimeters, patrol roads, surveillance cameras, electronic warning devices—and, for good measure, patrols of killer dogs. Upon approaching Palestinian cities, towns and neighborhoods, it becomes a wall of solid concrete 26 ft (8 m) high, more than twice the height of the Berlin Wall.

Unlike that other infamous wall, however, the Israeli barrier is not linear; it consists of a complex series of secondary and tertiary barriers entrapping Palestinians in dozens of tiny enclaves. A quarter-million people find themselves locked into bits of territory between the border and the Barrier, a hundred villages are separated from their agricultural lands. So, too, do another quarter-million Palestinian residents of East Jerusalem find themselves separated from the West Bank by a double system of physical barrier and restrictions of movement. With barrier gates permitting farmers only limited access to their fields, many have abandoned their farms and orchards. Thus forced to move into Areas A and B, this induced exodus from the land thereby paves the way for Israeli annexation of Area C.[24]

Nodes and Matrices

As today, Jewish settlements in the pre-state period were established strategically, the idea being that they would eventually define the borders of the Jewish state and secure its interior spaces. With the outbreak of the Arab Revolt in Palestine in 1936, they were defended by *homa umigdal* (wall and tower), a fortified perimeter that enabled dozens of new Jewish colonies to be founded in isolated and hostile areas far from other settlements, thus systematically extending the pre-state boundaries. As in the case of settlements and the Separation Barrier today, Sharon Rotbard notes that *homa umigdal* "was more an instrument than a place." It expressed in the clearest physical terms the relationship of Zionist colonists to the Palestinians (and Palestine): the *homa* (wall) creating spaced that excluded Palestinians while simultaneously, through the *migdal* (tower), observing and controlling them.[25]

The relevance of such an approach to counter-insurgency operations elsewhere is evident and noticeable. Notes the critical Israeli architect Eyal Weizman:

> The "Intifada" unfolding in Iraq is part of an imaginary geography that Makram Khoury-Machool called the "Palestinization of Iraq". Yet, if the Iraqi resistance is perceived to have been "Palestinized", the American military has been "Israelized". Furthermore, both the American and Israeli militaries have adopted counterinsurgency tactics that increasingly resemble the guerrilla methods of their enemies. When the wall around the American Green Zone in Baghdad looks as if it had been built from left-over components of the West Bank Wall; when "temporary closures" are imposed on entire Iraqi towns and villages and reinforced with earth dykes and barbed wire; when larger sections are carved up by road blocks and checkpoints; when the homes of suspected terrorists are destroyed, and "targeted assassinations" are introduced into a new global militarized geography—it is because the separate conflicts now generally collected under the heading of the "war on terror" are the backdrop to the formation of complex "institutional ecologies" that allow the exchange of technologies, mechanisms, doctrines, and spatial strategies between various militaries and the organizations that they confront, as well as between the civilian and military domains.[26]

Israel's approach to pacification through "Palestinization" was manifested most starkly, perhaps, in Guatemala during the 1980s, when the Israeli military presence was palpable. "In the post-massacre re-organisation of the landscape and permanent fragmentation of communities," writes Almond

> ... hundreds of thousands of refugees, mostly indigenous, had fled their homes during the worst periods of massacres. The "poles of development" were forced re-settlements of displaced indigenous in highly controlled and tightly regulated units. Their inspiration was taken from, to a significant degree, the principles of Jewish kibbutzes and moshav agricultural collectivities in an attempt to regain control,

both physical as well as ideological, of the rural population (one observer called them "a distorted replica of rural Israel.") One of the architects of the scheme, a Guatemalan Air Force Colonel called Eduardo Wohlers, was trained in Israel.[27]

The systematic incorporation of Judea, Samaria and Gaza into Israel "proper" began with Ariel Sharon's concept of linking the settlements—strong nodes (*ta'ozim*)—into an ever-thickening matrix that, connected by a maze of highways and infrastructure, would literally reconfigure the entire country, creating a Greater Land of Israel while eliminating any possible Palestinian state, at least one that would be truly sovereign, territorially coherent and economically viable. Adapting the strategy he employed so effectively against the Egyptians in the 1973 war, Sharon saw that

> ... a thin line of settlements along the Jordan would not provide a viable defense unless the high terrain behind it was also fortified." Consequently, he proposed to establish "other settlements on the high terrain ... [and] several east-west roads along strategic axes, together with the settlements necessary to guard them.

In 1982, a few months before the Israeli invasion of Lebanon, Sharon, then minister of defense, published his *Masterplan for Jewish Settlements in the West Bank Through the Year 2010*—later known as the "Sharon Plan." In it he outlined the location of more than a hundred settlement points, placed on strategic summits. He also marked the paths for a new network of high-volume, interconnected traffic arteries, connecting the settlements with the Israeli heartland. In the formation of continuous Jewish habitation, Sharon's plan saw a way towards the wholesale annexation of the areas vital for Israel's security. These areas he marked onto the map attached to his plan in the shape of the letter H. The "H-Plan" contained two parallel north–south strips of land: one along the Green Line containing the West Bank from the west, and another along the Jordan Valley, accepting the presence of the Allon Plan to contain the territory from the east.

These two strips separated the Palestinian cities, which are organized along the central spine of the West Bank's mountain ridge, from both Israel proper and from the Kingdom of Jordan. Between these north–south strips Sharon marked a few east–west traffic arteries—the main one connecting through Jerusalem, thus closing a (very) approximate H. The rest—some 40 percent of the West Bank, separate enclaves around

Palestinian cities and towns—were to revert to some yet undefined form of Palestinian self-management.

The small red-roofed single-family home replaced the tank as the smallest fighting unit. District regional and municipal plans replaced the strategic sand table. Homes, like armored divisions, were used in formation across a dynamic theatre of operations to occupy strategic hills, to encircle an enemy, or to cut communication lines.[28]

Sharon's strategy, carried out by all subsequent Israeli governments, even in the midst of "peace processes," called for massive expropriation of Palestinian land, part of a systematic campaign designed to dispossess, displace and confine Palestinians, mainly by employing law, administration and partisan planning as instruments of control. By simply not recognizing Ottoman or British-era deeds as valid, Israel "legally" expropriated a full 79 percent of the West Bank, providing a legal basis for Judaization and transforming the West Bank *de facto* into Judea and Samaria.[29]

Kitur/Encirclement, Isolation and Layered Defense Systems

In prisons, the authorities do not actually occupy the living space of the prisoners, but rather create controlled prisoner spaces (cells, visiting and work areas, the cafeteria). The enclaves in "east" Jerusalem, the fragmentation of the West Bank into Areas A, B, C, H-1, H-2, nature reserves and closed military zones, as well as concentrating Palestinian citizens of Israel in specific areas all replicate a prison structure.

Nowhere is this more in evidence than in Gaza, which has been literally reduced to a squalid open-air prison or warehouse. Thus movement of Palestinians inside Gaza *after* the removal of the settlers is severely limited, as has been their ability to use their tiny land's scarce resources. The Israeli authorities have declared an area extending 45 miles (71 km) along the border with Israel and 985 ft (300 m) deep into Gaza as a "buffer zone," though in reality Palestinians might be fired upon if they come closer than just under a mile (1,500 m) from the border, an area bulldozed flat and kept barren by the Israelis where 113 farms were leveled, irrigation systems and greenhouses destroyed, and 140,000 olive trees and 136,000 citrus trees uprooted. In this way, Gazan farmers are prevented from accessing their prime agricultural land, 35 percent of Gaza's scant arable land, many being shot when they do. A similar "no-go" zone extends the length of the seashore. Gaza fishermen, restricted by the Israeli Navy to a fished-out and sewage-saturated strip extending only 3 miles (4.8 km) into the sea (instead of the 20 miles (32 km) agreed upon in the Oslo process), are thus barred from 84 percent of their fishing waters. Between 2006 and May 2013, 544 shooting incidents were recorded in the Access Restricted Areas of Gaza, resulting in at least 179 civilian deaths and 751 injuries.[30] The three wadis that drain seasonal waters from Israel onwards towards the Mediterranean via Gaza have dried up due to their waters being diverted by Israel into the Negev, meaning that once-abundant Gaza is facing the prospect of desertification. Deprived of water, Wadi Gaza is today a thick sludge of sewage winding its way through populated areas and agricultural lands alike, polluting both the soils and the aquifer.[31]

High-tech observation posts constructed along the border allow soldiers to monitor movement 3.7 miles (6 km) into Gaza, day and night, recalling the wall and tower complex, a "constant panoptic observation policed by the vantage point of the 'tower' determined the overpowering relations" between the colonists and their surroundings.[32] Jonathan Cook describes one deadly panoptic system, Sentry-tech, developed by Rafael and deployed on the border with Gaza:

"Spot and Shoot," as it is called by the Israeli military, may look like a video game but the figures on the screen are real people—Palestinians in Gaza—who can be killed with the press of a button on the joystick. The female soldiers, located far away in an operations room, are responsible for aiming and firing remote-controlled machine-guns mounted on watch-towers every few hundred metres along an electronic fence that surrounds Gaza.

The system is one of the latest "remote killing" devices developed by Israel's Rafael armaments company ... The Spot and Shoot system—officially known as Sentry Tech—has mostly attracted attention because it is operated by 19- and 20-year-old female soldiers, making it the Israeli army's only weapons system operated exclusively by women ...

The women are supposed to identify anyone suspicious approaching the fence around Gaza and, if authorized by an officer, execute them using their joysticks. The Israeli army, which plans to introduce the technology along Israel's other confrontation lines, refuses to say how many Palestinians have been killed by the remotely controlled machine-guns in Gaza. According to the Israeli media, however, it is believed to be several dozen. Audio sensors on the towers mean that the women hear the shot as it kills the target. No woman, *Haaretz* reported, had failed the task of shooting what the army calls an "incriminated" Palestinian.[33]

Encirclement also facilitates military suppression of uprisings, just as "lock-downs" do in prisons, as well as enabling Israel to freeze financial operations vital to Palestinian life, cut communications and limit or stop the shipment of vital goods and supplies when the need arises. After Hamas won the elections in January 2006 (but a year before they took control of Gaza), the Olmert government decided that "the movement of goods into the Gaza Strip will be restricted; the supply of gas and electricity will be reduced; and restrictions will be imposed on the movement of people from the Strip and to it." In addition, exports from Gaza would be forbidden entirely.[34] Dov Weisglass, an adviser to Sharon and Olmert, is said to have commented infamously: "The idea is to put the Palestinians on a diet, but not to make them die of hunger."[35] In 2008, the Coordinator of Government Activities in the Territories (COGAT) drew up a plan, called the "Red Lines" Plan, to limit food consumption in Gaza, which had been made largely dependent upon the truckloads of food and other goods that Israel allowed in through the sealed crossings.[36] According to a model formulated by the Israeli Ministry of Health, a "minimal subsistence basket" was calculated, based on the Arab sector in Israel "adjusted to culture and experience" in Gaza, a nutritional value "that is sufficient for subsistence without the development of malnutrition."

The "Red Lines" formula calculated that, on average, each person in Gaza required a minimum of 2,279 calories per day, which translated into 2,575.5 tons of food for the entire population, or 170.4 truckloads per day, five days a week. COGAT then *deducted* 68.6 truckloads to account for the food produced locally in Gaza—mainly vegetables, fruit, milk and meat—plus another 13 truckloads to adjust for the "culture and experience" of food consumption in Gaza. It then added 34 tons per day to take into consideration "sampling" by toddlers under the age of 2. Altogether, COGAT concluded that Israel needed to allow 131 truckloads of food and other essential products into Gaza every day. About 90 per day have been allowed in, although the policy, still shrouded in secrecy, seems to have been liberalized over the past several years. Still, the security establishment maintains, in what it calls its "separation policy," sweeping and indiscriminate restrictions on the movement of goods and people between Gaza and the West Bank.[37]

In the end, what have played key roles in deterrence and control are

… the creating of territorial defensive shields through the establishment of multi-layered systems (including electronic fences, high-technology sensors, special rules of engagement, security buffer zones, and various delaying obstacles that slow would-be terrorists from reaching their targets) and an increasing number of professional units trained specifically to oppose the terrorist threat.[38]

Monitoring Movement/Surveillance

As in a prison, the IDF and police "guards" closely monitor Palestinian movement and activity. The daily life of Palestinians is closely filtered through a maze of physical obstacles to movement—some 600 checkpoints surrounding Areas A and B, separating Jerusalem from the West Bank and Palestinian parts of the city from Jewish ones, and allowing a controlled stream of trucks carrying approved food or materials into a besieged Gaza—all monitored through a panoptic web of surveillance systems. And as in prisons, the IDF has developed detailed protocols on operating checkpoints: different types of blockades, how many soldiers are needed for each kind, how to differentiate between civilians and militants, and so on. "These are details that only people who were involved in it for many years can know," says Eitan Ben-Eliahu, a former Israeli Air Force commander, "and other armies, like the U.S. military, haven't had … enough experience."[39]

Palestinian individuals wishing to enter Israel ("approved" men over the age of 16) are required to carry an electronic ID card containing biometric templates (fingerprints, retinal and facial measurements), personal and security information. The data is then fed into a biometric access control system installed in Israeli checkpoints—of 99 fixed checkpoints in the West Bank protected by advanced fencing systems, intrusion detection and electronic surveillance as of 2014, 59 were internal checkpoints separating Palestinian enclaves well within the West Bank. At hundreds of surprise and random "flying checkpoints" set up throughout the West Bank and East Jerusalem, personal data may also be processed on laptops.[40] The data control system is part of the BASEL project developed by EDS Israel, a Hewlett Packard subsidiary, and used to restrict Palestinian movement across checkpoints. (HP also produces Israeli biometric ID cards.[14])

Less technological barriers to movement such as permanent road barriers of concrete blocks, boulders, earth mounds and trenches, closed military areas and buffer zones are commonly found through the West Bank, Gaza and even blocking East Jerusalem neighborhoods. Ties between Palestinians in Gaza and the West Bank have been severed altogether. The cumulative effect is to create borders unilaterally, with no need for political negotiations or Palestinian input.

Creating a Legal and Administrative Environment Conducive to Control

The Matrix of Control employs a tight web of administrative and legal restrictions that trigger sanctions whenever Palestinians try to assert their national claims to self-determination, resist the Occupation or merely expand their life space.

Military Government/"Civil" Administration

In the first days following the 1967 war, the Israeli government accepted the fact that the Palestinians were now living under occupation and were therefore entitled to the protections afforded them by the Fourth Geneva Convention. A military government was established over the West Bank and Gaza on June 11, 1967, the day after the war ended. It was ready-made, its personnel and policies simply imported from the military administration Israel had imposed on its own Palestinian citizens immediately following the 1948 war, and which had been lifted just six months before. That regime

> ... operated as an instrument of despotic rule, as an occupation force in every respect, with the goal of preserving separation and ethnic superiority. Knesset protocols reveal its operations blatantly: expulsion of Palestinians across the border, internal exile from one village to another, collective punishments, a ban on freedom of movement, censorship, restrictions on political organizing, bureaucratic arbitrariness, constraints in free economic competition. Other measures included land expropriations, trials of Arab civilians in military courts ... and the use of organized violence, often resulting in fatalities—culminating in the wanton killing of 47 people in Kafr Kassim in 1956 and many other attacks.[42]

Almost immediately, however, political pressures emerged, especially from within the ruling Labor Party, to annex the Old City of Jerusalem and its surroundings, seize permanent control over the Jordan Valley, considered Israel's indispensable security border, reclaim the Etzion Bloc settlements that had been lost in 1948 and "resettle" Hebron. These specific demands were soon subsumed by a messianic urge, shared by orthodox Zionists, Greater Land of Israel supporters and not a few intellectuals of Socialist Zionist persuasions, to annex all of the occupied territory.

In short order, Meir Shamgar, the Military Advocate General, once a member of Begin's Irgun terrorist organization, acted to alter the status of the West Bank and Gaza. Declaring that the Geneva Conventions do not apply since there was never a sovereign authority over them (the doctrine of the "Missing Reversioner," which has been universally rejected), he assigned them the status of "administered" or "disputed" territories over which the military commander has the power to change, cancel, or overrule any local law.[43] East Jerusalem was annexed outright and came fully under Israeli law. During the subsequent decades, the West Bank became ever more incorporated into Israel. Israeli law was extended throughout Area C, the 62 percent of the West Bank fully controlled by Israel and where its settlements are found—now referred to by the biblical term "Judea and Samaria." By 1995, with the establishment of Areas A and B, Palestinians found themselves confined to an archipelago of tiny islands, plus the cage of Gaza, fenced in by Israel and isolated.

Still, because an Occupying Power is forbidden by international law to replace the local laws with those of its own and Israel wanted to arouse as little opposition to its occupation as possible, it instead imposed an entirely new layer of de facto laws in the form of some 2,500 military orders. When supplemented by Civil Administration policies, these military orders effectively constituted a corpus of law designed to keep the Palestinian population under strict control, thereby obviating the need to use the army on a daily basis to enforce order.

Military orders cover almost all aspects of Palestinian life: administrative, legal, political, economic, educational and even personal (Order 818 establishes how Palestinians can plant decorative flowers, and how many). Just to give you a sense of how minute and invasive Israeli control is, here are a few examples of military orders:

- Order 5 declares the entire West Bank a closed military area, with exit and entry to be controlled according to the orders and conditions stipulated by the military.

- Order 25 makes it illegal to conduct business transactions involving land and property without a permit from the military authorities, while Order 364 gives the military the power to appropriate land simply by declaring it "State Land."

- Order 101 prohibits all gatherings of ten or more persons "for a political purpose or for a matter that could be interpreted as political" or even "to discuss such a topic," unless they have received authorization in advance under a permit issued by the Israeli military commander in the area. Anyone breaching the order faces imprisonment for up to ten years and/or a hefty fine.

- Order 144 repeals the protection of civilians as ensured under the Fourth Geneva Convention.

- Order 224 declares that the Emergency Regulations installed by the British Mandate Authorities in 1945 are in effect in the West Bank.

- Order 291 stops the process of land registration, and since Israel refuses to recognize Ottoman- or British-era deeds, a full 72 percent of the West Bank could be classified as "state lands," making expropriation from their Palestinian owners a simple administrative matter.

- Order 270 designates a further million dunams (250,000 acres) of West Bank land as closed "combat zones," facilitating their transfer to settlement or infrastructure projects.

- Order 363 imposes severe restrictions on construction and land use in yet other areas zoned as "nature reserves."

- Order 393 grants any military commander in Judea and Samaria the authority to prohibit Palestinian construction if they believe it necessary for the security of the Israeli Army or to ensure "public order."

- Order 977 authorizes the Israeli Army or its agencies (such as the Civil Administration) to proceed with excavation and construction without a permit, providing an avenue for settlement construction, such as in the Jordan Valley, that bypasses legal and planning systems.

- Order 1651 allows for the imposition of a closed military zone, thereby declaring a certain area off limits for certain periods of time. This order is many times used to deny the right to peacefully demonstrate, or as a pretext to use violence to disperse demonstrators.

Other military orders severely infringe on individual human rights and the responsibility of the Occupying Power to safeguard the well-being of the population under its control:

- Order 30 gives military courts jurisdiction over all criminal cases in the Occupied Territories.
- Order 50 forbids the importing, distribution, or publishing of newspapers without the permission of the military authorities.
- Order 79 prohibits broadcasting without a military permit.
- Order 101 forbids meetings of ten or more persons "where the subject concerns or is related to politics," without permission from the Military Commander. It is also forbidden to raise flags, or distribute or publish political articles or pictures (including artwork): "No attempt should be made to influence public opinion in a way which would be detrimental to security." Soldiers may use force to apply this law. Punishment for non-compliance with this order is a prison sentence of up to ten years.
- Order 107 lists 55 books on Arabic language, history, geography, sociology, philosophy and Arab nationalism banned from being taught in schools (the list continues to grow).
- Order 132, used widely during the Intifadas, allows for the arrest and imprisonment of children between the ages of 12–14 years.
- Order 1015 requires the permission of the Military Commander for the planting of fruit trees (including olives).
- Order 892 establishes "Regional Councils" and municipal courts for Israeli settlements, thereby creating separate judicial and legal systems for Palestinians and Israelis residing in the Occupied Territories.[44]

Key to the administration of the Matrix of Control was Military Order 947 that established a "Civil Administration" in 1981. Despite its name, the Civil Administration constitutes a military government under the Ministry of Defense, but gives the impression of normal, proper administration of an integral part of Israel rather than a military regime. Indeed, it was created, says Order 947, "for the well-being and good of the population and in order to supply and implement the public services, and taking into consideration the need to maintain an orderly administration and public order in the region." Today it administers Area C, although it operates nine coordination offices with the Palestinian Authority.[45]

Planning and Zoning Regulations

Discriminatory zoning and planning are ideal vehicles for concealing Israel's political agenda under a facade of technical maps, "neutral" professional jargon and seemingly innocuous administrative procedures. Indeed, they enable Israel to claim that there is no occupation, merely the proper administrative authority of at best a "disputed territory." On the basis of two British Mandate planning documents—the Jerusalem Regional Planning Scheme RJ5 (1942) and Samaria Regional Planning Scheme RS15 (1945)—Israel has frozen Palestinian development in Jerusalem and the West Bank as it was in the 1940s. Some 48,000 Palestinian homes and livelihood structures (as of this writing) have been declared "illegal" and have been demolished. At the same time, Palestinians have been forcibly evicted from their lands in Area C and pushed into Areas A and B. A little-noted provision of British planning law, now part of the policies and power of the Civil Administration, provides the "power to grant a relaxation of any restriction imposed by this scheme." This enables the Israeli authorities to "legally" construct hundreds of thousands of housing units for Jews on lands zoned for agriculture, while strictly enforcing the Regional Schemes in the case of the Palestinians—all legal and seemingly non-discriminatory.[46]

Israeli administrations do not hesitate, when necessary, to adopt blatantly discriminatory policies, however. Already in 1967, the Israeli government adopted an explicit policy of maintaining a 72 percent majority of Jews over Arabs in Jerusalem. As a result, Palestinians, who constitute a third of the Jerusalem population within the city's gerrymandered borders, have access to only 11 percent of the city's urban space for residential, commercial and industrial purposes.[47]

Mass Detentions and Limitations on Civil Liberties

Israel added yet another layer of control by retaining the British Defense (Emergency) Regulations of 1945, once decried by Menachem Begin as "Nazi, tyrannical, immoral and illegal."[48] Under these regulations, which permit people to be held indefinitely and without charge, Israel has detained, arrested, or imprisoned hundreds of thousands of Palestinians adjudged to be security threats. According to Addameer, the Palestinian Prisoners' Support and Human Rights Association, 800,000 Palestinians have been detained by Israel in the Occupied Territories since 1967—

approximately 20 percent of the total Palestinian population there and about 40 percent of the total male Palestinian population. These figures include approximately a total of 10,000 women jailed since 1967, 8,000 Palestinian children arrested since 2000 and 14 members of the Palestinian Legislative Council.[49] More than 120,000 Palestinians were arrested during the six years of the first Intifada.[50] The numbers declined during the years of the Oslo peace process, but shot up again at the beginning of the Second Intifada; by April 2003, about 28,000 Palestinians were incarcerated.[51] By March 2008, Israeli civilian and military authorities held more than 8,400 Palestinians: 5,148 were serving sentences, 2,167 awaiting legal proceedings and 790 under administrative detention. As of September 2014, 6,200 Palestinian prisoners were being held in Israeli jails.[52]

Sorting People By Differential Rights And Life-Spaces

In accordance with Military Order 297, the Civil Administration consigns the Palestinian population of the Occupied Territory to a number of different categories—residents of the West Bank, Gaza, or East Jerusalem, subsequently of Areas A, B, C, H-1, H-2 and the Jordan Valley; children, youth, adults and seniors, also categorized by gender, each class having differing privileges and restrictions on movement; those with permits to enter Israel for varying periods; VIPs with special privileges; people confined to their homes or communities for security reasons. Moreover, each category is assigned a different ID card, sometimes in different colors, e.g., blue for Israeli citizens and permanent residents, orange/ green for Palestinians of the Occupied Territory.[53] The permit system induces economic impoverishment and thus emigration by excluding Palestinian workers from the Israeli job market. Thousands of Palestinians are classified as "infiltrators," even in the homes where they were born. According to Military Order 1650, issued in 2009, an "infiltrator" is anyone who enters the West Bank illegally, as well as anyone "who is present in the Area and does not lawfully hold a permit." Up to 35,000 Palestinians in the West Bank face immediate arrest or deportation without judicial review, especially people whose address is recorded as being the Gaza Strip, even if they live or were born in the West Bank.[54]

The census and population registries play key roles in the inclusion, exclusion and control of the Palestinian population.[55] Because Palestinians will outnumber Jews in the area between the Jordan River and the Mediterranean by 2020, Israel considers the "demographic bomb" the greatest threat to its hegemony. To counter this trend, Israel actively pursues policies of displacement facilitated by the partisan application of seemingly innocuous and technical head-counting. By revoking their residency rights for various and sundry reasons, Palestinians can be exiled, prevented from returning home, or barred from entering Israel. Whether one was in one's home at particular periods and what one's address is bears directly on a person's ability to live in a home (or in the country, for that matter), or to keep or lose lands passed down over generations. Who may marry whom, live where, have children "registered" or not, even where one may be buried, is determined by seemingly technical personal data—all within a political context in which the Israeli authorities formulate the differential rights associated with each of the myriad categories, with an eye to their declared policy of "Judaizing" the country. Tens of thousands of spouses and their families live apart because Israeli citizens who marry people from the Occupied Territory or Arab countries cannot get permits for "family reunification"—another law that applies to all citizens although it impacts exclusively upon the Palestinian population.[56]

The overall purpose of such policies is twofold. It renders a population "manageable," while making life so unbearable that those who have the wherewithal—the educated middle classes in particular—"voluntarily" leave, thereby further weakening Palestinian society and leaving it leaderless. Schemes of "transfer" have become an acceptable part of Israeli political discourse; they are found in the official platforms of several major Israeli parties, including Avigdor Lieberman's "Israel Is Our Home." Transfer is not only induced, of course; deportations, revoking of residency, or simply not allowing people back into the country are common.[57]

Blurring Civil/Military Lines in the Enforcement of Internal Security

Israel's fundamental concept of itself is of a nation-in-arms, whereby the body politic is so diffused with military and securocratic practices and values that little separates policing, domestic security, intelligence gathering and military operations, either juridical or operationally.[58] Its approach to securitization is borne out of its long experience in the entire gamut of securitization, itself arising out of its century-long conflict with the Palestinians and its half-century of occupation. In a domestic environment where a fifth of one's own population is considered "the enemy" and more than a third of the population under the state's authority have no civil rights, Israeli securitization embraces a strange amalgam of pacification and militarized policing. In Israel, the army, security agencies and police forces do not operate as distinct entities but as an integrated pacification system spanning civil and military authorities—the MISSILE complex as a model for emerging human security states.

Now this is not new in the military sphere. Pacification, after all, is the ultimate purpose of counter-insurgency. Israel's contribution, beyond its innovative tactics and weaponry, is in offering a model of an effective security regime that rests on a blurring of the civil-military distinction, effective not only against immediate threats but in creating mechanisms of long-term domination. Since liberal democracies of the Global North have always carefully separated external military from internal security and policing, they lack models and even weaponry and tactics that combine the two. By the same token but in reverse, repressive states of the Global South have long mixed the civil and military, but have been unable to develop agencies and policies for sustaining their control; hence their interest in the "training" provided by 250 Israeli security firms.

The Israeli military has always been highly integrated into Israeli political decision making. Indeed, in his book *Generals in the Cabinet Room*, Yoram Peri describes the IDF's Military Intelligence and Planning and Policy Directorates as "the political arm of the military."[59] In 1992, during the First Intifada, a Home Front Command was established, the IDF's fourth command, which divided the entire country into five districts under a unified framework of highly integrated military/security/police cooperation, with no distinction made between Israel "proper" and the Occupied Territories. Paramilitary units of the police—the Border Police, the Yasam special patrol unit, and Yamam, an elite SWAT and undercover COIN unit—actively engage in counter-insurgency alongside such specialized IDF units as Duvdevan. The dividing line between the military and police therefore passes deeply through the police sector into that gray area between normal law enforcement and "public security," defined by the Ministry of Internal Security as "the prevention and thwarting of terror acts planned by terrorist organizations [that the] police carry out through patrols, searches, raids and information campaigns designed to increase the level of public awareness."[60] (Tellingly, the Ministry of Internal (or Public) Security replaced the Ministry of Police.)

When the states of the Global North need an effective model of securitization, then, they turn to Israel, the "only democracy in the Middle East," yet one that has succeeded in retaining its democratic image while thoroughly militarizing.

8

Operational Doctrines and Tactics

Having surveyed the overall conception and structure of Israel's Matrix of Control, let's now turn to its more operational elements.

Interactive Intelligence Gathering

"The first priority," counsels Meir Dagan, a former Director of the Mossad, "must be placed on intelligence, then on counter-terrorism operations, and finally on defense and protection."[1] The fact that the IDF's Military Intelligence Directorate (Aman) holds the status of an independent service on a par with the army, air force and navy (the latter two having their own intelligence services as well) reflects the special place Israel gives to intelligence gathering. It is supplemented by other dedicated units: the Combat Intelligence Collection Corps specializing in urban warfare and border control; the Nesher (Eagle) 414 special unit called "HaNayedet" (The Moving), which operates on the Gaza Strip and the Egyptian border; the Shahaf (Seagull) 869 special unit known as "HaMovil" (The Leader), operating on the Lebanon border, and the Nitzan 636 special unit ("Zikit" or Cameleon) that operates in the West Bank. On a par with these military intelligence units are the General Security Service (better known as the Shin Bet or the Shabak), which deals with internal security threats, Mossad, responsible for foreign intelligence and covert operations, and the National Security Council, all under the Prime Minister's Office.

The Combat Intelligence Collection Corps briefs IDF ground units on salient enemy traits. It also contributes intelligence analysis into the process of planning the size, nature and deployment of forces, and above all strengthens intelligence collection capacities in all the regional commands. Combat intelligence troops engage in observation and the laying of ambushes on the forward lines. Hundreds of female troops, as I've mentioned, serve as lookouts in operations rooms where they operate a wide range of surveillance equipment and automatic firing ("see-shoot") weapons on the Gaza border.[2]

The intelligence community fields a wide range of high-tech equipment in its information-gathering activities, from "families" of spy satellites to surveillance drones and mini-UAVs. On the ground, the Israeli Intelligence Corps' Unit 8200, responsible for regional situational awareness, collects signal and open-source intelligence from within the Palestinian territories. A variety of instruments provide early warning or situational awareness to soldiers in the field: high ground-based masts, radars, observation points, portable ground systems, soldiers equipped with intelligence-gathering capabilities on foot and in vehicles.

For all that, Israel's approach to security insists that HUMINT—real-time human intelligence that is close, "in your face," personalized, the product of being embedded among the enemy—trumps technologically-generated intelligence. Only through human interactions can detailed information be gathered regarding who is involved in terrorism or insurgency on all levels, how their activities are organized and who the circles are that support these groups and individuals, plus details of financing, arms, infrastructure, ideology, planned attacks and the like. Security and undercover agents, Shin Bet or another associated agency such as the secretive Unit 504, together with their informers, are thus the finger on the pulse, able to detect movement, preempt actions, disrupt terrorist infrastructures, guide troops in arrests or retaliatory strikes and in general proactively manage and control events. Shin Bet agents knowledgeable about a particular locale will often join IDF units in the field.[3] In the first couple of years of the second Palestinian Intifada, Israeli agents prevented more than 340 suicide bombings from advancing beyond the planning stages and intercepted 142 would-be bombers.[4]

Towards these ends, Israel has recruited tens of thousands of Palestinian collaborators. Though deployed to disrupt the terrorist infrastructure, the practice also disrupts and undermines the very fabric of Palestinian life, sowing distrust within communities and families. Collaborators are infiltrated into political, religious, or resistance organizations and, willingly or not, provide crucial information that results in raids, arrests, or targeted killing. They act as intermediaries between the military administration and the local population, even assisting interrogators. But not all informants' tasks relate to "counter-terrorism." As middlemen, they play a major role in buying Palestinian-owned land for eventual sale to settlers or to the Israeli government.[5] Not infrequently, collaborators, privileged by their Israeli handlers, immune from the law and armed by the IDF, turn into violent "rogues" bedeviling their own people. Armed collaborators

> ... are those spies whose cover has been blown and who have become intermediaries or land dealers. In a state of isolation, however, they become fugitives and prepared to use arms against their own people. These collaborators terrorize the population. They guide Israeli forces or Israeli Special Forces (*mustaribin*) to the homes of activists and wanted persons or drive the cars that carry them.[6]

Even 20 years ago, it was estimated that 40,000–120,000 individuals had been turned unwillingly (and occasionally willingly) into collaborators through threats, extortion and "incentives," although the number is certainly much higher today.[7] In 95 percent of the cases brought against the tens of thousands of Palestinians tried for various offenses in the military courts of the "Civil" Administration, the detainees are "persuaded" to turn informant in return for a reduced sentence.[8] Since Palestinians are vulnerable to pressures to supply information to the security services, it is often difficult for them to resist, especially as their most basic needs require Israeli permission: obtaining a driver's license, for example, or a business license; acquiring a work permit, or a permit to build a house or even plant a garden; for travel abroad for business, pleasure, or medical care; for passing through a checkpoint to visit a relative or to pass through a gate in the Separation Barrier to tend to one's land; for receiving medical care in Israel or visiting a relative in prison, or for securing residency rights for a loved one. No opportunity for restriction is missed.

Complementing this army of collaborators "recruited" and operated by Shin Bet handlers are IDF special forces who, disguised as Arabs (*mist'arabim*, or "Arab-like"), operate both undercover and in the open, conducting ambushes or night raids. The best known of these units is Duvdevan, or "cherry," a reference to an innocuous-looking variety of Israeli cherry that actually packs a lethal poison, which specializes in operations against militants in urban areas. Driving modified civilian vehicles and wearing Arab civilian clothes, Duvdevan is authorized to operate independently in carrying out high-risk arrests, raids, targeted killing, kidnappings and other urban warfare operations. There have also been instances where they have actually acted as *agents provocateur*. In all their activities, the various undercover army units work with one clear political aim: "maximum weakening, in every possible way, of the Palestinian national collective."[9]

The Limited Use of Unlimited Force, Disproportionate Force, Cumulative Deterrence and Escalation Domination

Until the rise of the Likud to power in 1977, the surrounding Arab states were considered the source of existential threat to Israel, and the IDF prepared for conventional warfare abroad. Begin and Sharon, however, saw the conflict quite differently, i.e., not as an interstate Arab–Israeli conflict but an inter-communal one pitting Israel against the Palestinians.[10] Since both endeavored to create a Greater Land of Israel at the expense of even a truncated Palestinian state in the Occupied Territory, something the Palestinian could never accept, the Palestinians indeed became the ones that stood in the way and resisted, not the wider Arab world which was willing to comes to terms with the Jewish state. The Palestinians, then, had to be subjugated and ultimately either pacified or expelled.

The thrust of IDF engagement thus shifted from counter-insurgency (COIN) to counter-terrorism, a fine yet vital distinction. Palestinian resistance was seen as "a fact of life," irreversible, insoluble and permanent. The shift to counter-terrorism meant that military and security operations that in fact served to strengthen the Occupation could be justified by "security." Not only would the Israeli public, most of whom do not support the Greater Land of Israel project, accede to policies whose political aims they would not have accepted otherwise, but the international community as well has been induced to accept Israeli repression. After all, who can negotiate with terrorists? Had Israel framed its struggle with the Palestinians as counter-insurgency, it would have been admitting that there exists "another side;" granting the Palestinians the status of "insurgents" would paradoxically lend them and their resistance legitimacy. The disconnect between security measures and any attempt to resolve the conflict—or even pressure to resolve the conflict, be it domestic or foreign—led to what Catignani characterizes as "military and political adventurism," or what Maoz refers to as "the unlimited use of limited force."[11] For Catignani, the 1982 war in Lebanon, launched less than a year after Sharon became minister of defense, marked the turning-point from conventional warfare to warfare amongst the people.[12]

True, the IDF occasionally resorted to conventional warfare as a tool of pacification when it suited its purpose: against the Palestinians during the two Intifadas, in three major assaults on Gaza (2008/9, 2012 and 2014), against the PLO in Lebanon in 1982, Hezbollah in 1993 and 1996, and in the second Lebanon war of 2006. These "operations," as Israel labels them, were actually a form of reverse hybrid war, a state dressing pacification and displacement in a mix of conventional warfare and counter-terrorism. Under this conception, disproportionate military force—"limited use of unlimited force," to reverse Maoz's phrase—periodically destroys terrorist infrastructure to a degree that a return to previous levels of activity would take years, thus granting Israel a prolonged period of quiet.

By disproportionate force, Israeli strategists mean "a multilayered, highly orchestrated effort to inflict the greatest damage possible on the terrorists and their weapon systems, infrastructure, support networks, financial flows, and other means of support."[13] Israel, of course, has long employed disproportionate force against Palestinian resistance, going all the way back to the campaigns against the *fedayun*, or "infiltrators," in the 1950s, which were framed as "reprisal raids."[14] Indeed, "reprisal" became a major pretext for launching limited yet disproportionate attacks—witness the Qibya massacre, a "reprisal" operation that occurred in October 1953 when Israeli troops under Ariel Sharon attacked the village of Qibya in the West Bank, killing at least 69 villagers, two-thirds of them women and children, and demolishing 45 houses, as well as Sharon's attacks on Gaza in 1955, or other retaliatory actions.[15] Cordesman noted much more aggressive and effective IDF tactics on the ground between the two Intifadas, including curfews lasting weeks and even months, a forthright policy of targeted assassinations, mass arrests and the use of helicopters and stand-off precision weapons.[16]

A belief in the efficacy of disproportionate response has given rise to a number of controversial Israeli military doctrines. One is the Mofaz/Ya'alon doctrine, declared at the start of the second Intifada in September 2000. Prime Minister and Minister of Defense Ehud Barak, together with Chief of Staff Shaul Mofaz and General Amos Gilad, then the Coordinator of Activities in the Territories, viewed the outbreak of protests as an opportunity to use military means to force the Palestinians to accept Israeli dictates, as the Oslo peace process began to collapse. Thus, in response to Palestinian demonstrations in which no shots were fired, reports the late

Reuven Pedatzur, a senior lecturer at the Strategic Studies Program, Tel Aviv University,

> ... during the first few days of the Al-Aqsa Intifada soldiers in the territories fired 1,300,000 bullets. This astounding statistic embodies the entire story. In the conflict with the Palestinians, at the end of September 2000, senior IDF commanders adopted Gilad's assessment, which was based on his own perspective, and according to which Yasser Arafat's foray into negotiations was a scheme aimed at leading to Israel's destruction, and that he in no way plans to reach an agreement. This explains what took place once the intifada broke out, and the unrestrained shooting that ensued. Then-Chief of Staff Shaul Mofaz, with the support of his senior aides, did not plan to bring about the end of the conflict at its very onset. Having adopted Gilad's approach, he had an opportunity to finally "beat" the Palestinians, to "vanquish" them and lead them to negotiations in a weakened and exhausted state. This is the origin of the "burned into their consciousness" thesis, which became a cornerstone of the Israel Defense Forces' policy in the territories. We'll hit the Palestinians until the recognition of their weakness vis-a-vis Israel's might is burned into their consciousness. This is the only way they will understand that they are best off coming to terms with their inferiority and accepting Israel's demands.
>
> This gave rise to the objective defined by Mofaz, his successor Moshe Ya'alon, and their colleagues in the general staff: achieving military victory in what was at first described as a war with the Palestinians. This explains why the IDF began to use such massive firepower when the uprising broke out in the territories. This also explains why over a million bullets were fired in the first few days, even though there was no operational or professional justification. The intent was to score a winning blow against the Palestinians, and especially against their consciousness. This was not a war on terror, but on the Palestinian people. IDF commanders projected their viewpoint regarding Arafat's intentions onto the entire Palestinian society ...
>
> But this was not preparedness for alleviating the violence, but rather for escalating the conflict. Soldiers were given a free hand to shoot without limit. In the first three months of the intifada, the number of Israeli casualties was low, at which time the IDF proudly cited the large number of Palestinian casualties as evidence of the military victory and the correctness of the policy of massive use of force ... .[17]

The effect of the Mofaz/Ya'alon doctrine was immediately apparent in the high number of civilian casualties suffered in the Second Intifada—more than 3,300 Palestinians killed, at least 85 percent of them civilians. Some 650 were children and youths, half under the age of 15. In 88 percent of the incidents in which children were killed, there was no direct confrontation with Israeli soldiers. Another 50,000 Palestinians were injured, 20 percent of whom were children and youths. Some 2,500 civilians were permanently disabled.[18]

One of the most devastating assaults on Palestinian civilian population centers, framed as a reprisal attack, took place in March/April 2002, when Prime Minister Ariel Sharon unleashed Operation Defensive Shield. Initially, the operations focused on the sprawling refugee camp of Jenin. A 40,000 square meter area containing 140 multi-story housing blocks was demolished, leaving 4,000 people homeless; another 1,500 homes were damaged. The bulldozer drivers gleefully described the "football stadium" they had carved out of the densely packed camp.[19] The two-storey D-9 Caterpillar bulldozers, specially designed to demolish homes and buildings, then proceeded to destroy the urban infrastructures of virtually all the major Palestinian cities. Operation Defensive Shield revealed yet another part of the Mofaz/Ya'alon doctrine, one that Israeli military commanders call "constructive destruction:" "laying waste to the Palestinian Authority, reinstating full Israeli control of the kind that existed before the first Intifada, and reaching an imposed settlement with obedient canton administrators."[20]

During the week-long Operation Rainbow in May 2004, in the midst of the Intifada, 300 Palestinian homes were destroyed in the Rafah section of Gaza. In Operation Days of Penitence in northern Gaza in October 2004, over 160 Palestinian civilians were killed and over 500 injured and 90 homes demolished. A month-long assault on Gaza in June/July 2006, in response to the capture of the Israeli soldier Gilad Shalit, named Operation Summer Rains, resulted in the deaths of at least 159 Palestinians and wholesale destruction of the Palestinian infrastructure.[21]

Disproportionality, in the form of the Dahiya Doctrine, became a hallmark IDF doctrine during the second Lebanon war of 2006. During that war, the Israeli Air Force destroyed the Hezbollah stronghold of Dahiya, a densely packed neighborhood of Beirut. In explaining why it did so, Major General Giora Eiland stated that attacks against Israel will be deterred by harming

… the civilian population to such an extent that it will bring pressure to bear on the enemy combatants. Furthermore, this policy is intended to create deterrence regarding future attacks against Israel, through the damage and destruction of civilian and military infrastructures which necessitate long and expensive reconstruction actions which would crush the will of those who wish to act against Israel.[22]

Gabi Siboni, a colonel in the reserves and a member of a security think-tank at Tel Aviv University, laid out the Dahyia Doctrine in detail months before the 2008 Gaza "operation":

> With an outbreak of hostilities, the IDF will need to act immediately, decisively, and with force that is disproportionate to the enemy's actions and the threat it poses. Such a response aims at inflicting damage and meting out punishment to an extent that will demand long and expensive reconstruction processes. The strike must be carried out as quickly as possible, and must prioritize damaging assets over seeking out each and every launcher. Punishment must be aimed at decision makers and the power elite … attacks should both aim at Hezbollah's military capabilities and should target economic interests and the centers of civilian power that support the organization …
>
> This approach is applicable to the Gaza Strip as well. There, the IDF will be required to strike hard at Hamas and to refrain from the cat and mouse games of searching for Qassam rocket launchers. The IDF should not be expected to stop the rocket and missile fire against the Israeli home front through attacks on the launchers themselves, but by means of imposing a ceasefire on the enemy.[23]

"What happened in the Dahiya quarter of Beirut in 2006 will happen in every village from which Israel is fired on," declared Gen. Gadi Eisenkott, then head of the IDF's Northern Command and today the Chief of Staff. "We will apply disproportionate force on it and cause great damage and destruction there. From our standpoint, these are not civilian villages, they are military bases … This is not a recommendation. This is a plan. And it has been approved."[24] Or as Tzipi Livni, Israel's foreign minister during the invasion, put it frankly: "Hamas now understands that when you fire on its [Israel's] citizens it responds by going wild—and this is a good thing."[25] For its part, the Goldstone Committee concluded that

The tactics used by Israeli military armed forces in the Gaza offensive [of 2008–09] are consistent with previous practices, most recently during the Lebanon war in 2006. A concept known as the Dahiya doctrine emerged then, involving the application of disproportionate force and the causing of great damage and destruction to civilian property and infrastructure, and suffering to civilian populations. The Mission concludes from a review of the facts on the ground that it witnessed for itself that what was prescribed as the best strategy appears to have been precisely what was put into practice.[26]

After the brief but devastating operations of 2004–06, disproportionate force was applied to Gaza in four major subsequent "operations." Operation Cast Lead was a three-week assault on Gaza in late December 2008, in which more than 1,400 people were killed, mainly civilians, about $2 billion of infrastructure was destroyed and some 7,000 homes demolished.[27] In Operation Pillar of Cloud in 2012, some 1,500 sites were bombed and thousands of people were displaced, and in Operation Protective Edge in 2014, another 2,200 people were killed, two-thirds of whom were civilians, 12,000 people injured, a quarter of the Gazan population (475,000 people) displaced and 18,000 homes demolished.[28]

Another IDF policy based on disproportionate response is the "Hannibal Procedure." When Israeli soldiers are captured, it states, rescuing them becomes the main mission, even at the cost of hitting or wounding them. While originally intended to permit shooting in the direction of the captors with light arms in order to prevent their escape with the soldier, it knows no limits. When, in Operation Protective Edge, it was believed (falsely, it turned out) that an IDF soldier had been captured by Hamas in the Rafah area, the entire urban area came under massive Israeli artillery fire and air strikes in which hundreds of buildings were destroyed and at least 130 people killed.[29] Disproportionality, of course, constitutes a grave violation of international law, in particular Article 51(5)(b) of Protocol I of the Geneva Conventions and Article 8(2)(b)(iv) of the Rome Statutes. But in Israeli doctrine it represents a crucial element of cumulative deterrence: escalation domination, controlling the "tempo" of the conflict, if not its outcome. In this unilateral doctrine, preemptive and disproportionate force—seizing the offensive, engaging in surprise raids, undertaking clandestine targeted operations—is intentionally applied in order to intimidate the enemy and reduce their capacity to mount attacks.[30]

In between such operations, Israel follows a routine policy of continual preemptive actions (*p'ulot yezumot*), the "unlimited use of limited force," in particular against "terrorist infrastructure." Through constant harassment and arrests (including collective punishment), destruction of weapon factories, storage facilities and tunnels but also offices and cultural institutions, the demolition of homes, targeted assassinations, mass arrests, deportations, administrative limitations on movement and activity, permanent and surprise checkpoints, the recruiting of collaborators and much more, the IDF keeps insurgent groups off-balance and limits their ability to mount attacks—all the while "degrading" their capabilities, garnering intelligence and, over time, "teaching" the enemy the futility of aggression, perhaps even inducing more moderate behavior.[31] This is what hundreds of Israeli security experts sell to armies and security forces abroad. But unlike counter-insurgency which in the end aims to create conditions for coexistence (unless genocide is the plan), Israel has adopted counter-terrorism as its form of permanently controlling and pacifying the Palestinians.

This strategy of "cumulative deterrence," then, informs Israel's approach to conflict management, much of it readily applicable, as we shall see, to police operations as well. Eventually, Israeli strategists like General Doron Almog contend, a near-absence of direct conflict may pave the way to political negotiations and a peace agreement.[32] This claim is highly contentious. It assumes that the source of rebellion or insurgency is merely behavioral, as the term used to describe it, "terrorism," removes any legitimate political grievances. Military and securocratic repression may, indeed, "soften" the positions of one's adversaries and bring them to the negotiating table; it could be argued that that happened back in 1988 (if not well before) when the Palestinians accepted the two-state solution. Bringing them to the table did little to resolve the conflict, however, since *Israel* proved unwilling to make the concessions necessary for a true peace. What Almog seems to mean, then, is that effective repression as embodied in cumulative deterrence leads to "victory," the enemy's complete capitulation, a specious claim at best.

OK, says Almog, if the cumulative deterrence policy has brought neither peace nor submission, it has significantly strengthened Israel's overall strategic situation, having created a kind of military "normalization." The fact that neither the Palestinian Authority nor the Arab states continue to call for the destruction of Israel or prepare militarily towards that end vindicates the Israeli approach.[33] Amidror, citing the "quiet" that has prevailed in the West Bank since Operation Defensive Shield in 2002, agrees that Israel's aggressive COIN strategy is effective.[34] Israel maintains, then, that pacification through securitization is indeed possible, and it is this claim that so attracts hegemons to the "Israeli model," the Matrix of Control. Statistics indicate, however, that cumulative deterrence has not only failed but has exacerbated anti-Israeli violence.[35]

Aerial Occupation

The worst wing of Israel's occupation prison, its Supermax section, genuinely a warehouse, is Gaza. When attempts to maintain a settler fortress-within-a-prison-within-a-fortress proved unsustainable, Sharon's government decided to "disengage." In mid-2005, it removed both the settlers and the army from Gaza. Rather than actually abandoning control over the territory, however, Israel merely replaced traditional ground-based occupation with "aerial occupation"—"invisible occupation," "control without occupation" or, borrowing a term from the 1920s when the British first employed air power against recalcitrant elements in their Empire, "aerially enforced colonization." Says Weizman:

> Similar belief in "aerially enforced occupation" allowed the Israeli Air Force to believe it could replace the network of lookout posts woven through the topography by translating categories of "depth", "stronghold", "highpoint", "closure" and "panoramas" into "air defense in depth", "clear skies", "aerial reconnaissance", "aerially enforced enclosure" and "panoramic radar". With a "vacuum cleaner" approach to intelligence gathering, sensors aboard unmanned drones, aerial reconnaissance jets, attack helicopters, unmanned balloons, early warning Hawkeye planes and military satellites capture most signals emanating from Palestinian airspace. Since the beginning of the Second Intifada, the [Israeli] Air Force has put in hundreds of thousands of flight hours, harvesting streams of information through its network of airborne reconnaissance platforms, which were later placed at the disposal of different intelligence agencies and command-and-control rooms.[36]

Aerial control proved an effective alternative to the use of troops, who at any rate had refrained from entering Gaza's dense quarters. It allowed Israel to claim it was no longer the Occupying Power, thus able to cast any offensive campaign as mere "self-defense." The very deployment of drones serves to intimidate and terrorize the population into submission. Amassi, a father of eight children, relates:

> It's continuous, watching us, especially at night. You can't sleep. You can't watch television. It frightens the kids. When they hear it, they say, "It is going to hit us." Israel's military may not be on the ground anymore. But they are in the air — looking, always, at every square inch of Gaza. They don't have to be here in Gaza City to affect every aspect of the lives of Gazans.[37]

Targeted Assassinations

Targeted assassinations, euphemistically known as "executive action," "focused preemption" (*sikul mimukad*), "preemptive killings," "extra-judicial punishment," "leadership decapitation," "liquidation" (*khisul*), "selective targeting," "targeted killings," or "long-distance hot pursuit," have long been practiced by Israel. Already in 1948, on the basis of detailed "village files" compiled with the help of collaborators, men of each Palestinian village captured whose names appeared in the files—politically active individuals or those that had participated in actions against the British or the Zionists—were identified: "The men who were picked out were often shot on the spot."[38] This would be declared Israeli state policy in 2000, with the outbreak of the Second Intifada. By September 2014, about 466 Palestinians had been assassinated by snipers, helicopter gunships, drones and remote-detonated bombs, up to 40 percent of them innocent bystanders.[39]

Targeted assassinations are operationally effective. They weaken an enemy's ability to plan and execute operations, especially those of non-state actors that rest on a network of people rather than on high-tech equipment and a modern army:

> The killing of a key individual, much like the destruction of a command-and-control centre or a strategic bridge in "conventional wars" is intended to trigger a sequence of "failures" that will disrupt the enemy's system, making it more vulnerable to further Israeli military action.[40]

When combined with mass arrests, they can seriously disrupt communications, freedom of movement and planning, and sow distrust in the ranks.[41]

Assassinations often escalate conflict as well, but Israel turns this apparent shortcoming into an advantage. Conceived as a doctrine of "escalation dominance," killings can be strategically timed to frustrate diplomatic initiatives or attempts to unite factions. They have been used to eliminate moderate leaders such as Thabet Thabet or Ismail Abu Shanab, as well as those political leaders that Israel simply wishes to remove; in August 2003, the government authorized an open "hunting season" on the entire political leadership of Hamas.[42] Targeted assassinations can also be used to inflame "the ground" so as to justify new military initiatives as mere reactions, as happened in the lead-up to both Cast Lead and Protective Edge, when the killings of Hamas militants led intentionally to the outbreak of hostilities. Assassinations have been carried out to "restore order," to "sow chaos," or to "deliver a message." Militarily, as Esposito shows, they have been used to test new technologies.[43] And there are other reasons: "because too much money was already invested in the manhunt, because security forces enjoyed the thrill, [because the IDF and defense contractors] wanted to impress foreign observers … or [because the security forces wanted to] keep themselves in practice"—or for vengeance.[44] The fact that targeted assassinations invariably result in significant numbers of "collateral deaths" only adds to their deterrent effect. "The lesson of the most recent Israeli assault on Gaza, as in all previous assaults, is that civilians are not 'collateral' or accidental casualties of war between combatants, but the very object of a settler-colonial counterinsurgency," observes Laleh Khalili. "The ultimate desire of such asymmetric warfare is to transform the intransigent population into a malleable mass, a docile subject, and a yielding terrain of domination."[45]

Led by Israel, the core capitalist militaries and others have adopted targeted killings as integral and legal components of their own counter-insurgency strategy.

Urban Warfare

Over the years, the struggle against the Palestinians and subsequently against Hezbollah took the form of hybrid but mostly urban warfare. Israel faced irregular forces who utilized traditional guerilla tactics—hiding in complex terrain and "amongst the people"—yet who now had access to stand-off weapons such as short- and medium-range missiles, anti-tank guided missiles and human-portable air-defense systems. Their capacity to wage hybrid war allowed them to construct a battlespace to their advantage, whether in the towns and hills of southern Lebanon in the case of Hezbollah, or in the dense urban settings of refugee camps and cities in the case of the Palestinians. Despite overwhelming military advantages, conventional armies have been unable to convincingly defeat such irregular forces. This is true of the IDF as well. Israel may have won a stunning victory over several powerful Arab armies in just six days in 1967, but it achieved only an inconclusive ceasefire after 51 days of fighting Hamas in Gaza in 2014.

According to Weizman, the IDF's shift from conventional to urban warfare took place under the command of Ariel Sharon:

In 1971 Major General Ariel Sharon, commander of Israel's southern zone, turned his attention to Gaza's mushrooming insurgency. Perplexed about how to regain control of the enclave, Sharon walked much of the territory over a 2-month period, trying to devise a policy of eliminating guerrillas while not unduly inflicting harm on the population. General Sharon hit upon a unique method of sub-dividing Gaza and crippling movement and communication amongst terrorist units. On maps, he dissected the province into squares of a mile or two in area. General Sharon then trained "first-rate infantry units" for what he called "antiterrorist guerrilla warfare" whose tactics would create "a new situation for every terrorist every day …"

General Sharon assigned squads of elite soldiers to each zone, in which they were to learn intimately the paths, orchards, houses, and other features as well as the routine comings and goings of the inhabitants. Anything out of the ordinary aroused their interest and their deadly response. In the buildup camps, the troops compared the outside and inside measurements of houses to detect crawl spaces or false walls behind which terrorists hid. In rural areas, they looked for ventilation pipes from underground bunkers. Dressing soldiers as Arabs, planting undercover squads, turning captured terrorists into agents (called *shtinkerim* or stinkers), the IDF generated intelligence that led to dead or captured guerrillas …

Sharon also focused on making terrorists operate in the open, where their stealth was exposed to Israel attack. For this task, he employed bulldozers to widen roadways in the refugee camps, which facilitated patrolling and reduced unobserved movement. Bulldozers also dug up bunkers often located next to thick cactus hedges. IDF patrols of orchards often trailed bulldozers behind other vehicles for quick employment.

The purpose was to force underground cells into the open where they stood in Israeli crosshairs. These and other techniques substantially cranked down, although did not eliminate, terrorist incidences.[46]

As defense minister, Sharon refined the IDF's approach to urban warfare during the 1982 Lebanese War, particularly during the seven-week siege of Beirut.[47]

Weizman then relates in detail the story of OTRI, the IDF's Operational Theory Research Institute, established in 1996 by Generals Shimon Naveh and Dov Tamari, as a research institute and training center specializing in urban warfare, one of the "shadow world" of similar institutes that had come into being among core militaries following the end of the Cold War.[48] It was here where Israeli doctrines of urban warfare, now officially called LASHAB, the Hebrew acronym for *l'khima al shetakh banui* or "warfare on built-up terrain," and Close Quarter Combat (CQC) were honed and disseminated. By the time of the Second Intifada, OTRI was functioning in an environment uniquely suited for the wedding of theory and application. OTRI's director, Naveh, who has been described as "Michel Foucault on steroids,"[49] had developed a "System Operational Design" (SOD) for deploying troops and attacking complex urban terrain, one which, following the emergent concepts of "Network Centric Warfare," treats the operating environment in a holistic fashion, employing systems-thinking to non-linear relationships in the battlespace. In developing this approach, Naveh and his colleagues also had at their disposal a rich literature of critical post-colonial and post-structural theory from which they could draw useful concepts of space and cities that they could apply to urban warfare. Theory aside, Naveh & Co. also possessed what no other urban warfare institute did: a laboratory consisting of millions of people living in diverse settings, including cities and densely packed refugee camps, which was the occupied West Bank and Gaza.

Indeed, asserts Weizman, during Operation Defensive Shield, with Sharon now serving as prime minister, the West Bank became "a giant laboratory of urban warfare ... keenly observed by foreign militaries, in particular those of the USA and UK, as they geared up to invade and occupy Iraq."[50] The pitched battles in Nablus and especially in the Jenin refugee camp updated the "template" of Israeli urban warfare and militarized security.[51] From there, new technologies were regularly added, as evidenced in the three assaults on Gaza between 2008 and 2014. Weaponized UAVs and other forms of precise weaponry came into use, as did optics and robotics.

The Israeli Model

The main elements of the Israeli model of urban warfare began to assume a teachable form. *"Sufficient victory"* assumes that resistance will continue indefinitely although in a manageable form. Securitization thus begins, as Meir Dagan tells us, with *proactive intelligence*, be it the surveillance and wiretapping of units like 8200, more traditional intelligence as gathered by AMAN, the Military Intelligence Directorate or the Shin Bet, underground human intelligence gained through informants by *mist'arabim*, or operations as conducted by IDF Special Forces (*Sayeret Matkal* and other reconnaissance units), the Border Police, and their YAMAM/YAMAS units.

Proactive intelligence leads directly to *proactive actions of prevention, deterrence and interdiction*. A key tenet of Israeli counter-terrorism holds that if despite intelligence efforts and preventive measures terrorists cannot be apprehended, killed, or have their mission disrupted before they set off, then the security forces have failed to interdict them and they have succeeded.[52] Continual campaigns of *cumulative deterrence* serve to *dismantle the infrastructure* that supports terrorist, insurgent, criminal, or even political opposition groups, together with continual preemptive actions (*p'ulot yezumot*) to garner intelligence while keeping insurgent groups off-balance.

Through all this, Palestinians are confined to *security zones* which limit their ability to circulate and resist, but which also localize them into fairly manageable cells—the cells of Areas A and B, Gaza and pockets of "east" Jerusalem. When the IDF decides to embark on one of its campaigns to "dismantle the terrorist infrastructure," it merely *encircles and isolates* (kitur) *the specific target*, be it a city or an area of the city, which lies within a security zone that has already been partially securitized. It then sets into operation a series of progressively constricting actions that both reduce the area to be secured and fragment it into more easily managed units. Targeted by combined military-police actions, these zones become total battlespace. Although operations differ in certain ways, overall they share a common conception of urban warfare.

Once the sectors that constitute "ungovernable spaces "and "denied areas" are isolated, hermetically sealed and placed under curfew, drones and ground-based robots, equipped with weapons as well as surveillance devices, provide broad situational awareness and "control at a distance." Here is another form of *layered securitizing*, what Weizman calls "vertical occupation."[53] All along, Israel has based its system of occupation/

governance on *vertical layers of control*: control of the air, in the case of the Occupation surveilling Palestinian movements by satellites and UAVs and maintaining the ability and privilege of assassinating targeted individuals or hitting key targets; control of the ground, whether in the form of routinely circumscribing Palestinian life-space, monitoring that space through different forms of intelligence gathering, locating an armed presence in the midst of Palestinian life-spaces or launching a military attack. When the attack takes place, troops alternate, depending upon the battle conditions, among *control and engagement "at a distance"*, *massive assaults by bulldozers* on Palestinian positions and especially urban infrastructure, and *swarming* over the urban battlespace.

"Engagement at a distance" involves both saturation and precision bombing from the air, sea and land; precision missiles, the use of high-tech enhancements to long-range firing of snipers, tanks and remote-controlled weapons platforms alike and, lately, robotics. In order to eventually engage in Close Quarters Combat, the IDF has had to develop tactics of moving troops into densely populated areas with maximum force but a minimum of "friendly" casualties. In this, it relies on the Combat Engineering Corps of the IDF, whose motto is "Always First." While it carries out many routine operations—mobility assurance, road breaching, defense and fortification construction, counter-mobility of enemy forces, construction and destruction under fire, sabotage, explosives, bomb disposal and special engineering missions—a signature role of the Corps' Engineering Vehicle Operators is driving massive Caterpillar D-9 bulldozers into dense urban built-up areas, either to open passages for tanks, APCs and infantry, or to engage in massive demolition. *Swarming* involves attacking the "front," actually innumerable points of contact from every direction that cannot be effectively opposed. In Operation Defensive Shield, swarming was famously accompanied by "infestation," whereby soldiers break through the walls of homes and progress home to home, street to street through the protected inner spaces of the dwelling themselves, avoiding as much as possible direct exposure to enemy fire, and in fact surprising the enemy by emerging and engaging in unexpected places.

Effective as these tactics may be, such assaults invariably embroil the civilian population in the fighting. And here we return to a key element of Israeli securitization: *impunity*. The IDF places a greater value on the lives of its soldiers and the success of its military operations than it does on the lives of those it is fighting, including civilians of the enemy population, a central proposition of its "lawfare" campaign. Impunity combined with disproportionate force and zero tolerance lends Israeli military operations—and by extension its police tactics as well—*a degree of aggressiveness* that until recently was unacceptable in most core societies. Possessing an occupied territory is valuable in itself for perfecting warfare amongst the people, but the ability to test tactics and weaponry where attack, deterrence, demoralization and impunity towards civilians is unrestrained provides advantages not available in more conventional training and testing grounds.

Weizman documents explicit orders IDF commanders received from their political and military superiors during the Second Intifada to do anything necessary to kill Palestinian "terrorists" and pacify the entire people under Israeli control. He describes the "horrific frankness" of what was intended. Thus, in May 2001, Prime Minister Sharon summoned his Chief of Staff Shaul Mofaz, the head of the Shin Bet and their deputies to an urgent meeting in which he says: "The Palestinians … need to pay the price … They should wake up every morning and discover that they have ten or twelve people killed, without knowing what has taken place … You must be creative, effective, sophisticated." The next day, in what Weizman describes as "an atmosphere of indiscriminate killing," Mofaz told his field commanders that he wanted "ten dead Palestinians every day, in each of the regional commands"—orders he then conveyed directly to lower-ranking officers in the field. Naveh himself described to Weizman the IDF's frame of mind:

> The military started thinking like criminals … like serial killers … they study the persons within the enemy organization they are asked to kill, their appearance, their voice, their habits … like professional killers. When they enter the area they know where to look for these people, and they start killing them.[54]

Indeed, as Weizman relates, during the attack on Nablus in 2002:

> Kokhavi ignored Palestinian requests to surrender and continued fighting, trying to kill more people, until Mofaz ordered the attack over. It was the political and international pressure brought to bear in the aftermath of the destruction of Jenin that brought the entire campaign to a quick halt.

Nonetheless, his tactics were considered successful. He was congratulated by his superiors, including Sharon—although calls were also issued abroad that he stand trial as a war criminal.[55] Kokhavi subsequently served as director of military intelligence.

As the troops advance in one form or another, the cordoned areas are ever more tightened into ever smaller and disconnected zones. *House-to-house searches* are made, often aided by a hand-held, Israeli-developed imaging device that allows troops to "look through" walls by producing 3D renderings of people inside. *Mass arrests* follow such operations, the practice of *administrative detention*, a hold-over from the British Emergency regulation whereby people can be held indefinitely without charge (with the consent of a compliant court), making it possible to imprison thousands of people at a go.[56]

Finally, the element of *demoralization* characterizes Israel's approach to urban warfare and, beyond it, to the process of securitization in general. An important by-product of infiltration into an adversary's organization is to cause a sense of mistrust and insecurity, thus damaging the organization's morale and effectiveness alike. The same strategy accompanies policies of targeted assassinations and mass arrests.[57] Demoralization has two other elements as well: *despair and humiliation*, each intended to paralyze the population's ability to resist, a subtle but nonetheless powerful aspect of pacification. Despair has long been part of the Zionist strategy of forcing the Palestinians to submit to Jewish national demands. As Ze'ev Jabotinsky put it in his seminal work of 1923, *The Iron Wall*:

> Every native population in the world resists colonists as long as it has the slightest hope of being able to rid itself of the danger of being colonized. That is what the Arabs in Palestine are doing, and what they will persist in doing as long as there remains a solitary spark of hope that they will be able to prevent the transformation of "Palestine" into the "Land of Israel."[58]

Ben-Gurion, Jabotinsky's ideological rival, also articulated a policy of inducing despair after the outbreak of the Palestinian Revolt in 1936:

> A comprehensive agreement is undoubtedly out of the question now. For only after total despair on the part of the Arabs, despair that will come not only from the failure of the disturbances and the attempt at rebellion, but also as a consequence of our growth in the country, may the Arabs possible acquiesce to a Jewish Eretz Israel.[59]

The "Iron Wall" doctrine has remained a central element in pre-state and Israeli policy for 80 years. "An iron wall is the most reasonable policy for the coming generation," says Israeli historian Benny Morris approvingly:

> Ben Gurion argued that the Arabs understand only force and that ultimately force is the one thing that will persuade them to accept our presence here. He was right ... In the end what will decide their readiness to accept us will be force alone. Only the recognition that they are not capable of defeating us."[60]

Humiliation also plays a role in demoralization. The Israeli journalist Amira Hass described what happened when IDF troops occupied the Palestinian Ministry of Culture in the center of El Bireh during Operation Defensive Shield:

> On the evening of Wednesday, May 1, when the siege on Arafat's headquarters was lifted and the armored vehicles and the tanks had rumbled out, the executives and officials of the ministry who had rushed to the site did not expect to find the building the way they had left it ... But what awaited them was beyond all their fears ... In the department for the encouragement of children's art, the soldiers had dirtied all the walls with gouache paints they found there and destroyed the children's paintings that hung there in every room of the various departments—literature, film, culture for children and youth books, discs, pamphlets and documents were piled up, soiled with urine and excrement. There are two toilets on every floor, but the soldiers urinated and defecated everywhere else in the building, in several rooms of which they had lived for about a month. They did their business on the floors, in emptied flowerpots, even in drawers they had pulled out of desks. They defecated into plastic bags, and these were scattered in several places. Some of them had burst. Someone even managed to defecate into a photocopier.[61]

In the wake of "messy" invasions of Jenin, Nablus, Bethlehem and other Palestinian cities, the IDF sought to improve its "art of destruction," to move on to "*smart destruction.*"[62] Soon after Operation Defensive Shield, the IDF began work on a massive training facility, the Urban Warfare Training Center (UWTC). The largest mock-up of an (orientalist) Arab city in the world, it was constructed with the help of the US Army Corps of Engineers and located near the Tze'elim Base in the Negev.[63] Opened after the disastrous Second Lebanon War in 2006, when Israeli ground troops fared poorly against Hezbollah fighters, it consists of 600 buildings on a 7.4 square mile (12 square km) "campus." Among the structures of this simulated urban environment, called variously "Baladiya" ("city" in Arabic) or "Chicago," presumably because of the threats of violence under its calm exterior, are eight-story apartment blocs, public buildings, schools, commercial centers, market places, residential neighborhoods and shabby refugee-camp-like shacks. Its varied environments are adaptable to conditions in the West Bank, Gaza, Lebanon, Syria, Iraq, or anywhere in the Middle East. And it is intended not only for IDF training but also for joint exercises with the US Marines, NATO and the Special Forces of other militaries.

And, indeed, Niva traces the Israeli "imprint" on US counter-insurgency doctrine. He found the reality in Iraq at that time, a country "increasingly caged within an archipelago of isolated ethnic enclaves surrounded by walls and razor wire and reinforced by an aerial occupation," reminiscent of "Israel's urban-warfare laboratory in the occupied West Bank and Gaza Strip over the past decade"; not just reminiscent, he claims, but derivative, part of the "Palestinization" of Iraq.[64] He cites Mike Davis, who reports that in the wake of the Mogadishu debacle of 1993:

> Israeli advisors were quietly brought in to teach Marines, Rangers, and Navy Seals the state-of-the-art tactics—especially the sophisticated coordination of sniper and demolition teams with heavy armor and overwhelming airpower—so ruthlessly used by Israeli Defense Forces in Gaza and the West Bank.[65]

It was also around this time that the US Army Corps of Engineers constructed in Israel the Urban Warfare Training Center, where US troops received training before leaving for Iraq.

Perhaps the most emblematic policy coming out of the Israeli model, says Niva, was "the isolation of entire villages in 'hostile' areas, surrounding their residents in razor wire with strictly controlled entry and exit points." In the town of Abu Hishma, American units implemented what they had learned of Israeli tactics: the town was surrounded by barbed wire, its men were issued mandatory identification cards, and checkpoints were established. And during the second assault on Fallujah in November 2004

... the U.S. military used many tactics clearly modeled on the Israeli assault on the Palestinian Jenin refugee camp in 2002. For example, U.S. Marines and Iraqi forces, in what was called a "dynamic cordon," ringed the city with checkpoints in an attempt to fix the insurgents in place as remotely piloted surveillance drones circled overhead on the lookout for stockpiled car bombs. They led with tanks, which broke through enemy lines and drew out the insurgents, while D-9 bulldozers, a staple of Israeli actions in the West Bank, plowed through enemy positions. Infantry bypassed booby traps and snipers by traveling through holes in breached walls, another well-known Israeli innovation.[66]

From here it is but a short distance from the Matrix of Control to domestic securitization. Graham describes how the lock-down of the Jenin refugee camp characterizes the way Israeli security experts train local police in creating sanitized "security zones" and "perimeter defenses" around financial cores, government districts, embassies, venues where the G-8 and NATO hold their summit meetings, oil platforms and fuel depots, conference centers in "insecure" Third World settings, tourist destinations, malls, airports and seaports, sites of mega events and the homes and travel routes of the wealthy.[67] Jimmy Johnson examines Israeli securitization of international "mega-events" such as the World Cup and Olympics, and how they derive from Israel's occupation.[68] He also notes how Israeli and US enforcement mechanisms overlap on what he evokes as the "Palestine-Mexico border." Here, most visibly, the US government awarded Elbit a contract to provide both electronic detection systems and surveillance by its Hermes 450 drones; the Israeli firm Aeronautics Defense Systems supplies their Orbiter UAV and SkyStar 300 aerostat systems for further surveillance. Magna BSP, which provides surveillance systems surrounding Gaza and on the new barrier being built along the Egypt-Israel border, has partnered with US firms to enter the lucrative "border security" market, while NICE Systems provides CCTV for notorious anti-immigrant Sheriff Joe Arpaio's Maricopa County Jail system in Arizona.[69] Already in 2003, the US Department of Homeland Security established a special Office of International Affairs to institutionalize the relationship between Israeli and American security officials.

Creating a Regime of Economic Control and Dependence

Since the start of the Oslo peace process, a permanent "closure" has been laid over the West Bank and Gaza, severely restricting the number of Palestinian workers allowed into Israel and impoverishing Palestinian society, whose own infrastructure Israel has kept under-developed. Much of the structural imbalance that keeps the Palestinian economy highly dependent upon that of Israel derives from the Paris Economic Protocol signed in 1995 as an annex to the Oslo II agreement. It carefully preserves complete Israeli control over the Palestinian economy, including Israel's "right" to stop all shipment of goods for "security reasons" and to hold and check those goods for as long as it wants. This alone all but destroyed Palestinian commerce, Israel's "right" to impose closures on the movement of goods and workers dong the rest. Due to the economic closure of the past two decades, manufacturing amounts to only 10 percent of the Palestinian economy; nearly 90 percent of industrial enterprises in the Occupied Territories employ less than five workers each, 70 percent of Palestinian firms have either closed or have severely reduced production— and yet Palestinian workers have been prevented from accessing the Israeli economy.[70]

Thus unprotected from an Israeli economy 60 times its size, the deliberately de-developed Palestinian economy imports 90 percent of its goods from Israel while exporting to its economic master 88 percent of its exports. By the end of the Oslo "peace process," the per capita Palestinian GNP had fallen to about one-eighth of what it had been at the beginning, only seven years before. Seventy-five percent of Palestinians, including two-thirds of the children, live in poverty, on less than $2 a day, defined by the UN as "deep poverty." More than 100,000 Palestinians out of the 125,000 who used to work in Israel, in Israeli settlements, or in joint industrial zones have lost their jobs.[71] Israel also maintains control over utilities (such as water, electricity and phone services) in the Occupied Territories, charging exorbitant prices. Today the Occupied Palestinian Territory occupies third place on a list of the thirteen most urgent targets of international aid, all the rest being in Africa.[72]

We shall return to these elements of the Matrix of Control when we examine the "Israeli model" of securitization in Chapter 12.

Part V

Managing Hegemony Throughout the World-System

9

Serving the Hegemons on the Peripheries: The "Near" Periphery

In the next three chapters, we will turn our attention away from the core states to examine Israel's military and securocratic involvement with countries, elites and non-state actors on the peripheries of the world-system. In particular, we will look at Israel's role in helping maintain core hegemony over the peripheries, i.e., Hegemonic Task 2, whether by direct intervention or though various forms of support for "pliant" comprador elites, primarily through training and equipping the military and security forces of non-core hegemons. But, again, we must keep in mind that Israel's strategy of "serving hegemons" must be balanced with its security politics and its own political and economic agenda.

Israel is an important player on the peripheries of the world-system, although it is not a major one in terms of military sales. All totaled, the developing world bought $483 billion of arms between 2003 and 2010 (Saudi Arabia and the Gulf States accounting for about half of that amount). Israel's arms sales of $8.7 billion during that period amounted to only 2 percent of the trade, placing it seventh among the largest arms exporter to developing countries, behind the US, Russia, France, the UK, Germany and China, but ahead of Italy, Ukraine, Spain and Sweden.[1]

In 2012, the Israeli Defense Export Controls Agency (IDECA) issued 8,716 export permits for 18,000 defense commodities to 130 countries. According to IDECA, most Israeli companies focus on Poland, India, South Korea, Australia, Thailand, the US, Colombia, Brazil and Chile, though Latin America is seen as "a developing continent as far as security sales." Udi Shani, the director-general of the Israeli Defense Ministry, recommends focusing as well on Azerbaijan and Vietnam. At the same time, Israel's arms sales to Africa more than doubled from 2012 to 2013, continuing a multi-year upward trend. In 2013, it sold $223 million worth of arms to African countries, an increase from just $71 million in 2009.[2]

But the thrust of its security politics drives Israel into a degree of involvement in global security matters that, as I argued earlier, exceeds in extent, depth and quality the reach of any other country, including the United States. To be sure, Israel cannot compete with larger countries in producing and exporting major platforms, nor does it do the volume of business of larger arms exporters. Israel, after all, accounts for only about two percent of the world's arms sales and "only" three Israeli firms are found among the hundred largest arms exporting companies. Nor does it have bases or any permanent military presence abroad. Looked upon laterally, however, Israel's reach extends beyond a specific hegemon's spheres of influence. It possesses the ability to engage in the highest-level security projects, from Theatre Defense in space to the most sophisticated weapons development, yet also penetrates, trains, supplies and works with the deepest levels of countries' domestic security services, guided by the amoral axiom of former Prime Minister Shamir, "Israel is not free to choose its friends according to the nature of their internal politics."[3]

The story of Israel's security politics in the non-core countries, then, is a mixture of straightforward arms dealings and support, most of it covert or quiet, for the ruling hegemons. When it comes to the rulers of countries on the peripheries, Israeli involvement becomes more personalized, with Israeli business people-cum-military advisors, suppliers and trainers identifying up-and-coming leaders and currying relationships with them until they reach power, afterwards playing a key role in the security affairs of their countries. As the notion "pivotal" conveys, Israel is by no means the only player in each security realm in every place, but its presence across the entire securocratic spectrum is unique, if not unmatched.

Because earlier decades have been thoroughly covered in the publications mentioned above, the following survey of Israeli security politics will focus primarily on the contemporary picture.

Creating "Alliances on the Periphery" Through Arms Sales and Training

Israel's "thrust" into global security politics has two drivers: one, as I discussed earlier, is its need to garner support for its occupation policies;

the other, related but no less critical, is the need to counter the threats—military and diplomatic—that the Arab and Muslim countries can mount, especially given the interminable conflict generated in large part by the Israeli–Palestinian-Arab conflict. Israel's security strategy begins, as we explored in depth in Chapters 7 and 8, with a model of "sufficient pacification," whose operational principles, tactics and weaponry can be exported to other countries facing securocratic challenges. Moving further afield, Israel endeavors to outflank its regional adversaries with what was once known as the "alliance of the periphery," but which is a concept that has continued relevance.

The original attempt to forge an informal, even to a degree secret, "alliance of the periphery" began in the 1950s when it became apparent that the US would not extend a security guarantee to Israel. Ben-Gurion's government therefore sought to establish alliances with a series of states and peoples circling the hostile Arab core—Turkey, the Iraqi Kurds and Iran, Muslims but not Arabs, and Christian Ethiopia—building on their common fears of Nasser's pan-Arabism and the Soviet Union. In this way, Israel could lessen its isolation and enhance its international influence even while bolstering its deterrence. Over the years, this fluid concept broadened. In 1982, Israel equipped the Christian Phalange of Lebanon with advanced weaponry, including tanks. Besides using them to drive the PLO out of Lebanon (recall the Sabra and Shatila massacres) and, in fact, engineering the rise of Maronite ally Bashir Gemayal to take over Lebanon, they were to play a key role in Sharon's plan to use Israel's military power to establish political hegemony over the Middle East.[4] It also flirted with the Lebanese Druze. Israel even sided with the royalists in Yemen, and attempted to use the Copts in Egypt, as well as the Jewish communities remaining in Muslim countries, as wedges.[5] Still later, the de facto "alliance" extended to Christian rebel groups in southern Sudan and, most recently, to the Central Asian states of Georgia, Azerbaijan and Kazakhstan, from where Israel has access to Iran and where it may influence a "northern tier" of Islamic states, pitting them against the Iran and the Arab states to the south.[6]

Yet another circle, so to speak, is comprised of states with which Israel can establish some measure of hegemony or influence through its security ties, an alliance of a *political* periphery. Among these states I would number, in Africa, Uganda, Kenya, Rwanda, South Africa, Angola, the Congo, Cameroon, Nigeria, Equatorial Guinea, the Ivory Coast and Sierra Leone; in Latin America, Mexico, Brazil and Colombia (often referred to pejoratively as "the Israel of Latin America"); in Asia, South Korea and

China; in Southeast Asia, Vietnam and Singapore, plus Australia; in Southwest Asia, India and Sri Lanka; in Europe, Poland. Special mention might be made of two countries that Israel has long courted and who fit into the "Alliance" framework: Morocco and Oman.[7]

The "Alliance" then connects with two other blocs of global powers: Core Patrons, Germany, Italy and the UK in Europe, together with NATO, the European Union, and, above all, the US; and Counterhegemons (in fact or potentially) represented by the BRICS/MINT countries. Still, Israel never misses an opportunity to parlay its military ties with any country into a relationship that, no matter how tenuous, might bolster its international standing. Israel's security links thus extend far beyond those countries included in the different "alliances of the periphery." (See Figure 9.1).

Iran was a key part of the original "Alliance of the Periphery." In 1957, soon after the Shah of Iran established with the help of the CIA the notorious internal security force SAVAK, its head, General Taimur Bakhtiar, invited the Mossad to become actively involved in its affairs, which soon blossomed into open and much wider military and intelligence cooperation, including the sale of Uzis and other weapons to the Imperial National Guard. In 1958, the Mossad signed formal letters of cooperation with the National Intelligence Organization of Turkey and with the Iranian SAVAK. The tripartite agreement was named Trident, or "Ultra-Watt."[8] In 1963, Israel helped advise Iran's counter-insurgency operation against dissident tribes in the south.[9] By the 1970s, American interests and Israeli security politics had converged in the Nixon Doctrine, in which Israel and the Shah's Iran were considered America's two top cops in the region. In return for being one of the first states in the region to recognize it, Israel played a key role in organizing, training and equipping the SAVAK, the Shah's dreaded security apparatus, which also became an important source of intelligence information and a partner, with Turkey's security services as well, in operations serving all these countries and their American patron.[10]

The fall of the Shah in the Iranian Revolution of 1979 only strengthened and extended Israel's influence. One American "cop" might have been lost, Chomsky relates, but

Israel's position became even stronger in the structure that remained. Furthermore, by that time, Israel was performing secondary services to the United States elsewhere in the world. It's worth recalling that through the '80s especially Congress, under public pressure, was imposing constraints on Reagan's support for vicious and brutal dictatorships. The

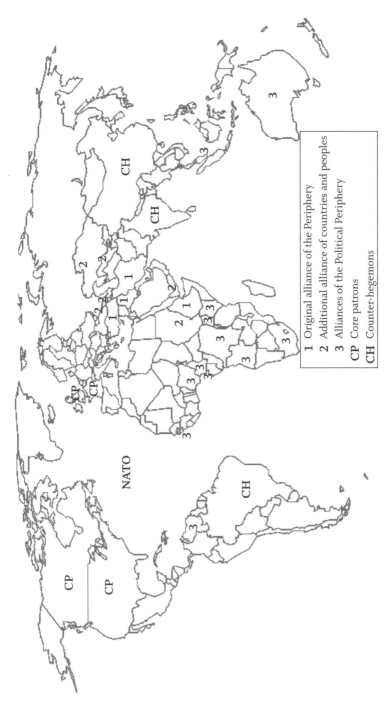

Figure 9.1   Circles of Israeli Security Politics

1 Original alliance of the Periphery
2 Additional alliance of countries and peoples
3 Alliances of the Political Periphery
CP Core patrons
CH Counter-hegemons

governments around the world—say Guatemala, which was massacring people in some areas in a genocidal fashion up in the highlands—the U.S. could not provide direct aid to Guatemala, because Congress blocked it. Congress was also passing sanctions against aid to South Africa, which the Reagan administration was strongly supporting and continued to do so right through the 1980s. This was under the framework of the war on terror that Reagan had declared. The African National Congress— Mandela's ANC—was designated as one of the more notorious terrorist groups in the world as late as 1988. [So] that it [could] support South African apartheid and the Guatemalan murderous dictatorship and other murderous regimes, Reagan needed a kind of network of terrorist states to help out, to evade the congressional and other limitations, and he turned to, at that time, Taiwan, but, in particular, Israel. Britain helped out.[11]

Israel's role as American surrogate was highlighted most notoriously in its involvement in Irangate, which also indicated that Israeli military relations with Iran did not end with the Islamic Revolution. The Revolution left Iran in possession of American arms but no spare parts; moreover, the Israeli government attempted to maintain discrete contacts with the Iranian military, with which it had worked closely and which it supported over the Iraqis in their 1980–88 war, in the hopes of eventually overthrowing (or at least moderating) Khomeini. When the war with Iraq broke out in the 1980s, Israel discreetly supplied more than $30 million in military equipment and parts to the Khomeini regime, in clear violation of the American arms embargo and despite the Carter Administration's appeal not to do so until the hostages were freed. The Israeli-Iranian channel subsequently proved useful (if ultimately embarrassing) to the Americans when, in what became known as the Iran-Contra scandal of 1986, Israel, at the behest of the Reagan Administration, secretly supplied arms and spare parts to Iran out of its own stocks, which the US promised to replenish, in an attempt to free the American hostages. The proceeds from that sale were then used to bypass a congressional ban on funding the Contras, using Israel as a surrogate. Indeed, after Congress finally forced the Reagan Administration to end its involvement with the Contras, Israeli advisers supplying training and Israeli weapons replaced the Americans.[12]

"We are going to say to the Americans," said Ya'akov Meridor, the chief economic coordinator in the Israeli cabinet at that time:

"Don't compete with us in [apartheid] South Africa, don't compete with us in the Caribbean or in any other country where you can't operate in the open. Let us do it." I even use the expression, "You sell the ammunition and equipment by proxy. Israel will be your proxy," and this would be worked out with a certain agreement with the United States where we will have certain markets ... which will be left for us.[13]

Israel, in fact, continued to supply the Khomeini regime with military equipment and ammunition at least until 1987.[14]

The Middle East

Turkey was, of course, a key to the Alliance of the Periphery. Turkey had de facto recognized Israel already in 1949 and, after Ben-Gurion made a secret visit to Ankara in 1959, the two countries agreed to help each other obtain arms and economic assistance from the US while Turkey, a NATO member since 1952, would help Israel join the Alliance. By the 1990s, Israel and Turkey were drawing closer, united by common concerns over Iran and its ally Syria, and both were key players in Washington's Middle East order after the end of the Cold War and the outbreak of the First Gulf War of 1991. Moreover—and this is a recurrent theme in Israeli security politics—Israel could provide military technology that the West was reluctant to sell to Turkey because of its war against the Kurdish insurgency. In 1992, Turkey upgraded its diplomatic relations with Israel to the ambassadorial level, and in 1996, the two countries signed a formal military pact.[15]

According to Lebanese General Moustapha Sleiman, in that pact

... the ammunition industries in the two countries concluded an agreement [for] the manufacture of Popeye surface-to-air missiles; the sale of Israeli Python 4 air to air missiles to Turkey; Turkish manufacture of the Galilee infantry rifle; the formation of defensive doctrines against ballistic missile attack; eventual Turkish participation in the production of Israel's Arrow anti-missile system; and joint manufacture of the jet-propelled 400 kilometer range Delilah cruise missile. It was reported that the Turks voiced great interest in intelligence and other data transmitted by the Offek satellite Israel recently fired into space. An Israel firm has contracted to modernize 54 Turkish F-4 Phantoms and 48 F-5s, at a cost of some $900 million and ... Turkish planes are to undergo structural improvements and be fitted with radar systems, computerized aeronautical systems, navigational systems, electronic warfare systems, and armaments to improve their performance in bombing missions … The offer to sell Israel's Merkava Mark-3 tank and to modernize Turkey's Patton (M-60A3) marks the two countries' growing interaction in relation to ground forces, including improvements in artillery capabilities both in range and in penetration power.[16]

Sleiman also mentions mutual military visits, joint training and exercises, and staff exchanges. Moreover, the Israeli Air Force could access Turkish air space and bases in its operations against Iran and Syria, while Israel provided Turkey with military hardware and upgraded its fleet of American Phantoms. In the context of the Oslo peace process, this suggests that this agreement with Turkey ended any chance of Syrian-Israel peace.[17]

Operation Cast Lead in 2008–09 triggered the sharp decline in relations between the two countries as the Erdoğan government grew ever more hostile to Israeli policies vis-à-vis the Palestinians, in the context of wider regional politics. Turkey blocked Israeli participation in joint US, Turkish, Italian military exercises in June 2010, after the IDF violently boarded the Turkish ship *Mavi Marmara*, which was attempting to bring humanitarian aid to Gaza through the Israeli blockade, and killed nine Turkish activists. Turkey suspended defense contracts worth $56 billion, including a $5 billion deal for a thousand Merkava Mk-3 tanks, and dropped a $2 billion bid for IAI's Arrow-2 anti-ballistic missile system.[18] Netanyahu's apology for the attack in March 2013 did not measurably un-freeze relations. It remains to be seen how Israel's disposal of its natural gas finds—of prime interest to Turkey, yet also bringing the Cyprus issue into the equation—will influence relations, together with Israel's growing military closeness to Greece and the Iraqi Kurds as a counterweight to Turkey.

The Kurds as well have always been a key part of the Alliance of the Periphery, a non-Arab people embedded as they are primarily in northern Iraq, a geopolitically crucial region of the Middle East. Indeed, the prospect of a Kurdish state raises concerns over a "second Israel" in the Arab world, based on traditionally strong political and even military relations between the two peoples. Support for the Iraqi Kurds is often generated by the large (150,000+) Kurdish-Jewish community in Israel, as well as by AIPAC.[19] In 1965, at the height of the Kurdish rebellion against Baghdad, Israel supplied the Kurdish forces with arms, including Soviet arms captured from Egypt and Syria, training and funding, all funneled through Iran, so that they could mount a major offensive against the Iraqi Army; several IDF platoons served in a training and at times command function.[20] Kurdish national leader Mustafa Barzani visited Israel twice, in 1968 and 1973, as did his sons Idris and Masoud. The latter has been the President of the Kurdish Regional Government since 2005.

Reports of continued but discrete Israeli military involvement with the Kurds surface periodically.[21] Israel is said to conduct covert operations from the territory of Iraq using the organizations in the Kurdish-populated areas of Iran as part of its "Kurdish strategy." Besides destabilizing the Iranian regime, Israel, together with the Americans, is attempting to obstruct Iran's nuclear program by aiding Kurdish fighters of the United Front of the Eastern (Iranian) Kurdistan in infiltrating into the Iranian Kurdistan where, among other operations, they lay surveillance devices. By laying this groundwork of training and cooperation with the Kurds, Israel is positioning itself to take advantage of changes in the Iranian or Iraqi regimes.[22]

When it comes to the broader Arab world, the notion of an Israeli–*Arab* conflict appears shaky. While its true that Israel is constantly embroiled in wars or more limited military operations, in surveillance and all means of striking overtly or covertly against targets of all kinds, in rapidly shifting alliances and interests, its relations with many countries of the region have also been characterized by often close if discrete military and political ties, some extending from before the establishment of the state.

From the standpoint of security politics, Israeli concerns at different times over Soviet influence, pan-Arabism, radical Islam, liberation movements and even uprisings demanding democratic reform have been shared by most of the members of the Arab League, as well as France, Britain and the US. Israel has often served as a conduit for American and European military aid and intervention. Even its military or covert security interventions have won the appreciation of particular Arab regimes at particular times—although encouraging inter-Arab fighting and factionalism was as much a part of the equation as supporting conservative regimes. In the 1950s and '60s, Israel trained the security services of the Moroccan king so that he could consolidate his position vis-à-vis the country's restive political parties, and in the 1970s prevented a coup against the king.[23] It joined with Saudi Arabia and Iran in supporting the royalists against the Nasser-backed republicans during the 1962–70 Yemeni civil war, coordinated with the US. During the 1970s, Israel assisted Sultan Qaboos ibn Said's totalitarian regime in Oman in its battle with insurgents in Dhofar province. In 1970,

Israel protected Jordan from a possible Syrian invasion, while in 1976, Israel created the South Lebanon Army and invested more than $150 million in military supplies and training for the (fascist) Christian Maronite Phalange militia in anticipation of the 1982 Lebanon War.[24] More recently, Israel sold weapons to the Saleh regime against which the Yemeni people had been rebelling since 2011[25] and aids the al-Sisi government in its struggle against the Muslim Brotherhood. Israel even cooperates with the Saudis over plans to attack Iran and other regional issues.[26]

Even a conservative Israeli political analyst with strong criticism of Arab politics admits that

> ... in spite of the grassroots enmity toward Israel, almost all Arab leaders have formulated some sort of functioning cooperative relationship with Israel to advance their national or personal interests. However, due to the Arab public consensus against such policy ... even today, a significant majority of such communication is unknown to the general public ... The study of Israel in the Middle East is not only an analysis of the various wars; rather, it is a study of the various coalitions, regimes, leaders, and leaderships in the region and their motivations to make coexistence or peace with Israel possible.[27]

This reveals the political logic, often hidden, of security politics, and certainly would not hold true with Israel's military clout. "Everything is underground, nothing is public," says General Amos Gilad, director of the Israeli defense ministry's policy and political-military relations department:

> But our security cooperation with Egypt and the Gulf states is unique. This is the best period of security and diplomatic relations with the Arabs. The Gulf and Jordan are happy that we belong to an unofficial alliance. The Arabs will never accept this publicly but they are clever enough to promote common ground.[28]

The Arab Peace Initiative, formulated by the Saudis and approved unanimously by the Arab League at its meeting in Beirut in March 2002, reveals the degree to which Israel is considered an important ally of conservative Arab regimes—to the point where they would welcome it as a regional hegemon. In that initiative, the Arab League offered Israel peace, recognition and full normalization, including integration into the region, in return for the establishment of a Palestinian state in the

Occupied Territories and acceptance of the refugees' right of return, although in numbers agreed upon by "mutual consent." The subtext of the Saudi Initiative, I suggest, was (and very much still is) this: We want you to take your place alongside us, the undemocratic Arab regimes fearful for our own survival in the face of the Arab Spring and its local, simmering manifestations, a resurgent Islamic fundamentalism and growing Iranian influence, as a regional power. We need (and admire) your military prowess, and appreciate your ability to bring to our part of the world greater American involvement (i.e., weaponry and political support). So please, let's come to a quick resolution of the Palestinian problem so we can move onto more pressing regional agendas.

As General Gilad says, everything is underground when it comes to arms transfers and mutual support between Israel and the conservative Arab regimes. The British Department for Business, Innovation and Skills, which oversees all of that country's military and security exports, offered a tiny glimpse when it reported that Israel had sold military and security equipment to four Arab countries (Algeria, Egypt, the United Arab Emirates and Morocco), in addition to Pakistan, between 2008 and 2012. In 2010, the Israeli government asked for permits to sell HUD (head-up cockpit displays) systems with British parts, to a number of countries, including Morocco and Egypt. It also requested permits, in 2009, to export to Algeria aerial observation systems, helmets for pilots, radar systems, military communication systems, navigation systems, drone components, and systems that disrupt ballistic equipment, optical target acquisition systems and airborne radars. In the same year, Israel asked for permits to sell HUD systems to Morocco, in addition to asking for permits to supply the United Arab Emirates with components for drone, aerial refueling systems, ground and airborne radars, helmets for pilots, parts for fighter jets, thermal imaging and electronic warfare, and systems that disrupt missile launchers. Morocco deploys Israeli-made Delilah cruise missiles and Python 4 air-to-air missiles.[29]

Mention should be made of Cyprus, arguably a part of the Alliance of the (Near) Periphery, but with added importance since the discovery of massive reserves of natural gas in the eastern Mediterranean. Since the gas fields cross territorial boundaries undersea, they have provoked major conflicts, some connecting to other issues and carrying military threats, among the countries of the region—Greece, Cyprus, Turkey, Lebanon, Israel and the Palestinians (gas fields extend into Palestinian offshore waters). As relations with Turkey decline, Israel has boosted its security ties with Turkey's arch-adversaries, Greece (the impact of the 2014 elections is as yet unclear) and Cyprus. Israel and Cyprus are both currently exploring oil resources off the southern coast of the country. In 2012, Israel signed an agreement with Cyprus (that Israeli papers have noted "is reminiscent of Ben-Gurion's alliance") that allows the IDF to deploy naval forces and airplanes in Cyprus's territorial waters and airspace to defend natural gas sites against Turkish threats to either countries' offshore installations. For its part, Turkey insists that any natural resource discovery involving Cyprus must benefit Turkey as well and be exploited cooperatively, because of its claims and interests in the northern part of the island, which it controls. The Turkish President Tayyip Erdoğan has threatened Cyprus with military action if it pursues its offshore drilling program with Israel. Israel and Cyprus have conducted a number of joint military exercises in the past several years, and Defense Minister Ya'alon has stated that Israel intends "to improve the preparedness of its navy in the Mediterranean to protect the gas facilities of Israel and Cyprus."[30]

Central Asia

The Caucasus represents one of the regions where, for all intents and purposes, Israel's "Alliance of the Periphery" continues to function. "The pursuit of diplomacy with Central Asian republics (CARs) such as Kazakhstan and Turkmenistan, and Azerbaijan in the Caucasus—which were not only Muslim but offered more stable alternatives to volatile Middle Eastern energy—was effectively a recast of Ben-Gurion's 'periphery doctrine,'" write two Israeli political analysts. "On the whole, Muslim Central Asia is significant to Israel for economic, diplomatic, and security reasons. This also sheds light on why a relatively distant Israel saw it a matter of strategic necessity to project is own influence into the region."[31] "In the post-Cold War period," adds another:

Israel was compelled by changes in the international environment to seek new allies and to re-invent itself by finding a new role in the American global strategy. Israel sought to build its new alliances in areas that included the South Caucasus and Central Asia against its new enemy—the Islamic regime in Iran, and was successful in establishing good relations with Azerbaijan and Kazakhstan. In this strategy, Israel pursued the advancement of the shared interests with the United

States regarding the Newly Independent Muslim states (preventing the penetration of radical Islam, nuclear proliferation and ensuring the energy security of the West.) In the 1990s, Israel desired to serve as a "subcontractor" when the United States sought to outsource the conduct of its foreign policy in these regions. Thus, in the early 2000s, Israel pursued a policy of advancing bilateral ties with the above-mentioned countries."[32]

No less than nine interlocking foreign policy objectives have been put forward to explain Israel's keen interest in keeping Central Asia part of its "Alliance":

- Prevent the spread of Iranian influence in the region,
- Minimize the influence of the Arab world,
- Divert attention from the Israel–Palestine conflict,
- Expand the strategic relationship with the US,
- Curb the emergence of hostile regimes and foster the creation of "moderate" Muslim states,
- Curb the development of WMD,
- Develop an economic hinterland,
- Develop the Israeli arms industry and Israeli military effectiveness through the sale of military hardware, and
- Ensure the protection of local Jewish communities.[33]

To that we add others: moderating the dangers of the decline in relations with Turkey in that strategic region, and helping its core allies ensure that Iran or other radical Islamic forces do not fill the geopolitical vacuum in the southern periphery of Russia—or, indeed, that that strategic region not be re-absorbed into a new Russian Empire. This also addresses the fears of the Central Asian states themselves, plus bolstering their authoritarian regimes against yet another threat: democratization. The Arab Spring scared the hell out of them.[34]

Azerbaijan and Israel have had close relations since Azeri independence in 1991. Early on, Israel supported the Azeris in their conflict with Armenia in the early 1990s, supplying them with Stinger missiles.[35] The constant strengthening of Israeli-Azeri relations, a base from where Israel surveils Iran and from which it could launch an attack, only augments Iran's sense of encirclement.[36] Indeed, on an official visit to Baku in 2012, Israeli Foreign Minister Avigdor Lieberman quipped that "Azerbaijan is more important for Israel than France." And don't forget oil: 70 percent of Israel's oil currently comes from Azerbaijan and Russia, making the region of added strategic importance to Israel.[37]

For its part, Azerbaijan has sought to use Israel to break out of its geographic and diplomatic isolation, squeezed as it was between Russia and Iran. An extremely authoritarian regime with a terrible human rights record, the Azeri government has also used Israel to plead its case in Washington, by means of the Jewish lobby:

> The Jewish advocacy coalition serves as an essential pillar in this relationship between Azerbaijan and the US. This role is appreciated by the ruling elite in Azerbaijan. Indeed, it appears that access to the Jewish lobby in the United States was one of the reasons for creating an axis with Israel.[38]

Ties with Azerbaijan, oiled by Israeli weapons, advance Israeli interests in other ways as well. Azerbaijan receives a significant amount of oil via the Baku-Tbilisi-Ceyhan pipeline and in return it represents a ready market for Israeli arms. Azerbaijan, whose annual defense budget tops $4 billion, an increase of 493 percent in one decade, has risen to the top ranks of Israeli export markets, having purchased nearly $4 billion in Israeli arms between 2011 and 2014. Israel Aerospace Industries has sold at least $1.6 billion worth of UAVs, radars, intelligence systems and air defense missiles. This includes a Barak-8 SAM system, 75 Barak 8 SAMs, a Green Pine Air search radar, Gabriel-5 anti-ship missiles, five Heron UAVs and another five Searcher UAVs and TecSAR, the IAI spy satellite that has been deployed in support of Azerbaijani military operations in the mountainous terrain of Nagorno Karabakh, where it has been described as "indispensable" in the conflict against Armenian insurgents. Elbit, which opened a subsidiary called Elbit Systems of Azerbaijan in 2009, won a $56 million contract to upgrade Azerbaijan's Soviet T-72 tanks, which will be carried out by Elbit Systems Land and C4I, Tadiran and Elop. Rafael has sold the Azerbaijani military Spike anti-tank missiles and targeting systems.[39]

According to the 2011 SIPRI Arms Transfers Database, Azerbaijan had acquired about 30 drones from Israeli firms Aeronautics Ltd. and Elbit Systems by the end of 2011, including at least 25 medium-sized Hermes-450 and Aerostar drones, plus 6 Lynx self-propelled multiple rocket launchers and 50 Lynx missiles, 5 ATMOS 155-mm self-propelled guns, five 120-mm self-propelled mortars, and 10 Sufa aircraft, American-built but Israeli-modified F-16s.[40] In October 2011, Baku signed a deal to license and domestically produce an additional 60 Aerostar and Orbiter drones. Its most recent purchase from IAI in March 2012 reportedly included 10 high altitude Heron-TP drones.[41] The Azeri Ministry of Defense Industries has created a joint venture with an Israeli company, Aeronautics Defense Systems, to produce UAVs, currently being manufactured and assembled by the Baku-based Azad Systems Company in Azerbaijan. In June 2013, Azerbaijan showcased its military advantage to its regional rivals, Armenia and Iran, by publicly demonstrating its new locally produced UAVs, as well as the Israeli-manufactured Hermes and Heron UAVs during a military parade. Azerbaijan purchased the EXTRA Israeli tactical missiles during Operation Protective Edge; their test-fire was broadcast on Azerbaijani television.[42]

To counter a bolstered Iranian presence in the Caspian Sea, Azerbaijan completed assembling the two high-speed border patrol 3rd Class Shaldag V boats under licensing from the Israel Shipyards in July 2014. Azerbaijan is also in the process of negotiating a purchase of Israeli Sa'ar-4.5 missile boats. Azerbaijan also employs Israeli security companies for providing services of a sensitive nature. In 2001, the Israeli firm, Magal Systems, was granted a contract to construct a security fence for Baku's Bina airport, one of Azerbaijan's key strategic assets, and to train its security personnel.[43]

In September 2014, Israeli Defense Minister Moshe Ya'alon visited Azerbaijan, which was hosting ADEX-2014, its first international arms exhibition. There, 16 Israeli arms firms offered a wide variety of air, sea, land and space systems, plus cyber-security, in which Baku has shown interest. The Azeri military is also negotiating the purchase or co-production of Namer APCs.[44] Indeed, over the last 25 years, Azerbaijan and Israel's ties have expanded to include broad cooperation in the military and security fields, as well as the exchange of intelligence information, with Israeli intelligence operatives participating in collecting human intelligence about extremist Islamist organizations in the region and monitoring troop deployments of Azerbaijan's neighbors—especially Iran.[45] In the end, commented one military analyst, "Azerbaijan is considered a favorite destination for the Israeli arms industry, and there are existing partnerships between the military institutions of the state with almost every Israeli defense industry."[46] This, asserts Murinson, is proof-positive of the effectiveness of Israeli security politics:

The proof of the reliability and longevity of the Azerbaijani-Israeli ties came at the cusp of Israel's Operation Protective Edge against Hamas in the summer of 2014. When the majority of Muslim states accused Israel of humanitarian crimes and Europe marked a significant spike in anti-Semitism, a Muslim Azerbaijan stood out as a beacon of support born out of the country's self-interest and commitment to its Western identity.[47]

Another key player in the Central Asian "periphery" that allows Israel to circumvent its "hostile near abroad" is Kazakhstan, whose human rights records rivals Azerbaijan's in its steady deterioration, hostage to the ruling Nazarbayev clan.[48] "Since Israel's independence," write Feiler and Lim,

> ... the threat emanating from its Arab neighbors has necessitated the optimization of ties along its periphery and beyond. Furthermore, Israel's dependence on oil and gas imports, the production and trade of which are still heavily dominated by the Muslim Middle East, has rendered it vulnerable. Thus, when the Soviet Union dissolved in December 1991, Israel hastened to reach out to the emerging republics in Central Asia and the Caucasus, Kazakhstan and Azerbaijan chief among them. In the following two decades, the form and substance of bilateral relations have evolved significantly and have extended to sensitive security cooperation.[49]

Kazakhstan and Uzbekistan, both with small if significant Jewish communities, are the only two Central Asian states to have embassies in Israel. Among other reasons for promoting relations with Israel is the threat posed by radical Islam to Kazakhstan. Its economic dynamism make it the most vulnerable of the Central Asian states to the "three evils" so feared in the region's politics: religious extremism, separatism, and terrorism.[50]

Israeli companies such as Elbit, Israel Aerospace Industries, Israel Military Industries and Gilat Satellite Networks have participated in the Kazakhstan Defense Expo trade fairs held in Astana in 2010 and 2012. On January 2014, Kazakhstan's Defense Minister Adilbek Dzhaksybekov visited Israel and signed a military cooperation agreement formalizing military and defense ties. Kazakhstan's military contacts with Israel have concentrated on three areas: upgrading Soviet-era equipment, purchases of advanced weaponry, and joint production of military equipment. Kazakhstan is particularly interested in cooperating with the Israeli military and defense companies in the areas of unmanned systems, border security, command-and-control capabilities and satellite communications. IMI produces weapons systems, along with modernizing and integrating them into the armed forces; while Elbit Systems develops and modernizes various weapon systems, UAVs, avionics, radars and reconnaissance satellites. Rafael produces various missile and aircraft technology defense systems and tactical missiles. Israeli companies have upgraded Kazakhstan's 600 Soviet T-72 tanks as well as the avionics of the Kazakhstani Air Force's Sukhoi-25 fighters. Kazakhstan currently builds, under Israeli license, self-propelled mortars, multiple rocket launch system and howitzers, which it plans to sell to other Central Asian countries.[51] Significantly, Kazakhstan has granted Israel access to Baikonur Cosmodrome as part of a joint space program, where a series of telecommunications satellites built by IAI has been launched, the most recent being the Amos-4 in September 2013.[52]

Surprisingly, according to Bouceck, "Uzbekistan enjoys perhaps the greatest cooperation with Israel of all the central Asian republics when it comes to military and security matters," revolving primarily around the threat of Islamic fundamentalism emanating out of Iran and Afghanistan.[53] And, indeed, in the 2000s, the Uzbek government asked for Mossad's assistance in eliminating local Islamist groups.[54]

Again, ties to the Central Asian states advance Israel's security politics. When Iran sought to utilize its chairmanship of the Organisation of Islamic Cooperation (OIC) to censure Israel, they did not support the move. And in the wake of the Goldstone Report investigating Israel's role in Operation Cast Lead in Gaza, the CARs abstained from voicing a vote at the UN. Israel has also prevailed upon Kazakhstan to halt its sale of uranium to Iran.[55]

As in other parts of the world, the role played by Israeli arms deals and "businesspeople" in currying relations with Central Asian states is crucial. "Person-to-person relations between Israel and Central Asia are probably Tel-Aviv's leading means of influence in the region," is the way Laruelle puts it. And here Israel has a major advantage: many of the "Israeli" brokers are themselves indigenous to the region or to the wider former Soviet Union, e.g., Bukharan Jews and Russian-, German- and Yiddish-speaking Ashkenazi communities. Lev Leviev, the "king of diamonds" in Israel, Africa and Europe, is a native of Uzbekistan and is president of the World Congress of the Community of Bukharan Jews. He is personally acquainted with Uzbek President Islam Karimov and Kazakh President Nursultan Nazarbayev, and "is an indispensable ally for anyone wanting to establish themselves in Central Asia." Former Israeli Minister of Foreign Affairs Avigdor Lieberman, a native of Moldova, has been campaigning for stronger ties to Central Asia, particularly to Tashkent, since the 1990s. In Kazakhstan, oligarch

Alexander Mashkevich who heads the holding Eurasian Natural Resources Corporation also has Israeli citizenship and acts as a central intermediary for business. He chairs the Eurasian Jewish Congress, one of five branches of the World Jewish Congress, and has the ear of President Nazarbayev.[56]

Due to its strategic ties with Russia, Israel tends not to intervene directly in the affairs of other countries in the region closer to Europe, where tensions are high between NATO and Russia. In fact, in 2014, Israel angered the US by avoiding support for its sanctions on Russia over the Ukraine, while also canceling a planned sale of UAVs to the Ukraine over fears of alienating Russia.[57] Georgia represented a partial exception to this policy. At the time of the Russia invasion in 2008, Israel was a dominant force in the Georgian defense establishment; in fact, the Georgian Minister of Defense, Davit Kezerashvili, was a former Israeli, and many Georgian immigrants worked in Israeli arms plants. Over the years, Israel sold Georgia UAVs, rocket launchers, anti-tank mines, and cluster bombs.

In a bizarre episode, Israeli General Gal Hirsch (a failed general who resigned from the IDF after exhibiting poor leadership in the 2006 war in Lebanon) became involved in an arms deal—in fact, he promised the Georgians that if they followed his advice and purchased the military equipment he recommended, they would actually defeat Russia in a war over the self-proclaimed pro-Russian breakaway republics of South Ossetia and Abkhazia. This, despite the fact that Israel, not wanting to harm its relations with Russia, approved only "non-offensive" weapons. At the same time, another Israeli General, Israel Ziv, tried to drum up business for his arms firm Global CTS in Abkhazia, hoping to break into a previously inaccessible market and, beyond it, Russia itself. After beating up Georgia and displacing 192,000 people, Russia occupied the two provinces, where it remains today. Since then Israel has considerably lowered its profile there.[58]

Africa

Africa represented yet another sphere in Israel's "Alliance of the Periphery." Of particular importance to Israel's geo-strategic posture were the countries of the Horn of Africa—Ethiopia, Kenya and Sudan—which control the shipping lanes to Eilat and are close to Egypt, Yemen and Saudi Arabia. This also gave Mossad agents and Israel Defense Forces officers an excuse to be involved in the internal affairs of African regimes. According to various publications, Israelis were involved in *coups d'état* in Uganda and

Zanzibar, or at least had prior knowledge of them.[59] Israeli involvement in Ethiopia was well-known and fairly public, going back to the 1950s. Israel aided Ethiopia in its war against Eritrean secession. Even after Haile Selassie's overthrow in 1974, it maintained military relations with the Derg military junta, training Mengistu Haile Mariam's Presidential Guard and the Ethiopian police. According to the Eritrean People's Liberation Front (EPLF), the Mengistu regime received $83 million worth of Israeli military aid in 1987, and Israel deployed some 300 military advisers to Ethiopia. Additionally, the EPLF claimed that 38 Ethiopian pilots had gone to Israel for training. Nonetheless, immediately upon independence in 1993, Eritrea opened itself to Israeli development and military projects. Israel has small naval teams in the Dahlak archipelago and Massawa and a listening post in Amba Soira, a small but focused and significant presence aimed primarily at monitoring Iran and countering its inroads into East Africa, especially into Sudan.[60]

The Alliance aside, over the years Israel has expended considerable efforts and resources to woo as many of the sub-Saharan African countries as possible—utilizing its military prowess fully in the service of its security politics. During the period of de-colonization, the 1950s and '60s, Israel invested enormous resources and efforts in currying relations with the emerging African states. Israel's decision to do this, explains Chazan, a noted Israeli expert on Africa,

> … was guided by several fundamental considerations. The first, and by far the most prominent, was political. The sheer number of African countries with voting rights in international bodies, and especially in the United Nations, meant that they could determine the difference between Israel's isolation and acceptance in the global community. Closely linked to this motive was a strategic concern: Reaching out beyond the immediate ring of hostile Arab states would create a security net, especially in the Horn of Africa and its eastern coast. Economic factors also intruded: The geographic proximity of Africa made it a potentially attractive source of raw materials and a new and growing market for Israeli products …
>
> During the heyday of the Israeli-African relationship, in the mid-1960s, Israel reaped significant benefits both on the bilateral and multilateral levels … At the United Nations, the African vote provided a firm cushion against repeated attempts to isolate Israel.[61]

Israel also maintained relations—and possibly more—with rebel leaders in Angola, Mozambique, Portuguese Guinea and Southern Rhodesia during the 1960s and '70s, as well as groups fighting the Federal Government of Nigeria, UNITA in Angola, Idi Amin as he rose to power and, of course, the rebel movement of South Sudan.[62]

For most years since 1975, according to SIPRI, Israel has ranked generally just below the ten largest exporters of major weapons. In the period 2006–10, Israel delivered major weapons to nine sub-Saharan states— Cameroon, Chad, Equatorial Guinea, Lesotho, Rwanda, the Seychelles, South Africa and Uganda, with Nigeria being the largest African importer of Israeli weapons, accounting for almost 50 percent of Israeli deliveries to sub-Saharan states, amounting to some $500 million between 2006 and 2009, rising to $318 million in 2113 alone—although imports from Israel made up less than a quarter of Africa's total arms imports.

Deliveries consisted mainly of small numbers of artillery, unmanned aerial vehicles, armored vehicles and patrol craft. However, in addition to major weapons, Israel also supplied small arms and light weapons, military electronics and training to several countries in the region. The presence of Israel Weapon Industries (IWI), the main Israeli producer of small arms, in Africa is indicative of the importance of Africa for Israeli small arms and light weapons (SALW) exports. While IWI provides no data on its customers, its website includes a map indicating three IWI office locations in Africa, the highest number for any continent. Its Galil and Tavor rifles, Negev machine guns and Uzi sub-machine guns are used by many African armed and security forces, mainly by the elite presidential guards or special forces.[63] Overall, Israel is one of only about a dozen countries that export $100 million or more in such weapons.[64]

10

Security Politics on the "Far" Periphery

Here we turn to another circle in Israel's expanded alliance of a *political* periphery: those countries of the peripheries and semi-periphery that are geographically far from Israel, but with which it can establish some measure of hegemony or influence through its security ties.

South and East Asia

In terms of security politics, the motivating force behind the original Alliance of the Periphery, some key countries in Asia could be considered integral parts of an extended Alliance. We might begin with one of the earliest and most successful of Israel's security projects: building the armed forces of Singapore. After that city-state gained its independence in 1965, an Israeli military delegation headed by Major General Ya'akov Elazari arrived under a veil of secrecy and started to build the various branches of the armed forces. Israeli military advisers set up the defense and internal security ministries, while a team under Maj. Gen. Yehuda Golan established the military infrastructure on the model of the IDF. Today, Singapore's army is considered the strongest and most advanced military in Southeast Asia. That alliance continues; security ties between the two countries remain strong and Singapore is now one of the biggest customers for Israeli arms and weapons systems, as well as being a partner. The Gil anti-tank missile, which is manufactured by Rafael, for example, was developed jointly with Singapore, as was the anti-armor weapon Matador and various high-tech systems, including surveillance. The first tangible political fruits of this relationship was Singapore's decision to abstain in the UN General Assembly vote condemning Israel for acts of aggression after the 1967 war. In 1968, as many other countries in Asia and Africa were severing diplomatic ties with Israel, Singapore established them.[1]

Since then, Israel has sold many systems to Singapore, including AWACs airplanes. The Singapore Army is reportedly operating a 52-man IAI Searcher-2 UAS in Afghanistan. Singapore was the first regional Spike user after it ordered a thousand of them in 1999. The Singapore Army integrated twin Spike launchers onto Light Strike Vehicles.[2]

Israel is a major military supplier to the countries of southern Asia, with exports to the region amounting to $3.9 billion dollars in 2013.[3] That year Israel was the fourth largest arms supplier to India, after Russia (nearly $30 billion), France ($20 billion) and the US ($15 billion), but in some years Israel has been second to Russia and its influence seems to be overtaking that of France and the US. Indeed, Israel has become one of the world's top arms exporters—its arms exports increased by 74 percent since 2008—largely due to deals signed with India, to whom its has sold some $10 billion in military equipment in the decade after 2000.[4] It has become the main supplier of UAVs to the Indian military, which have used them operationally for some time, notably in Kashmir and on the border with China (China also uses UAVs extensively to monitor activity on the border). The Indian armed forces operate at least 150 UAVs—this includes the Navy, which has land-based UAVs for maritime surveillance. Several dozen IAI Searcher I and II UAVs are in service with the Indian Army and Navy. The latter has at least a dozen Heron I/IIs operating alongside its Searchers. These were ordered in 2005. The Indian Air Force also has some Heron Is in service. Other Israeli UAVs fielded include the Harpy, 30 of which were delivered from 2005, and the IAI Harop loitering munition. Ten were ordered by the IAF in 2009 for $100 million, with deliveries from 2011.[5]

Since Indian Prime Minister Narendra Modi came to power in May 2014, defense and technology ties between Israel and India have gone into overdrive. Modi, a Hindu nationalist who is expressly anti-Muslim and pro-Israel, visited Israel in 2006. India is now the largest buyer of Israeli military equipment, while Israel is India's largest customer after Russia. In the first nine months of 2014, bilateral trade reached $3.4 billion. With a staff of six, Israel's military delegation in India is second only to that of the United States. India is steadily catching up with China, as it buys more Israeli defense and cyber-security technology, an area where China is limited, since the United States frowns on Israel dealing too freely with Beijing in defense matters.

Prime Minister Modi's cabinet cleared a long-delayed purchase of 262 Barak-1 missiles, which will be delivered over the course of about five years, starting in December 2015. These will be deployed on the country's 14 battleships. In October, India closed a $520 million deal to buy 8,356 Spike anti-tank guided missiles, human-portable "fire-and-forget" anti-tank missiles that lock on to targets before shooting produced by Rafael, and more than 321 launchers, chosen over a rival US offer of Javelin missiles for which Washington had lobbied hard to place. The jointly developed Israeli-Indian Barak-8 aerial defense missile system passed a major trial, which India called a "milestone." The Barak-8 is considered a versatile medium-range missile system capable of intercepting warplanes that can also be installed on missile boats, thereby providing an answer to coastal missiles—Russian Yakhont supersonic missiles in particular, that have been passed from Syria to Hezbollah—threatening Israel's natural gas platforms, its naval vessels and even its ports in the Mediterranean Sea. The mutual interests in developing the missile were clear: without the $1.5 billion Indian investment, Israel would have been left with great technology but no product. As it was, the system was developed mainly by IAI in collaboration with India's Defence Research and Development Organisation.[6] And, of course, Israeli companies are upgrading India's Russian-made tanks and aircraft.

The Indian minister of defense visited Israel for three days in July 2014 and talked with top Israeli officials about additional weapons deals, among them a control system for the Indian Air Force. Israel is also interested in selling India defense systems such as Iron Dome, though it has not been successful so far. In 2013, the Indian government approved the purchase of 15 Heron unmanned aerial vehicles produced by IAI, and IAI is angling to sell up to 40 UAS systems for monitoring the India-Pakistan border. India is also said to be deliberating about purchasing Israel-made Phalcon AWACS surveillance aircraft worth $1 billion, which are also operated by the Singapore Air Force.[7]

Other joint products are also coming down the pipeline. Hindustan Aeronautics Limited (HAL) is working on a prototype of an unmanned helicopter for the Indian Navy, based on the locally made Chetak helicopter, with IAI developing the flight control system. Rafael and IAI will also partner with Indian manufacturers to jointly build an integrated anti-missile system to be deployed against Chinese nuclear and conventional missiles (although Israel also supplies the Chinese Army). In order to more deeply penetrate the huge Indian market, IAI has established with Tata Advanced

Systems a joint venture company called Nova. It specializes in the development, manufacturing, marketing and support of defense products in India, particularly unmanned aerial systems (UASs), missiles, radars and electronic warfare systems.[8] Overall, Israel is eagerly taking advantage of India's willingness—nay, insistence—that it transfer military technology to local companies so that they may produce "Made in India" products. At a meeting with Modi at the UN in September, 2014, Netanyahu expressed his country's readiness and willingness "to discuss transfer and development of technologies with India. Israeli industries, including the defense industries, could contribute to the 'made in India' project, and thereby reduce costs of manufacturing products and systems developed by Israel."[9]

At Defexpo 2014, New Delhi's annual military and homeland security fair, SIBAT brought 21 Israeli arms companies to display their wares. Besides the large firms, the list of participants offers a glimpse into the range of military and security technologies which Israeli companies offer. They included:

- ACCUBEAT, which provides Accurate Frequency and Timing solutions for combat planes, UAVs, helicopters, ships and missile platforms;
- Beth-El Industries, a company owned by German "Christian Zionists," which manufactures CBRN (chemical, biological, radiological, nuclear) air filtration systems and claims a customer base of more than 60 armies and civilian authorities around the world.
- CONTROP, a company specializing in the field of EO/IR defense and homeland security solutions;
- DSIT SOLUTIONS, which specializes in sonar and acoustic solutions for the naval, homeland security, and commercial markets;
- ESC BAZ, manufacturers of Video Surveillance and Observation and Communication systems for the military and police;
- Meprolight, specialists in electro-optical and optical sights for armed forces, law enforcement agencies, and civilian markets;
- PALBAM Defense, providing metal technologies for rockets and missiles, and
- Verint, whose "communications and cyber-intelligence solutions help law enforcement, national security, defense forces and other government agencies neutralize terror and crime.[10]

Again, the impact of these ties on Israel's security politics seems clear. In December 2014, the Indian government indicated that it may shift its traditionally pro-Palestinian position in the UN and simply abstain on votes having to do with the Israeli–Palestinian conflict, a shift Indian newspaper *The Hindu* says "could amount to a tectonic shift in the country's foreign policy."[11]

Nearby, in Sri Lanka, General Vernon A. Walters, ambassador at large and former deputy director of the CIA, established an Israeli interests section within the US embassy in Colombo in 1982, thereby facilitating Israeli military involvement in the war with the Tamil Tigers—despite the fact that Sri Lanka and Israel had previously broken off diplomatic relations. Agents of Israel's General Security Services (the Shabak, or Shin Bet) trained the Sri Lankan Army, its Special Task Force and police in COIN warfare. Over the years, Israel also equipped the Sri Lankan Air Force with Kfir jet fighters, IAI Scout and Searcher drones, six Super-Dvora and 38 Shaldag fast naval patrol craft and Gabriel anti-ship missiles; Israel also trained the Sri Lankan technicians maintaining both the Israeli aircraft and the Russian MiG-27s, and supplied ammunition. In 2003, Rafael won a contract worth $10.8 million to upgrade 15 fast-attack naval craft, and the testing of nuclear-capable Israeli cruise missiles from submarines in Sri Lankan waters was also reported.[12]

In 2000, the two countries established full diplomatic relations. Immediately after the defeat of the Tamil Tigers (which has led the UN to investigate Sri Lankan Army for war crimes), Donald Perera, the Sri Lankan military's chief of staff, was appointed his country's ambassador to Israel. "I was familiar with Israel before coming here," he told the newspaper *Yedioth Ahronoth*:

> In the framework of my previous positions as air force commander and chief of staff, I had a great relationship with your military industries and with Israel Aerospace Industries. For years Israel has aided our war on terror through the exchange of information and the sale of military technology and equipment. Our air force fleet includes 17 Kfir warplanes, and we also have Dabur patrol boats. Our pilots were trained in Israel, and we have received billions of dollars in aid over the past few years. This is why I asked to be assigned to Israel—a country I consider a partner in the war against terror."[13]

There are potentially important political implications to Israel's proximity to Sri Lanka. Sri Lanka has moved out of the Indian orbit closer to China, which played a key role, militarily and diplomatically, in the government's victory over the Tamils. Indeed, that active involvement signaled a shift from China's "peaceful rise" as a world hegemon to a more assertive policy. Given the continued tensions between India and China, Israel's position as the #4 provider of weapons system to the first and #2 to the latter, as well as supplying a Chinese ally on the southern border of India, reveals skillful security politics. Widening the circle, having such close security relations with two BRICS countries, one of which (China) is decidedly anti-Western, reveals a certain assertion of Israeli arms independence, especially as its patron, the US, begins its defensive/aggressive "Asian pivot" to confront China. The Indian Ocean is seen as a key arena in twenty-first-century jockeying for influence among the US, India and China:

> India cannot help but be wary of the growing capability of China's navy and Beijing's growing maritime presence. Then there is the strategy known as a "string of pearls" which has involved China building bases in Myanmar, Bangladesh, Pakistan and Sri Lanka encircling India in the process. In Sri Lanka, the port at Hambantota sits directly astride the main east-west shipping route across the Indian Ocean denying India the advantage it had hitherto taken for granted.[14]

Israel is playing its role, but not necessarily as an ally committed to US hegemony.

At the far end of the Asian "Alliance" are Australia and South Korea, two strategically important allies, both geographically and political, as well as significant weapons customers. The former needs little security politics manipulation in order to reside in the "pro-Israel" camp: as a country whose foreign policy is coordinated with the United States and even to a significant degree dictated by it, Australia has always been one of Israel's closest allies. Both countries participate in the "Five Eyes" Echelon satellite program, monitoring international communications. In 2010, Elbit was awarded $298 million for the supply, integration, installation and support of a Battle Group and Below Command, Control and Communications (BGC3) system for the Australian Army's Land 75/125 program. A key to Australia's network-centric warfare strategy, the BGC3 is a Battle Management System (BMS) that links soldiers, and their commanders mounted in virtually any combat vehicle, and Command Post staff.[15]

Military relations with South Korea suffered momentarily when Israel chose Italian training aircraft over South Korea's after a heated competition, but they have returned to normal. South Korea has purchased around $400 million of Israeli defense systems, including the IAI's Green Pine long-range radar and systems made for the T-50 aircraft. The IAI's Heron UAS has been selected for the corps-level UAV upgrade project of the Republic of Korea Army.[16] South Korea is also said to be very interested in Rafael's Iron Dome missile interceptor. IAI has also submitted a bid for a $1.38 billion contract to provide air refueling tankers.[17]

Many of Israel's military exports to Asia are, of course, secretive. Elbit, for whom Asia represents 25–30 percent of its sales, was awarded contracts by "several customers in Asia" to supply "many dozens" of observation systems for maritime patrol aircraft, vessels and observation towers, as well as a contract valued at $32.7 million to supply an undisclosed regional army with advanced training systems for its armored and infantry forces, and another $20 million contract to supply an Asian country with dozens of CoMPASS (Compact Multi Purpose Advanced Stabilized System) payloads for maritime patrol aircraft to protect its coastlines—which has been installed onboard hundreds of platforms abroad, including Unmanned Aircraft Systems.[18] It has also been awarded a $290 million contract by "a customer in the Asia-Pacific region" to provide its tanks with night operation capabilities by supplying a variety of advanced systems, such as gunner sights and fire control systems.[19]

Latin America

In the 1970s and '80s, when it already had the ability to offer high-quality military assistance, Israel pushed aggressively to create alliances with regimes in Latin America; Brazil, Argentina, Nicaragua and Guatemala in particular could have been considered a part of the "far periphery" at that time. Latin America in general, by 1986, accounted for half of all Israeli arms sales.[20] In his book *Israel and Latin America: The Military Connection*, written in the mid-1980s, Bishara Bahbah puts forward a number of reasons why Latin America became a major Israeli market for arms and security equipment or, more precisely, what Israel offered those countries that so attracted them. It had to do, he contends, with the "suitability" of Israeli arms to the kinds of conflicts characteristic of Latin America (and, by extension, to other regions of the periphery as well), namely small wars and insurgencies, social unrest and crime related to poverty and an indiscriminate policy of arms exports and training, coupled with Israel's surrogate role vis-à-vis the US. This way of viewing Israeli arms sales continues to be relevant and useful, and not only for Latin America.[21]

Despite these affinities, Israeli military influence crumbled along with the military regimes in many South American countries (as well as in Central America) in the late 1980s and throughout the 1990s. With the return of a constitutional government in Argentina in 1983, no new arms deals were signed with Israel; in fact, in an effort to make a break with legacy left by the junta, President Alfonsin ended all military ties with Israel. While several scattered deals were made with Brazil (1994 and 1996), Uruguay (1997) and Venezuela (1990, 1999), nothing in this period rivaled the relationships forged during the years of military dictatorships.[22]

It is only in the past few years, then, that Latin America has again risen on the Israeli horizon. As Latin American economies grow, led by Brazil and Mexico, the militaries are also expanding and modernizing, creating a major arms market. Despite certain territorial disputes among these countries, however, instances of inter-state warfare are rare, the last one being a brief border clash between Ecuador and Peru in 1995. Indeed, one of the glaring contradictions in the political life of the region is the prominence of the military despite the lack of threats from neighboring states. Instead, the major source of threat and conflict is securocratic, stemming from social unrest and crime linked to poverty, and the operations of major crime organizations, drug cartels in particular. Together they generated insurgency, in some cases political, as with the Zapatistas in Chiapas, Mexico, in others a mixture of the political and criminal, as with the FARC and drug cartels of Colombia.[23] Whether to secure everyday life or the major mega-events that bring prestige and, to some, money—the 2011 Military Defense Games, the 2014 World Cup and the 2016 Olympics, all held in Brazil, being the main examples—the concerns of the human-security states of Latin America, where the boundaries among militaries, security forces, police forces and paramilitary units are blurred at best, create an affinity with what is considered the model of a human-security state: Israel.

Given the traditional support of Israel that has characterized Latin American governments and peoples all the way back to its establishment by the UN in 1947, Israel hardly needed to push its security politics. For all that, given the increasing unpopularity of Israeli policies towards the Palestinians in Latin America, "weapons diplomacy" is still called for. Brazil, for example, is the prime arms market in that region yet one of the most vociferous in its criticism of Israel, pushed by both popular opinion and well-organized protests.

Weapons diplomacy seems to carry the day in many cases, however. The Brazilian armed forces opened an office in Tel Aviv, and a few years later the Israeli daily *Ma'ariv*[24] crowed: "Defense Industries Take Brazil." "An historic agreement for security cooperation" between Brazil and Israel opens up "a market valued at billions of dollars" to Israeli defense industries, it reported. "There are already several giant deals on the table between Israel Aerospace Industries (IAI), Elbit and Rafael with Brazil."

Brazil, whose defense budget of $31.5 billion in 2013 accounted for 48 percent of South American arms purchases, is also the fifth largest importer of Israeli arms.[25] Although there were no extensive military ties between the two countries before 2000, since then the Israeli government and Israeli arms companies have developed close relations with the Brazilian military. Many arms sales are direct government-to-government transactions: Rafael, for example, which is government-owned, has sold 400 Python-3,200 Python-4 and 200 Derby missiles to the Brazilian Air Force.[26] But Israeli arms companies have also opened subsidiaries there in order to better integrate into the country's arms industry. IAI has formed a joint venture called EAE with Brazil's Synergy Group, and will provide maintenance and customer support services for IAI's various systems in use in Latin America, including UAVs. IAI Chairman Yair Shamir estimated that Latin America now accounts for only about 5 percent of IAI's overall sales, which reached $3.6 billion in 2008. But IAI expects substantial business growth, with the new joint venture with Synergy alone possibly delivering more than $100 million in new sales.[27] Bedek, an IAI subsidiary, provides comprehensive maintenance services for aircraft, engines and components, including heavy maintenance, modifications, upgrades, conversions and development programs in Israel and Brazil. It uses TAP M&E Brazil maintenance and production centers in Rio de Janeiro and Porto Alegre airports. IMI has given Taurus, a Porto Alegre-based small arms manufacturer (with a branch in the US), the license to produce its Tavor rifles in Brazil. The Brazilian Army is considering the Tavor as its new service rifle.[28]

Elbit has bought three Brazilian arms companies: AEL, Ares Aeroespecial e Defesa and Periscopio Equipamentos Optronicos. Elbit has also teamed up with Embraer, the Brazilian aerospace conglomerate that is the world's third largest producer of commercial, military, executive and agricultural aircraft. That partnership won a $230 million tender to upgrade F-5s in

2001 and provided systems for super Tucano ALX planes, and in 2008, they won a tender worth $187 million to upgrade AMX planes.[29] One of the primary goals of the joint venture is to promote Elbit's Hermes 450 and 900 UAVs in the Brazilian Air Force (the latter deployed for the first time in the 2014 assault on Gaza).[30] In fact, in 2014, Elbit announced that it has signed a contract with the Brazilian Air Force for Hermes 900 UAVs which, together with the 450s now in service, will be "equipped with a new and advanced intelligence gathering system considered as a breakthrough operational solution, will be operated by FAB in combined missions with the Hermes 450 fleet, already in operational use." For its part, IAI is said to have signed a $350 million contract to provide the Brazilian national police with Heron UAVs in order to secure the World Cup and the 2016 Olympics.[31] In order to stress the point that in the absence of warfare in Latin America the military becomes an extension of internal security (and vice versa), Elbit clarifies that both the Hermes models

> … will carry safety and security missions in the 2014 FIFA World Cup Games … Joint flight operations, using both the Hermes 450 and the Hermes 900, [provides] a unique solution for intelligence missions, border protection, perimeter control of infrastructure and critical sites, as well as Safe City programs and large scale events.[32]

Just to show how convoluted and intertwined is "defense" business, yet another Elbit subsidiary, Elbit America, announced that it had subcontracted with an American company to upgrade four Grumman C-1A aircraft for the Brazilian Navy. The subcontract is valued at $106 million. Elbit's Brazilian subsidiary, located in Porto Alegre, Brazil, will provide in-country contractor logistic support services for the program as a subcontractor to Elbit Systems of America.[33]

Elbit is also involved in a major modernization program of the Brazilian military, the development of a new locally produced APC, the Guarani. A key component of the new APC will be a variety of remote-controlled weapon stations for additional firepower, including Elbit's, with its 30mm cannon and ability to carry anti-tank missiles, which can be fitted on the vehicle. Ares, Elbit's Brazilian subsidiary, developed the remote weapon station called REMAX as part of a $25 million contract. (Through Ares, Elbit also recently signed a contract to supply 5,000 optical sights for the Brazilian Army's assault rifles.) As a part of the Guarani project, Elbit's AEL subsidiary won a $260 million contract for unmanned vehicle gun turrets. The new turrets mount 30mm automatic cannons including a coaxial mount for a 7.62mm machine gun, an advanced fire control system with automatic target tracking, ballistic computing, sensors management and displays.[34]

Not all is rosy in Brazil, however, especially as opposition mounts to Israel's occupation policies. In October 2013, Elbit announced that its AEL subsidiary had presented a model for the first Brazilian microsatellite for military applications—the MMM-1—whose launch it projected for December 2015. Produced in AEL/Elbit's Center for Development and Industrialization of Aerospace Equipment in Porto Alegre, the $16 million project was to position the state of Rio Grande do Sul "to be a space and technological modernization center for the defense segment" according to the state's governor. "The Center will contribute towards strengthening the Brazilian defense industry," said AEL's vice-president:

> We will have the capacity to produce avionics and develop unprecedented defense systems in Brazil, such as the electronic war systems, unmanned aerial vehicles, electro-optical technology and weapons guidance systems and space systems. The microsatellite will be the first major project.[35]

Unfortunately for AEL and Elbit, Porto Alegre is also where the World Social Forum is held as a main venue in which grass-roots organizations the world over congregate to "make the world a better place." In 2012, the Brazilian peasant movement had even convened a special WSF on the issue of Palestine. When they got wind of the AEL/Elbit project, Brazilian social movements and trade unions protested Elbit's role in the construction of Israel's apartheid Wall in the occupied West Bank and its close relationship with the Israeli military—and forced the state authorities to cancel the project. The rector of the university leading aerospace research in the region had declared that the university would not work with Elbit Systems on any research that could have military research, which also cast doubt on the project's viability. (In 2009, the Norwegian state pension fund divested from Elbit Systems as well.)[36]

In fact, Israeli arms companies seem to be somewhat on the run. Because of a virtual break in relations with Turkey, once one of Israel's largest arms partners, it has shifted its attention to Brazil, aided by a 2010 agreement that enables Israel to sell Brazil a wider range of weapons systems than had previously been possible. As a result, Israeli firms have become fixtures at the bi-annual Latin American Aerospace and Defense and Security Exposition (LAAD) in Rio de Janeiro, sponsored by no less than Embraer.[37] Thirty firms exhibited their wares at the 2013 fair, but their conspicuous position also drew protestors from dozens of Brazilian civil society organizations.[38] Whether that played a role in the cancellation of the AEL/Elbit military satellite project is debatable (though plausible). Elbit cancelled its exhibit at the prestigious Rotterdam arms fair due to local protests.[39] Still, Elbit's operations in Brazil between 1994 and 2009 totaled $750 million, and it is projecting a 30 percent annual growth in business there in the coming years.[40]

Brazil, of course, has the largest economy in Latin America and is the continent's primary arms producer. The close integration of Brazilian and Israeli arms firms, from joint projects to partnerships to wholly owned Israel companies in Brazil provides the Israeli arms industry with an entry to other markets in the region. In a recent interview, Rafael's vice-president, Lova Drori, commented on this:

> Rafael has a wide presence in some of Latin American armed forces, primarily Colombia, Chile and Peru. Some of our systems are also flying with the Brazilian Air Force ... In recent years LAAD evolved from a local Brazilian event into a regional exhibition; therefore, we address the entire region with a different focus. Regarding Brazil, evolving into a major power on a regional as well as global scale, we emphasize various aspects of security and defense, including air-defense, maritime and coastal security, leveraging our command, control and intelligence technologies for security management over vast regions of land and sea, utilizing derivatives of our military systems.[41]

Perhaps Israel's closest friend and staunchest military partner in Latin America is Colombia, largely because its prolonged counter-insurgency campaigns against both political opponents and criminal gangs fits well into the range of military goods and tactics offered by Israel.[42] In an interview with a senior editor at *Ha'aretz*, Yishai Halper, President Juan Manuel Santos was asked about criticism coming from former Venezuelan President Hugo Chavez, who called Colombia "the Israel of Latin America," partly because of its defense cooperation with Israel. "If somebody called my country the Israel of Latin America," he responded, "I would be very proud. I admire the Israelis, and I would consider that as a compliment."[43]

Colombia has Latin America's second largest military budget ($9.1 billion in 2013). In 1989, it purchased twelve revamped 1970s vintage delta-winged Kfir C-2 fighter aircraft as they were being retired from the IAF. Since then, they have been upgraded to the C-7 variant, a vastly improved model that includes an improved engine that significantly increased maximum take-off weight, two more weapons chambers, better avionics and in-flight refueling capability. The planes, armed with Israeli-made Python-3 AAMs, are mainly used in ground-attack missions during counter-insurgency operations. In 2008, Colombia signed a $150 million contract for an additional 24 Kfir aircraft upgraded to C-10 standards. This entails adding the Elta radar that provides information to a fire-control system in order to calculate a firing solution, head-mounted display capability and multi-function display panels. The refurbished Colombian version of the aircraft is termed Kfir COA. Israel has also supplied Derby and Python-5 missiles for the aircraft.[44] A similar process of upgrading has been done on Ecuador's Kfir fleet of twelve aircraft, one of which shot down a Peruvian Air Force plane during the 1995 Cenepa War. The Ecuadorian version of the C-10 upgrade is called Kfir EOA. Argentina is negotiating the purchase of 18 Kfir C-10s for $500 million, much to Britain's consternation.[45] IAI is attempting to sell a batch of 50 retired IAF Kfirs upgraded to C-10 standards; Bulgaria is a leading prospect.[46]

Ever mindful of the connection among arms sales, military assistance and its security politics, Israel pressured Colombia intensively to oppose the Palestinians' bid for recognition at the UN, and in 2012, Colombia abstained in the UN vote on Palestine.[47] In an interesting development, Jacques Wagner, a prominent member of the Brazilian Jewish community, once active in a Zionist youth movement, was appointed minister of defense in late 2014.[48] Whether that will play a role in Israeli security politics remains to be seen.

Mexico, Latin America's third largest military spender ($7 billion in 2014), is also invested in Israeli arms, though primarily for use against drug trafficking. In 2009, it purchased $233 million worth of Hermes 450 UAVs, most likely to locate marijuana and opium in the northwestern states of Sinaloa, Durango and Chihuahua. Still, Israeli military personnel have been reported in Chiapas, including the representative of the Israeli Ministry of Defense for Mexico, Honduras and the Dominican Republic.[49]

To round off the discussion, we should also make mention of Chile, not a major customer of Israel overall, but a purchaser of high-tech armaments nonetheless, and a potential market Israeli companies are keeping an eye on.[50] Chile has received from Israel Litening target pods for airborne missile systems, 60 Derby and 280 Python-4 missiles, 2,200 SPIKE anti-tank missiles, and a $50 million Hermes 900 UAV systems sale.[51]

What emerges from all of this is the range of hegemons served by Israel, from the US first and foremost, to Europe, India and China, then to the other states of the semi-periphery and on to Equatorial Guinea, Sri Lanka and Uzbekistan. Once we plug in private arms dealers and security firms, however, the extent of Israel's global reach, as it extends down deeply into the internal working and conflicts of countries as well as across the globe, becomes even more evident.

11

The Private Sector

Some 6,784 Israelis deal in security exports, some representing the 1,006 companies and 312 independent businesses engaged in the arms trade, others as freelancers.[1] *Ha'aretz* asks, however, why so many Israelis are arrested over illegal arms deals worldwide? They begin by suggesting a common profile based on seven Israelis then in jail in four countries:

> Even though it is doubtful whether those in jail know one another, they have quite a lot in common. All are men in their fifties or sixties. All are well to do (or were in the past), having made most of their money in international arms dealing or in exporting security services and equipment from Israel. They served in the Israel Defense Forces and reached mid-level ranks (from captain to lieutenant colonel), and when they were arrested, they denied the charges. Friends who came to their assistance described them, naturally, as "the salt of the earth."
>
> All seven are familiar faces in the corridors of the defense establishment, and at one time received arms dealing permits from the Defense Ministry. All sought to "expedite procedures" in violation of local or international laws, and did so out of pure greed. Due to this covetousness, they also fell into traps and can expect to face many years in jail.[2]

Private and Semi-private Arms Dealers

Yossi Melman, then the military correspondent for *Ha'aretz*, reported on a visit of Israeli Foreign Minister Avigdor Lieberman and an entourage of dozens of businessmen, most of them arms dealers, as well as security advisers and representatives of the military industries, to five African countries in August 2009. "It is a sad truth" he comments,

> … that with the exception of a few civilian enterprises in agriculture, communications, infrastructure and diamonds, almost all-Israeli activity on the African continent is related to weapons exports. "The ugly Israeli" in the guise of the arms dealer (mostly former intelligence and military officials), who promotes weapons sales on behalf of Israeli military industries, with the backing of the defense establishment, have given Israel a bad name world-wide. Israelis have been involved in civil wars (in Angola, Liberia, Sierra Leone and the Ivory Coast) and in aiding dictatorial regimes such as in Equatorial Guinea and the two Congo republics.[3]

According to Sarah Lieberman-Dar, an Israeli journalist with extensive experience in covering military issues in Africa, some 20 Israeli "business people" pull the strings in Africa. These are a mix of genuine business people—official representatives of Israeli arms firms and frequently of other Israeli companies or government projects in such areas as agriculture, infrastructure, communications, construction and security; business people—private arms dealers and private "security advisers" often engaged in shady activity, and rogues—private arms dealers, "trainers" and suppliers of death squads, militias and even criminal or terrorist groups and mercenaries. "The influence of the presidents' confidants is so great," says Lieberman-Dar

> … that "their president," as some of them call the president of the state which they work, makes sure to get their advice on almost every issue. They help him to foil revolts and to identify internal enemies, they equip the army, train the Presidential Guard, build buildings and pave roads that glorify the name of the president, some of them are even responsible for the public relations of the presidents in the world. The producer Arnon Milchin helped the public relations system of South Africa during apartheid. Meir Meyuhas helped the Zairian dictator Mobutu Sese Seko improve his image in the United States … Most of the president's confidants are not disturbed by the corruption and violations of human rights for which some of the continent's leaders with whom they work are responsible.[4]

Indeed, "brokering" is a major part of Israel's security relationship with Africa, and it is here where influential Israeli "business people" play a key role. "Israeli expatriates living in African states have long been instrumental in arranging arms deals for Israeli companies," reports SIPRI in a careful, understated manner:

> An Israeli businessman living in Nigeria [Amit Sadeh, a partner in a large shopping mall in Lagos], who was also involved in the controversial sale of air and sea drones by the Yavneh-based Aeronautics Ventures, to the Nigerian defense ministry organized the large deal for Israeli surveillance systems in 2006 and the sale of two Israeli patrol craft in 2008. This same person, like other Israeli expatriates, has also been reportedly involved in arranging arms deals that have no further connection with Israel, for example the sale of aircraft from Ukraine to Nigeria. Another Israeli expatriate brokered the 2008 sale of patrol craft to Equatorial Guinea.
>
> There have also been occurrences of Israeli involvement in illegally organizing or selling weapons or services to several African states. For example, in January 2010, four Israelis working for small "military and defence" companies (including two in the United States) were among 22 persons indicted in the USA for violating anti-corruption laws ... In June 2010 an Israeli "defence consultant" was among several persons indicted in the USA for attempting to sell 6000 AK-47 rifles to Somaliland using a falsified end-user certificate for Chad.[5]

The Israelis, Lieberman-Dar relates, generally prefer to concentrate their businesses in one country. Hezi Bezalel is the dominant Israeli figure in Rwanda, having begun his African career in Uganda (where he continues to do business and is a confidant of President Yoweri Museveni). There he befriended Paul Kagame, a Tutsi refugee from Rwanda, a former officer in the Ugandan Army, who headed the Tutsi Rwandan Patriotic Front that entered Rwanda during the 1994 genocide and ended it, with the help of arms supplied by Bezalel. Whether or not Bezalel was involved, starting in 1992, Israel sold arms and later provided training to the Hutu-dominated Rwandan military and to the Hutu militias that in 1994 perpetrated the genocide, continued to send arms during the genocide and then supplied arms to the Tutsis thereafter. Human Rights Watch reported: "Arms dealers in Israel, the United Kingdom, South Africa, and Albania had no scruples about selling weapons to authorities who were executing a genocide" and millions of dollars of ammunition was shipped from Israel to Rwanda in the midst of the genocide.[6] Kagame then took control of the country, initially as minister of defense, and remains its ruler until today. The end of the Rwandan civil war did not end the need for arms, however, as Kagame initiated two large counter-insurgency campaigns against Hutu rebels in the Congo, the Rwandan Army joining forces with that of Uganda. Although a ceasefire was declared in 2003, fighting continues.

Bezalel himself, the honorary consul of Rwanda in Israel, remains the main actor in maintaining close ties between the two countries; indeed, Rwanda has been called "the Israel of Africa." He sells military equipment to Rwanda and even plays a role in building its army, as well as being involved in the local cellphone industry, waste disposal and other enterprises (including a business relationship with Ehud Barak, Israel's former prime minister, defense minister, chief of staff and not an insignificant arms dealer himself). He is also said to be behind the recent deal to deport African asylum seekers in Israel—mainly from South Sudan and Eritrea—to Rwanda and Uganda in exchange, though they have no arranged status in these countries, are not granted basic rights and, for the most part, they do not have any official documents or permits. These countries agree to take them in return for arms—a clear case of arms-for-refugees human trafficking.[7]

Sami Meyuhas, one of the most influential Israeli "business people" in Africa, concentrates his activities in Cameroon. He inherited his position from his father, Meir Meyuhas, the former Mossad agent who had been active in Zaire and Cameroon since the early 1960s. Meir was a close confidant to Mobutu; he had an official position as Mobutu's "business adviser" and developed contacts between him and the American Jewish community, and especially with Jewish members of Congress. Meyuhas kept up relations with Mobutu even during the years when Zaire, like most other African countries, cut their diplomatic ties with Israel in 1973. Predictably, Zaire was the first African country to re-establish ties with Israel in 1982, leading the way for the others, but only after Meyuhas arranged a secret meeting in Zaire in 1981 between then-Defense Minister Ariel Sharon and Mobutu. There, Sharon signed a five-year agreement under which "Israeli military advisers will restructure Zaire's 20,000-member armed forces"—and train Mobutu's 7,500-member Presidential Guard. Israel's visible military presence, according to a senior Zairian official, represented not only a "weapon of dissuasion" to countries and forces bordering on Zaire, but "also a dissuasive force against the opposition and even a force of intimidation regarding the population who say to themselves that Mobuto is supported by a powerful ally."[8] He also promised Israel would intervene on Zaire's behalf with the American government. Immediately upon the re-establishing of ties, then-Foreign Minister Yizhak Shamir also visited Zaire. In Cameroon, where Meyuhas had the official title "Special Adviser to the Presidency of the Republic," he had his office in the presidential quarters.[9]

Meir's son Sami is a close confidant of Cameroon President Paul Biya, known as "the Qaddafi of Black Africa," who leads a lavish lifestyle and has amassed a fortune estimated in the hundreds of millions while ruling as a dictator for more than three decades over one of the poorest countries in the world. Indeed, so corrupt is Biya's regime that even the Israeli Ministry of Defense decided to withdraw its delegation there, though Meyuhas continues business as usual. He is reported to make up to 25 percent on each arms deal.[10] In 2010, Colonel Avi Sivan, a military adviser to Cameroon's president in charge of training the Presidential Guard and an associate of Meyuhas, was killed in a helicopter crash in Cameroon. He had been a founder of the elite IDF counter-insurgency unit Duvdevan, the head of the Defense Ministry's delegation to Cameroon and subsequently a private security adviser to the Cameroon government.[11]

Corruption, cozy business relationships between rulers and foreign entrepreneurs, the free-for-all looting of national resources, hundreds of millions of profits to be made by all concerned, suppression and the impoverishment of the local population—all this requires Presidential Guards, elite special ops units, exaggerated militaries, ubiquitous security forces and the infusion of arms. Easily dismissed as part-and-parcel of "failed states," there is *agency* here, both local and international. Profits are there to be made, power to be wielded by classes of people who have vested interests. "International warlordism" best describes this world-system. Its closed loop of transnational corporations, their commercial and military agents "on the ground," corrupt politicians and ruling-class collaborators, security forces and local warlords enforce "order" and keep everything moving—while suppressing the groaning masses.[12]

These workings of transnational capitalism as mediated through the comprador elite are nothing if not a form of pacification, a return to colonial-era "Native Administration" where the ruling classes of the periphery, acting as agents of the core, pacify the people.[13] They run their countries as client states for foreign interests, ensuring the smooth and inexpensive extraction of valuable resources, as well as access to local and regional markets. Besides supplying cheap and unprotected labor to outsourced core corporations, the comprador classes offer corporate investors subsidies, land grants, tax breaks and "industrial quiet;" in return, they enjoy direct subsidies and land grants, access to raw materials and cheap labor, light or non-existent taxes, few effective labor unions, no minimum wage or child labor or occupational safety laws, and no consumer or environmental protections.[14]

This casts additional light on the activities of Israeli "business people" in Africa and elsewhere, especially where the diamonds and minerals of West and Central Africa get mixed in with arms, security and profits. Rough and polished diamonds, in fact, are Israel's main export category, greater even than arms or security. Israel's gross diamond exports represented 30.5 percent of the country's total exports of $67.8 billion in 2011, 41 percent of its exports to the US, 41 percent of its exports to Asia (mainly India and China) and almost 20 percent of its exports to Europe.[15] Despite attempts to control the sales of "conflict diamonds" (or "blood diamonds"), that industry remains mired in severe human rights violations; what's more, Israel's diamond industry contributes in taxes more than $1 billion to Israel's military and security industries.[16]

In a provocative article entitled "Israelis and Hezbollah Haven't Always Been Enemies," Jimmy Johnson reveals the convoluted relationship between arms dealers in West Africa, the diamond trade and the violence they generate. Diamonds, he explains, have become the currency of choice for organizations like al Qaeda, the Taliban and Hezbollah, since they can be easily transferred across borders. "Blood diamonds" from West Africa have been particularly tied to war crimes and crimes against humanity perpetrated by former Liberian President Charles Taylor and his Revolutionary United Front (RUF), a rebel group backed by Taylor that was seeking power in Sierra Leone. Not only is the involvement of Israeli "businessmen" and arms dealers of note, but their routine interactions with such figures as Ibrahim Bah, the official arms and diamond broker for both the RUF and Taylor with links to al Qaeda. In January 2006, relates Johnson,

… retired Israeli Defense Forces Colonel Yair Klein was invited to Liberia by Simon Rosenblum, an Israeli businessman formerly based in Abdijan, Ivory Coast. During Taylor's reign [in Liberia], Rosenblum was a member of his inner circle. He carried a Liberian diplomatic passport, owned logging and road constructions interests in Liberia and his trucks were used to carry weapons from Liberia to the border with Sierra Leone. Klein arrived in Liberia after Taylor had been deposed, but when his presence became known he was forced to flee the country, and with good reason. From 1996 until 1999, Klein provided material and training to Liberia's Anti-Terrorism Unit and, in violation of the UN embargo [on blood diamonds], to the RUF as part of a diamonds-for-arms operation involving Klein. In January of 1999 Klein was arrested in Sierra Leone on charges of smuggling arms to the RUF ...

Klein's Anti-Terrorism Unit, a group widely criticized for gross abuses of human rights, was headed by "Chuckie" Taylor, the president's son, but Klein and Rosenblum weren't the only Israelis involved with the Taylors and Bah. Along with the $500,000 worth of diamonds in his possession, in a briefcase searched upon his August, 2000 arrest in Italy, Leonid Minin, a Ukrainian-born Israeli member of the "Odessa Mafia," was found to be in possession of correspondence detailing his sale to the Liberian government of millions of dollars worth of arms in exchange for diamonds and timber concessions. Minin had extensive dealings with Bah, but perhaps the most interesting item found in Minin's briefcase was that End-Use Certificate for 113 tons of ammunition and arms that exactly matched the End-Use Certificate found in the apartment of Hezbollah operative Samih Ossailly.

Hezbollah's activity in diamond trading has mostly been limited to Sierra Leone, Liberia and the Democratic Republic of the Congo (DRC). Israel, too, has long had ties in the area. Back in 1983, Israel was contracted to train and equip Mobutu Sese Seko's presidential guard, the notorious *Division Speciale Presidentielle*. It was during this time that Shimon Yelnik, an Israeli army officer in charge of Seko's presidential guard, became acquainted with Aziz Nassour. About a decade later, in late 2000, when Nassour needed arms to ensure his continued diamond enterprises in Liberia and Sierra Leone, he contacted his friend Yelnik, by then brokering arms in Panama, as revealed in an investigation by the Organization of American States into Yelnik's involvement with Colombian paramilitaries. The investigation also uncovered faxes between Bah and Yelnik and attempts to both avoid and make fraudulent End-Use Certificates in order to break the UN arms embargo. Investigative journalist Douglas Farah quotes one European intelligence agent as saying, "The likelihood these types of weapons were going to the RUF rebels in the bush is very hard to believe," leading to speculation that the weapons were actually destined for the Taliban in Afghanistan.

The contact between Israeli diamond dealers, extending beyond Sierra Leone and Liberia to the Democratic Republic of the Congo and Angola, and their counterparts in Hezbollah and al Qaeda is well summed up by an Israeli diamond dealer, who regularly did business with buyers he knew were Hezbollah and some he suspected were al Qaeda: "Here it is business. The wars are over there."[17]

And so it goes. Arcadi Gaydamak, a Russian-French-Israeli oligarch who ran unsuccessfully for the Jerusalem mayoralty and the Knesset, brokered an $800 billion arms purchase in 1990 for the then-UN sanctioned government of Angola. In so doing, he teamed up with the Israeli company LR Group, today the largest Israeli company operating in Angola, for supplies of aerial radar, unmanned aircraft, helicopters and other arms—even though Israel itself supported the UNITA opposition forces and LR sales to the Angolan government actually helped finance the purchase of arms used against it. Drones supplied to the Angolan Army that were manufactured by the Israeli firm Aeronautics Defense Systems and supplied by LR not only played a key role in killing UNITA leader Jonas Savimbi but exposing the illegal sale of "blood diamonds" by Israeli diamond dealers.

Gaydamak, who also travels on an Angolan passport, also gave another Russian-Israeli oligarch, diamond merchant Lev Leviev, his entrée to the lucrative diamond and mineral market of Angola at the height of its civil war, when the government of President José Eduardo dos Santos was desperate for hard currency to buy arms, and was more than willing to sell its diamonds and other resources to do so. By under-valuing and under-invoicing the diamonds, the Angolan diamond trade yielded at least $1.2 billion of profits in every year between 2001 and 2008—$100 million per month—which went to compensate Gaydamak for his re-arming of Dos Santos's army between 1992 and 1998 in defiance of UN sanctions. Over the past two decades, Israeli companies have sold about $300 million in arms and defense equipment to the Angolan government.[18] De Santos, by the way, is Africa's richest ruler, his personal fortune pegged at $20 billion, while 70 percent of his people survive on less than $2 a day.[19]

Israeli General Israel Ziv of Abkhazia fame, and David Tzur, the former Tel Aviv police commander, became involved in Guinea following a military *coup d'état* by Capt. Moussa Dadis Camara, who took power in December 2008 and immediately suspended the constitution and clamped down on freedoms in the country. Growing distrustful of both his own soldiers and the old Presidential Guard, Camara began looking for a security expert who would train his own guard of loyalists. He was introduced to Ziv and his company CTS Global, which he hired to establish, train and arm a new Presidential Guard. As part of a $10 million contract, Ziv also initiated the training of a larger force composed of members of the president's tribal loyalists. (One bizarre add-on to the contract provided for a CTS Global-sponsored "strategic workshop" for "increasing awareness of democratic values among Guinean decision-makers.") At around the same time, September 2009, Camara's Presidential Guard massacred (the term used by Human Rights Watch)[20] 157 opposition supporters who had gathered in the soccer stadium in Conakry to protest conditions in the country. The soldiers raped dozens of the women and hundreds of demonstrators were beaten. Finally the French government, together with the UN, appealed to Israel to re-examine the involvement of Israeli military advisers in Guinea.[21]

Faced with an embarrassing situation, the Israeli Foreign Ministry accused Ziv & Co. of signing the contract to train and arm the Guinean Army without having obtained the proper permits. Ziv brought in two other partners to argue that the contract should not be cancelled: Ephraim Sneh, a former deputy defense minister and Prof. Shlomo Ben Ami, the foreign minister during the Oslo peace process. "Veteran officials at the ministry," reports Melman

> ... were especially surprised by Ben-Ami's participation in the session. "We couldn't believe that a social democrat sensitive to the matter of human rights would be involved in this type of situation, and even more so, in a country like Guinea," one of them said. In what must be the most outrageous justifications for arming such a murderous dictator, Sneh and Ben Ami claimed, "If we had been there, we could have prevented the massacre."[22]

Another Israeli "confidant" to a dictator described by *Foreign Policy* magazine as the "worst of the worst,"[23] Teodoro Obiang Nguema Mbasogo, president of Equatorial Guinea these past 35 years, is Boas Badikhi.[24] A former officer in an IDF counter-terror unit, Boas is the son of Moshe Badikhi, an Israeli Air Force pilot sent to help Idi Amin establish an air force in Uganda in the early 1970s, and who became one of Amin's closest advisers. Through Badikhi, Israel has sold extensive quantities of arms and military infrastructure—more than $100 million worth—to Equatorial Guinea, Africa's third-largest oil producer. Besides supplying Shaldag patrol and escort boats and a Sa'ar missile boat, Israel Shipyards Ltd. and Israel Military Industries Ltd. (IMI) are reportedly building a dockyard in the country. IMI and another Israeli firm Aeronautics are involved in a multi-million dollar deal for building a fleet of drone scout vehicles for that country's military. And of course Badikhi and Israeli security companies have contracted to train Equatorial Guinea's elite Presidential Guard and local security forces. US law enforcement agencies revealed several years ago that Obiang had an account at the Washington, DC-based Riggs Bank containing some $700 million.[25] (Badikhi also sells arms to Southern Sudan together with David Ben Uziel, nicknamed "Tarzan," a former member of Ariel Sharon's notorious Unit 101, who personally trained Mobutu when he won his paratroopers wings in Israel in 1963.)[26]

But that doesn't exhaust the Israeli presence in Equatorial Guinea. Yardena Ovadia is an Israeli businesswoman commonly known as "the long arm of Obiang." She played a key role in the Israel Shipyards/IMI deal.[27] Just to illustrate how convoluted the ties are among minerals, arms, African dictatorships, Israeli security politics and broader international relations, it was a Jerusalem-based "think tank," the Institute for Advanced Strategic and Political Studies, closely associated with Jewish neo-con think tanks in Washington, that brokered the re-establishment of relations between Equatorial Guinea and the US, broken off in 1996. Obiang was feted by Condoleezza Rice, President Bush and later by President Obama. The reason: "West African oil is what can help stabilize the Middle East, end Muslim terror, and secure a measure of energy security."[28]

Gabi Peretz, another retired colonel from an IDF counter-terror unit, sells arms to Burundi, ranked the 167th poorest country in the world out of 177, and is close with its president, Pierre Nkurunziza. Barak Orland is Israel's man in Uganda, close to President Yoweri Museveni. Yair Gaon focuses on Gabon. After Simon Rosenblum was accused by the International Criminal Court of being in Charles Taylor's inner circle, working closely with Leonid Minin, his place in Liberia was taken by Yaakov Angel.[29]

Amit Sadeh is the Israeli point-person in Nigeria. Close to Yayale Ahmed, a former defense minister who today serves as the cabinet secretary, Sadeh brokered a $250 million sale of drones and unmanned boats, followed by other large arms deals. One was the sale of two Shaldag boats made by Israel Shipyards to the Nigerian Navy for $25 million—more than double the cost of these ships, which is an estimated $10 million combined. The Nigerians later claimed they were promised new boats, but instead received used ones from the Israeli Navy surplus that had been upgraded.[30] Melman had Sadeh in mind when he wrote about "the ugly Israeli" arms dealers. Not only did the Nigerian defense ministry pay Israel Shipyards and Sadeh an inflated price for old boats, but, says Melman, "these deals have put Israel in the position of interfering in an internal Nigerian dispute that could lead to civil war. The boats and intelligence equipment are intended for the use of Nigerian forces against rebels in the Niger River Delta region."[31] In an interview with *Ha'aretz* (Melman's paper at the time) a spokesman for the rebels warned Israel not to go ahead with the sales. It did.[32]

The "security" context to which Israeli companies pitch their sales and services is not merely a technical matter. In Africa as elsewhere, securitization is related to money and politics, especially in the context of resource wars most often waged against the masses of disenfranchised poor by their own comprador elites. Even where rebel forces resist, or when the situation deteriorates into a kind of gang warfare, pitting warlords and their supporters against all comers in the pillage of their country, the militaries and police of the state constitute just another looting force, engaged more in suppression than actual combat. In this sense, Israeli business people are merely partners in the general looting. "The military involvement or the security involvement is often the entrée to these countries," says Peter Hirshberg, an Israeli journalist who covers the country's mercenary firms,

> ... and that the real interests are in things like diamonds and other raw materials in certain countries, lumber for instance, that are much more lucrative. That is where the real money is, not in training some presidential guard for some dictator in Africa. The real money is in things like diamonds and lumber.[33]

This is the dark and largely undocumented underbelly of Israeli (and other) business dealing in Africa and elsewhere, the "shadow world" of the arms trade. In order to lend their commercial enterprises an air of legitimacy, Israeli business people tend to hide their arms dealings under resource extraction. Lev Leviev, Dan Gertler, Beny Steinmetz, the Herzliya-based LR Group and others own, control, extract from, sell and profit massively from diamonds, copper, iron ore, cobalt and other minerals throughout West and Central Africa, but are seldom linked to arms.[34] Feinstein does link Gertler to a diamonds-for-arms operation in support of the Revolutionary United Front (RUF), the gang responsible for atrocities in Sierra Leone and a puppet force of Charles Taylor, in violation of an UN arms embargo.[35]

Occasionally business and arms are visibly linked, as in the case of Gaydamak and Minin. Perhaps the most visible—and notorious—Israeli arms dealer-cum-businessman is Yair Klein, Israel's "best known mercenary." A former lieutenant colonel and special forces commander in the IDF, Klein established a private mercenary company called Spearhead Ltd., duly licensed as a "security firm" by the Israeli Ministry of Defense, through which he provided arms and training to armed forces in Latin America, Lebanon and Sierra Leone. Klein and his company have been accused of training the death-squads of drug traffickers and right-wing militias in Colombia in the 1980s. In 1989, he became a central figure in what was called "the Guns for Antigua scandal," an arms-for-drugs operation.

With the financial and logistical backing of two Israeli entrepreneurs resident in Antigua, Klein proposed to the Antiguan government that his security company, Spearhead Ltd., would establish a mercenary training camp designed to train "corporate security experts, ranging from the executive level to the operational level, and bring them to the highest professional capacity in order to confront and defuse any possible threat," with the idea of also using the camp as a cover for laundering weapons. In 1989, he and his associates placed a fraudulent order with Israeli Military Industries in the name of the Antiguan government for 100 Uzi submachine-guns, 400 Galil assault-rifles and 200,000 rounds of ammunition, worth $324,205. He then diverted the consignment to the Medellin drug cartel headed by Gonzalo Rodríguez Gacha. (One of the guns was used to assassinate Presidential candidate Luis Carlos Galán.) Klein is also suspected of involvement in the explosion of a Colombian airliner in November 1989. Tellingly, he also trained and equipped the infamous Carlos Castano's paramilitary groups, ostensibly with the knowledge and agreement of the Colombian and Israeli governments. In other words, Klein served all sides: the government, the paramilitaries and the drug cartels.

Back in Israel, Klein faced trial on three counts of exporting military equipment and expertise without the requisite licenses. He pleaded guilty and paid a fine of $13,400. A Columbian court convicted him *in absentia* for providing paramilitary training and arms to drug lords running international cocaine cartels. Although sentenced to ten years in prison, Klein successfully evaded attempts to extradite him.

Klein subsequently made his way to Africa where he linked up with the Liberian warlord Charles Taylor. In 1989–90, during the Liberian civil war initiated by Taylor, Klein provided Taylor's "Anti-Terrorism Unit" with materiel and training. He also smuggled arms to the Taylor-backed RUF, which carried out mass atrocities in Sierra Leone, in return for blood diamonds, for which he spent 16 months in a Sierra Leone prison between 1999 and 2000. He was released at the intervention of the Israeli and American governments.

On April 3, 2007, Interpol issued an international arrest warrant for Yair Klein and two other Israeli collaborators on charges of criminal conspiracy and instruction in terrorism. Klein was captured by Russian police in Moscow. The government of Colombia asked for his extradition, but again he was saved by a bizarre turn of events. Although Russia agreed to extradite him, the European Court of Human Rights ruled that that be suspended, since returning Klein to Colombia would violate his rights and liberties. Russia allowed Klein to return to Israel, where he lives quietly today.[36]

Private Israeli Security Firms

Klein's case reveals the central role played by private security firms like his company Spearhead Ltd. in providing weapons, training and security services to countries on the periphery. Reflecting on the relationship of the Israeli state to independent arms dealers during the height of Israeli military involvement in the "dirty wars" of Latin America in the 1970s and '80s, Almond writes:

> The close relationship between the Israeli state and the "independent" arms dealers and mercenaries it tried, in response to human rights concerns, to distance itself from, is another interesting factor in these activities. The intimacy that existed between the Israeli government, arms firms and the ex-military personnel that supplied and trained death squads and drug cartels, further complicates the notion of state sovereignty as being based on the exclusion of non-state actors. It shows how political decisions in Tel Aviv and Jerusalem were taken in collusion with allegedly independent actors. Of course, state figures such as Peres and Sharon openly visited and contributed to regimes such as those in Nicaragua and Honduras (Shimon Peres in 1957, Ariel Sharon in 1984). However in many other ways, the Israeli state supported the whole spectrum of legal and illegal activities in Latin America ...
>
> However, the most striking aspect of this intimacy is the extent to which some of the most notorious gunrunners and mercenaries involved—such as Mike Harari, Pesakh Ben Or, and Yair Klein—were directly connected with the highest echelons of the Israeli establishment. The trainer of paramilitaries in Colombia and South Africa, Yair Klein, operated under an official Israeli government license; Colonel Leo Gleser, a former Israeli commando, sold arms to Honduras through an

Israeli firm (ISDS) publicised by the Israeli Ministry of Defence; and former Mossad operator Mike Harari, who sold guns to the Panama regime in the 1980s, was the brother-in-law of Israel's attorney general [later Supreme Court Justice], Dorith Beinish. Israeli mercenaries, in other words, were not rogue outlaws, but rather semi-autonomous agents who could not have operated as efficiently as they did without the backing and the endorsement of the Israeli state.[37]

TAR Ideal Concepts illustrates the intimate relationship among the Israeli Ministries of Defense and Internal Security, local arms manufacturers, the private firms that sell security goods and the former but still-influential politicians and senior military/police officials who represent the commercial arms interests both at home and abroad. On its website, TAR Ideal Concepts presents itself as a "world leader in supplying military and police equipment and training," its expertise deriving from the fact that it is "a leading supplier to the IMOD," equipping Israeli ground forces, and the navy and air force, as well as serving as "a leading supplier of equipment and technology to Israel's Law Enforcement Divisions." Established in 1990, its "One Stop Shop" catalogue offers a transport helicopter, wheeled and tracked APCs, a wide range of SALW weapons, attack dogs, a range of optics and high-tech rifle sights, and force protection accessories. It also specializes in riot control, offering customers "the ultimate riot control vehicle" produced by the BAT company of kibbutz Beit Alfa, batons, a wide assortment of handcuffs, skunk repulsive liquids, communication devices and protective gear. Other TAR catalogues sell products for anti-terror and SWAT teams, urban warfare, homeland security, the "safe cities" program with its layered surveillance systems, intelligence, perimeter defense (for which it provides entire computerized control rooms for cities, ports, or airports, various kinds of barriers and road blocks, fencing, gating and illumination), armoring and bulletproofing, and more. It even has a Defense Academy that provides consulting services and specialized security training for local teams deployed in high-risk environments.[38]

Klein's company, Spearhead Ltd., no longer has a website, but many others do that provide extensive training to armies, security forces and elite units of countries on the periphery. "Since the 1950s," says SIPRI,

... Israelis and Israeli companies have been involved in training African armed forces, including special forces and Presidential Guards. Israeli instructors, either working for Israeli companies or for foreign companies, have trained the presidential guard of Equatorial Guinea since 2005 and special forces were reportedly trained in 2009 in Israel and by an Israeli company in Nigeria. Israelis have also been reported as training Guinean forces after the December 2008 military coup by Moussa Camara. The Israeli company Global CST won a $10 million order in 2009 that included the training, arming and equipping of Camara's presidential guard ... When the Israeli Ministry of Defense (MOD) learned of the contract, Global CST reportedly transferred the security element of the contract, probably including the Israel instructors, to a South African company ... [The Israeli MOD] commented that the Israeli Government could do little to prevent Israelis—employed by non-Israeli companies or working as private persons—from doing business in conflict zones.[39]

Tellingly, adds the SIPRI paper,

Israeli weapons, trainers and brokers have been observed in numerous African trouble spots and may play a bigger role than their numbers imply ... Issues like human rights and potential diversion or misuse of delivered weapons seem to have gained importance, but deliveries to conflicts and undemocratic regimes continue. While the African arms market is small, its commercial aspect is an important driver for Israel's arms sales.[40]

In Latin America, if less so in Africa, the Israeli mercenaries of the 1970s and '80s have been replaced by respectable private firms, "private military and security contractors" (PMSCs), all having links, more or less official, to the Ministry of Defense and the major Israeli weapons companies. Ziv's Global CTS advertises itself as "an Israeli based company for providing defense and security services to governments and significant international organizations." It specializes in complex and large-scale security projects, solving national security crises, establishing military forces and national law enforcement units, training military and special forces units and "taking down major crime organizations." Among its senior personnel is General Yossi Kupperwasser, director general of the Israeli Ministry of Strategic Affairs, but its senior staff includes, as we've mentioned, Ephraim Sneh and Shlomo Ben Ami, currently the vice-president of the Toledo (Spain) International Centre for Peace.[41]

Global CTS was awarded a $10 million contract to provide security consultancy and equipment to Colombia's Special Forces, and was instrumental in the 2008 rescue of 15 hostages held by the FARC. According to Melman:

> The Israeli activity, involving dozens of Israeli security experts, was coordinated by Global CST, owned by former General Staff operations chief, Brigadier General (res.) Israel Ziv, and Brigadier (res.) Yossi Kuperwasser. "It's a Colombian Entebbe operation," Ziv said Thursday when he returned from Bogota. "Both regarding its national and international importance. Betancourt [the presidential candidate who had been captured six years before] has become a symbol of the struggle against international terror. This is an amazing operation that wouldn't shame any army or special forces anywhere in the world."
>
> Asked about the Israeli involvement in it, Ziv said there is "no need to exaggerate." "We don't want to take credit for something we didn't do," a company source said. "We helped them prepare themselves to fight terror. We helped them to plan operations and strategies and develop intelligence sources. That's quite a bit, but shouldn't be taken too far." Israelis may not have taken part in the rescue, but they advised and guided, sold equipment and intelligence technology ...
>
> Israel has over the years sold Colombia planes, drones, weapons and intelligence systems. At the Defense Ministry's suggestion, Global CST won the $10 million contract to work with Colombia.[42]

Other reviews of Global CTS and Ziv's activities in Latin America are more mixed. In a cable released by Wikileaks, the American ambassador to Colombia reports that

> General Oscar Naranjo, Director of the Colombian National Police (CNP), told the Ambassador on November 24 that Defense Minister Gabriel Silva was souring on the Defense Ministry's relationship with Israel. Naranjo said that the CNP's relationship with retired Israeli Major General Yisrael Ziv and his firm Global CST had been a "disaster." Naranjo said he understood Ziv was trying to make inroads in Panama and Peru—and that he had shared his concerns with authorities in Panama and would do the same with Peru if asked. He noted that Silva overruled Colombian Armed Forces Commander General Freddy Padilla's decision to purchase Israeli UAVs. Government of Colombia (GOC) officials described their experience with Global CST under the "Strategic Leap" process as mixed.[43]

More than mixed, in fact. Another cable reveals that an employee of Global CST stole classified Colombian government information and attempted to sell it to the FARC:

> GOC officials have expressed security concerns about Global CST in the past, and found it difficult to work with a private firm on national security matters as they were prevented from sharing USG intelligence with them. In February 2008, CNP sources reported that a Global CST interpreter, Argentine-born Israeli national Shai Killman, had made copies of classified Colombian Defense Ministry documents in an unsuccessful attempt to sell them to the Revolutionary Armed Forces of Colombia (FARC) through contacts in Ecuador and Argentina. The documents allegedly contained high value target (HVT) database information. Ziv denied this attempt and sent Killman back to Israel.[44]

Yet another cable throws additional light on the workings of Global CST:

> Over a three year period, Ziv worked his way into the confidence of former Defense Minister Santos by promising a cheaper version of USG [US government] assistance without our strings attached. We and the GOC learned that Global CST had no Latin American experience and that its proposals seem designed more to support Israeli equipment and services sales than to meet in-country needs. Global CST was not transparent with us, and tried to insert itself into our classified discussions with the GOC. Given the GOC's experience with Global CST, it is no surprise that the Defense Ministry is pulling back from them and warning neighbors that their deals are not as good as advertised.[45]

All this aside, Israeli security training and protection firms have become respectable, and Big Business. International Security and Defense Systems (ISDF), the Israeli company that won the contract for securing the 2014 Olympics in Rio, advertises itself as "a worldwide influential, sophisticated security consultant and integrator" in areas such as homeland security, defense, maritime and aviation security, and securing infrastructure, multinational enterprises, mega-events and, as a part of the Safe Cities program, entire urban areas. Led by Leo Gleser, a major Israeli arms dealer of Brazilian origin who was featured in the film *The Lab*, ISDF serves primarily Latin America, with offices in Mexico City, Lima, Rio,

Buenos Aires, Tegucigalpa and Panama City, plus New Jersey. It also brings influential military, security and political visitors to Israel.[46]

Each Israeli firm has a niche of its own, but all stress that their operatives and services come of "years of experience" in the IDF. Max Security Solutions, for example, is based in Tel Aviv but has three regional offices—in Lagos, Vicenza and Mumbai—from which it operates in some one hundred countries. Max Security specializes in "enabling business continuity in the world's most volatile operating environments through proactive, client-tailored security measures": intelligence and risk assessment services, VIP protection and secure transportation. Like many other Israeli firms, it runs its own "academy," Max Security Academy, which trains local operatives, "whether it is establishing a new special forces unit, or training a multinational corporation's security staff or private security professionals." Max Security programs "apply Israeli knowledge and methodologies for counter-terrorism."[47]

Taking the term "academy" in its genuinely academic sense, ISCA, the International Security & Counter-Terrorism Academy, promotes "innovative research and projects" together with the usual security training programs. It seeks no less than "to address the security of societies by advancing practices and policies while maintaining the importance of democratic values and freedoms in everyday life." Thus it concentrates on being "both theoretical and practical," ISCA's research focusing on deviant behavior, mass crowd security, radicalization, crime prevention, counter-terrorism, community policing, and crisis management—a classic conflation of securitization and control. "Our practical strengths," says ISCA's website, "include negating ethnic profiling from security practices, detecting abnormal behavior, urban terrain analysis, and local key indicators." Its particular program, Search Detect React, specializes in proactively identifying illicit intentions before they come to fruition by using heightened awareness, the human factor, and local social and cultural norms.[48] ISCA participates in the SAFIRE project (SAFIRE stands for Scientific Approach to Finding Indicators of and Responses to Radicalisation) which "addresses the processes that underlie radicalization from moderation to violent extremism ... to improve the design and implementation of programs directed at preventing, stopping, and/or reversing the process of radicalization toward violent extremism." It links ten "research partners" in Europe specializing in securitization (including RAND).[49]

The Golan Group specializes in securitizing corporations and their avenues of business (transporting staff or products, securing meeting and conference venues, etc.) so that they may penetrate markets in the Third World that would otherwise be "out of reach" or not cost effective. Their training includes Krav Maga, tactics for law enforcement (instinctive shooting, law enforcement driving), dignitary protection and airport security. The Golan Group then adds another twist: having provided your company with a secure operating environment, it can also source innovative products and technologies for you to manufacture or sell, thus providing cheap sources of production for Israeli companies as well as new markets.[50]

Not only do Israeli security firms send their IDF-trained personnel to teach, advise and secure governments, corporations, vital facilities and events throughout the world, but the IDF itself plays a similar role, a useful extension of its security politics. Its Foreign Training Branch brings soldiers, commanders and would-be military heroes (Idi Amin, Mobutu and Samuel Doe come immediately to mind) to Israel for training and *hasbara*. "Most of the foreign soldiers go away feeling a strong connection to their Israeli counterparts and having a much better understanding of the threats facing Israel and the methods that must be used to face those threats," according to the Israeli newspaper *Israel Today*. A special attraction is the Tze'elim/Baladiya/Chicago urban warfare facility in the western Negev.[51]

Israel and the UN Arms Trade Treaty

Global military expenditures exceeded $1.8 *trillion* in 2014, or 2.3 percent of the world GDP.[52] Much of this trade is unsupervised or flies in the face of international law; it enables both state and non-state actors to commit massive violations of human rights with no fear of sanctions. Attempting to promote accountability and transparency, an Arms Trade Treaty (ATT) has been making its way through the UN system. It seeks to establish legally binding common standards for the international trade in conventional weapons (SALW as well as major weapons systems, but not ammunition) and to reduce the illicit arms trade. In particular, the ATT prohibits governments from exporting conventional weapons to countries where they know they will be used for genocide, crimes against humanity or war crimes, thus holding the sellers responsible for the "end use" of their arms. The ATT went into effect on December 24, 2014, after having been signed by 130 nations and ratified by 61.

While representing a major step forward in bringing some degree of control and transparency to the arms trade, the ATT nevertheless still leaves some major loopholes. It is not an arms control or disarmament treaty, and does not place restrictions on the types or quantities of arms that may be bought, sold, or possessed by states, including nuclear arms. Neither does it affect a state's domestic gun control laws (or lack of them) or, perhaps most seriously, sales by or to non-state actors.[53]

Like the US, Israel signed the ATT but will not ratify it. A chief reason given by 50 US senators in a letter to President Obama for Congress's refusal to ratify is two problematic clauses in the treaty. One requires governments to assess whether recipients of arms are likely to "commit or facilitate a serious violation" of IHL or human rights law; the other is a requirement to assess whether the arms deal could "contribute to or undermine peace or security" before a sale is approved. This, says Congress, constitutes "language that could hinder the United States from fulfilling its strategic, legal and moral commitments to provide arms to key allies such as the Republic of China (Taiwan) and the State of Israel."[54] The Israeli Defense Ministry agrees. The Defense Minister's chief of staff, Haim Blumenblatt, hinted that ratifying the treaty could indeed affect arms sales to and from the US, as well as with other countries. Minister of Defense Moshe Ya'alon opposes Israel's ratification of the treaty, as does the US, Russia and China, three of the world's leading arms dealing countries.[55]

Part VI

Domestic Securitization and Policing

12

Serving the Core's Ruling Classes "At Home"

In this chapter, we finally turn to internal security and policing, the "ISSILE" of the MISSILE Complex. Here we look at how Israeli methods of pursuing securocratic wars are applied by the ruling political and corporate classes within the core and semi-periphery in order to ensure their domestic hegemony. I suggest that Israel offers a coherent, thought-out and field-tested model of control that it actively propagates as an integral part of its security politics, together with appropriate weaponry. The "Israeli model" effectively addresses the endemic problem of "securing the insecurities" of an inherently polarized capitalist system, and for that reason law enforcement around the world seeks Israeli know-how. All of which brings us back to the issue of pacification.

The core states find themselves gripped by a permanent emergency of their own making, one exacerbated by the very excesses of their own neo-liberalism and "austerity." They find themselves in a paranoiac frenzy (which they also exploit for their own ends) around the need to identify and combat those sources of "contamination" that, they contend, lie behind the social unrest: insurgents, terrorists, dissidents, the working poor, marginalized minority populations, "Muslims," immigrants, a "desire" to bring down Western civilization, cyber-threats, the contamination of the water or air, birthrates, gender "confusion," multi-culturalism and myriad other unspecified threats to their hegemony. The urban centers of the core, targeted by but also increasingly inhabited by such sources of subversion, become both the source of the threat and the focus of militarized human-security states. Armed for the first time with totalizing securocratic technologies, the ruling classes, their militaries and their police finally glimpse the prospect of governing cities with high-tech omniscience and rationality. They find it possible to utilize "militarized techniques of tracking and targeting [to] permanently colonize the city landscape and spaces of everyday life in both 'homelands' and domestic cities of the West as well as the world's neo-colonial frontiers."[1]

In such an enterprise, where "Western security and military doctrine are being rapidly re-imagined in ways that dramatically blur the juridical and operational separation between policing, intelligence and the military," Graham explicitly references the model provided by Israel's security regime. Central to his analysis, as I alluded to earlier, is the "Palestinizing" of control, whether in a military sense, as in the war in Iraq or in counter-insurgency operations in Afghanistan, or in the domestic securitization of borders, airports, city streets surveilled by video cameras, or the way the police dismantle Occupy Wall Street protests. Graham, like Weizman[2] and Collins,[3] evokes a "Global Palestine," a Palestine writ-large that is infused with all the civilizational threats imperiling the core (and by extension "life itself"). In devising militarized responses to the threats emanating from the Palestinian microcosm, Israel is in fact blazing the path for civilizational gatekeepers the world over to deal with "their own" Palestines and Palestinians. Aware of the potency of its "model" for its security politics, Israel effectively parlays its campaign of control and pacification towards the Palestinians to lead its core allies in the crusade to defeat counter-hegemons and anti-systemic forces. On the way, it also promotes its weapons and tactics on the open market. Israel has become, Graham contends, "the ultimate source of 'combat-proven' techniques and technology."[4]

Propagating the Israel Model

"Since 9/11," AIPAC reports on its website

> ... the United States and Israel have intensified their homeland security cooperation. Israel shares priceless information about terrorist organizations with the United States and is one of five countries participating in the U.S. Counterterrorism Technical Support Working Group.[5]

In fact, the foundations for that cooperation, the transformation of American police and domestic security agencies from a professional civilian force entrusted with maintaining public order and protecting the community into a militarized force began well before 9/11, as Balko well describes.[6] "High intensity policing" indeed intermingles with "low intensity warfare" in a common securocratic "battlespace." Balko entitled his book *Rise of the Warrior Cop*, the term "warrior" or "warfighter" being applied equally to soldiers and police. After 9/11, the Global War on Terrorism became, indeed, global. In its first four years, more than 80,000 people around the world were detained without trial by the US.[7] And in this shift to militarized securitization, who better to turn to for training and inspiration than the most militarized and admired police and security forces in the Western world: Israel?

In 2002, the American organization Jewish Institute for National Security Affairs (JINSA), which holds that there is no difference between the national security interests of the US and Israel, inaugurated its Law Enforcement Exchange Program (LEEP). Partnering with the Israeli National Police, the Israeli Ministry of Internal Security, and the Israeli Security Agency (Shin Bet), and supported by the International Association of Chiefs of Police, the Major County Sheriff's Association, Major City Police Chiefs Association and the Police Executive Research Forum, LEEP brings US law enforcement executives to Israel for "education." Over a two-week period, police chiefs, sheriffs, senior law enforcement executives, state homeland security directors, state police commissioners, federal law enforcement leadership, deputies and others observe Israeli methods of coping with public security issues: preventing and reacting to acts of terrorism, border and perimeter security, restructuring their police forces and departments, exploring ways of cooperating with private security firms and sharing information—all with an eye to contributing to Israel's security politics by planting advocates deep in the American security community.[8] Over 9,500 law enforcement officers have participated in twelve conferences thus far.[9]

Over the years, other programs between Israeli and American police forces have sprung up as well, many mediated by US Jewish organizations. In 2002, less than a year after 9/11, the Bnai Brith's Anti-Defamation League (ADL) created an Advanced Training School that offers a program in counter-terrorism held twice a year in Washington, DC. The three-day seminar provides law enforcement executives and commanders from across the country with the latest information and resources to increase their capabilities in combating domestic and international extremist and terrorist threats, including training by the Israeli police. In its 2011 session, the program featured a presentation by Micky Rosenfeld, Superintendent of the Israeli Police. ATS has trained 970 law enforcement professionals, representing 245 federal, state and local agencies.[10]

In 2004, the ADL created its National Counter-Terrorism Seminar (NCTS) in Israel, bringing law enforcement executives from across the US to Israel for a week of intensive counter-terrorism training. NCTS connects American law enforcement officials with the Israeli National Police, the IDF and various experts from Israel's intelligence and security services. More than 175 law enforcement executives have participated in twelve NCTS sessions since 2004.[11]

In the militarized, anti-Arab/Muslim atmosphere of the Global War on Terror when the mission, modes of operation and "mindsets" of the police began to undergo a fundamental transformation, these programs have affected American law enforcement. In the plethora of laudatory testimonies to be gleaned from participants in the LEEP program and others, the deep penetration of Israeli security doctrines into US law enforcement is tangible. "The knowledge gleaned from observation and training during the LEEP trip," effused Colonel Joseph R. (Rick) Fuentes, Superintendent of the New Jersey State Police, "prompted significant changes to the organizational structure of the New Jersey State Police and brought about the creation of the Homeland Security Branch."[12]

Surveying how the securitization strategies, tactics and organization of the two countries "dovetail," Zunes notes that the first articulated notion of a "global war on terror" emerged from the influential policy paper, *A Clean Break: A New Strategy for Securing the Realm.*[13] Formulated for then-Prime Minister Netanyahu by a group of pro-Israeli neo-cons headed by Richard Perle, a future head of the Pentagon's Defense Policy Board under the Bush Administration, the paper advocated using force to reorganize Middle East geopolitics in line with American interests, beginning with the removal of Saddam Hussein and creating a regional "peace through strength" based on a strategic US-Israeli partnership.[14]

A Clean Break became a leading policy document as the Bush Administration geared up for the invasion of Iraq. What's more, "globalized Israeli security doctrines" guided the emerging Global War on Terror, particularly the notion that terrorism is the main enemy and that the world can be divided simplistically into "terrorists" and "anti-terrorists." Israel also inserted its campaign of "lawfare," arguing that international law does not apply to certain "gray zones" controlled by "terrorists," thus eroding the protections IHL affords non-state actors and individuals. The Israeli claim that certain categories of people—terrorists, jihadists, "unlawful combatants" and otherwise stateless persons—could be rounded up, imprisoned indefinitely and tortured dovetailed with the American claim that certain countries that posed threats to it or were "failed states" had forfeited their rights to sovereignty.

On an operational level, the "new urban warfare doctrine" adopted by the American Joint Chiefs of Staff borrowed heavily from Israeli tactics employed in the onslaught against Palestinian cities in Operation Defensive Shield.[15] The "Palestinization" of Iraq was evident in the ways Baghdad and other Iraqi cities and towns were secured just a year later.[16] From there the Israeli model found its way into doctrines of "asymmetrical warfare," counter-insurgency and counter-terrorism, eventually helping define core homeland security and police approaches to militarized urban securitization.[17] In terms of weaponry, the US and Israeli militaries have jointly developed the use of drones, totalized surveillance systems, sensors, robotics and "non-lethal weapons" in domestic policing, together with overtly militarized weapons systems, uniforms, language and tactics.

In the end, Graham concludes

> ... integration is underway between the security-industrial complexes and the military-industrial complexes of Israel and the United States. Even more than this, the emerging security-military-industrial complexes of the two nations are becoming umbilically connected, so much so that it might now be reasonable to consider them as a single diversified, transnational entity.[18]

Moreover, both the tactics and weaponry of these intertwined complexes and their dependence upon a permanent war/securocratic war economy are, Graham contends,

> ... firmly based on the generalization of doctrines and technologies forged during the long-standing lockdown and repression of Palestinian cities by Israeli military and security forces ... There is thus a danger of Israeli urban hypermilitarism being normalized across transnational scales, carried along by the US War on Terror as it targets cities and quotidian city life at home and abroad.[19]

And, as in the case of the Palestinians writ large, Israeli models of securitization serve not only Israeli security politics but the interests or the ruling hegemons of the core and beyond, "a perceived association of suspects to violence, disruption or resistance against the dominant geographical orders sustaining global, neoliberal capitalism."[20] As a "Global

Palestine" expands, militarized urbanism becomes just one expression of "global Palestinization."

Israeli security firms specialize in what Americans refer to as "homeland security," but they extend it into "homeland defense," protecting one's sovereign territory and population against external threats. This reflects Israel's security situation in which internal security, occupation and localized wars have given rise to the all-purpose concept *bitakhon*, "security," as in this official presentation of its homeland defense industry:

> Positioned at the forefront of today's homeland security technology, Israel has initiated and implemented state-of-the-art homeland security solutions based on guidelines, experience, and expertise acquired over decades of combating internal security and terror threats. As a small country, Israel's existence depends on its vigilance and providing an effective, measured response to evolving domestic and foreign threats. These requirements have challenged Israel's defense and security industries since their establishment in the late 1940s. Over the years since then, innovative systems and solutions have been created in order to meet these goals. Today, these advanced, fully-developed and tested capabilities are also securing many of Israel's allies and partners throughout the world, employing unique operational concepts supported by effective training and support, and providing a high level of security while maintaining a high quality of life for ordinary citizens. Israel's domestic security is largely self-reliant, depending mainly on homegrown defense and information technologies.[21]

The "umbilical" US-Israel security relationship is by no means the only one. Similar agreements and programs exist with other police and domestic security forces as well. Canada under Stephen Harper, a self-described "Christian Zionist," has gone a step further than his American compatriots. The Canadian-Israeli Public Safety Act signed in 2008 gives Israel extraordinary access to Canada's internal security and police apparatus covering broad but vague areas from border management and security measures (including biometric applications) to Canada's correctional services and prisons, crime prevention, critical infrastructure protection, emergency management, illegal immigration, law enforcement cooperation with Israel, organized crime, counter-terrorism and terrorist financing and trafficking in persons. Signed as merely a "declaration of intent" between the two ministers, the agreement was able to avoid undue parliamentary oversight, public discussion and media coverage.[22]

Chossudovsky raises a number of key questions regarding the Declaration of Intent. What type of border security and control of immigrants is involved? How does this impinge upon Canada's immigration procedures? Since Israel is not part of North America and the two countries do not share a common border, what is the underlying agenda? Will Canada assist Israel in policing its border with Lebanon, Syria and the Palestinian territories? Conversely, will Israeli officials assist Canada in ethnic profiling of people (including biometric applications, which is mentioned in the agreement) who visit Canada from the Middle East? Will Israeli officials have access to confidential files of Canadians? Given that Israel is a country on record for its numerous violations of human rights in Palestine and Lebanon, what role would it play, what changes would it propose, in Canadian public security, in particular in the ethnic profiling of Muslim Canadian citizens? What type of cooperation is envisaged in the areas of prisons and law enforcement, and what about "interrogation techniques" specifically mentioned by Dichter? Are Israeli consultants going to help Canadians reorganize their own correctional services? Will Israeli officials assist their Canadian counterparts in the domestic "war on terrorism", which in the post-9/11 period has led to arbitrary detentions on trumped-up charges, and what will that mean for those actively supporting Palestinian rights? If the pact is mutual, will Canadian police be directly involved in assisting Israel's police in suppressing Palestinians in the Occupied Territory? How much and what is Canada contributing to building the Palestinian security services as part of its contribution to the "peace process," especially in light of the fact that under the Declaration of Intent, Canada cannot exercise "neutrality," but must act as a partner of Israel in all issues of public security in the Occupied Territories?

Israel's reach, as we have noted, extends deep into internal security and policing of a great many of the countries of the world, both core and periphery, as we have seen over the course of this book. But again, why Israel? What in the Israeli model of security and policing is so innovative, or so effective, that it is sought out from Washington DC to Malabo?

The Israeli Model

Just as we described the Matrix of Control over the Palestinian territories as a coherent system that can be (and is) conveyed and exported—Ganor's protestations aside—so, too, can we perceive an Israeli model of civilian securitization and policing deriving from it. We must again identify the various pieces of the "puzzle" and fit them together.

Operational Assumptions

Many elements of Israel's approach to securitization derive from its fundamental yet structural insecurity. Israeli Jews must constantly assert their domination over another people, the Palestinians, for whom there is no legitimate place. Indeed, the Arabs represent half the people in "Greater Israel," yet Israel has no intention of either incorporating them as equal citizens or allowing them a state of their own. And the Palestinians who represent half of the population of the country under the domination of the Israeli Jews are themselves only half of a larger Palestinian people displaced in 1948 and claiming the right to return. Israel's dilemma is that it can only sustain its character as a "Jewish state" (plus "Judea and Samaria") by suppressing the right of the Palestinians to self-determination. For their part, the Palestinians can never accept permanent subjugation, which is all Israel can offer. Their endemic century-old insurgency has created, as we discussed earlier, the nation-in-arms that is Israel, whose very culture is infused with "civilian militarism."[23]

By definition, then, the "Arabs" under Israeli control (Israelis seldom use the term "Palestinians" as they refuse to recognize them as a national group) are viewed as a threat by Israeli Jews. "Arabs" embody fears over security, political instability, the legitimacy and sustainability of the "Jewish" state, biological dilution, a demographic challenge and fears of "Levantization."[24] For its entire existence and back into the pre-state period, Israel has been living officially under a permanent emergency; the Defense Emergency Regulations promulgated by the British in 1945 are still in effect, incorporated into Israeli law. They confer on the authorities powers to establish military tribunals for trying civilians without the right of appeal, conduct sweeping searches and seizures, prohibit publication of books and newspapers, permit the demolishing of houses as deterrence or punishment unconnected to convictions of suspects, imprison individuals administratively for an indefinite period, seal off particular territories, and more. Although the Israeli Knesset once intended to repeal them as contradictory to the basic principles of democracy, they have been retained because they provided a legal (or extra-legal) means of dealing with security, especially when it came to the Arab population both within Israel and, later, in the Occupied Territory—and they are frequently employed.[25]

Given this context, the Israeli police force is far from being merely a civilian agency charged with maintaining law and order. It is a paramilitary organization, operating under the Ministry of Internal Security, which works closely with the military and military security agencies under the state of permanent emergency. Tellingly, in listing its functions, the official police website begins with "prevention of acts of terror, dismantling of explosive devices and deployment in terrorist incidents," before moving on to such routine police matters as maintaining law and order, fighting crime and traffic control.[26]

For Israelis, the rise of terrorism reached a climax in 1974 when a school group in the Galilee town of Ma'alot was attacked and 22 children were killed. It was then that the Israeli police were formally declared a "dual purpose police" in which its traditional policing role was broadened to include ensuring national security within the state's borders. Consequently the police houses three overtly paramilitary units. The Border Police, originally the Frontier Police, was an IDF unit charged with protecting the state's borders and rural areas until it was incorporated into the police force in 1953; it numbers 7,500, a third of the police force. After 1967, it took on a leading role in law enforcement and anti-terror tasks in the Occupied Territory, most visibly as a militarized presence at checkpoints, providing security to settlements, conducting raids and arrests on Palestinian targets, and confronting protests. The Border Police also provide a military presence in East Jerusalem since the government prefers not to deploy the army in what is considered Israeli territory.

A second paramilitary unit, the Yamam or "Special Police Unit," exists within the Border Police. An elite counter-terrorism unit, it responds to terrorist attacks and hostage crisis situations, conducts SWAT operations and, as an undercover unit, works closely with the Shin Bet, the General Security Service, or Shabak, Israel's internal security service. For its part, the Shin Bet is the overall body responsible for security inside Israel. Answering directly to the prime minister's office, it is divided mainly into an Arab Affairs Division that conducts political subversion among, and surveillance of, Arab groups suspected of subversive or terrorist tendencies, and a Protection and Security Division that safeguards Israeli government buildings and embassies, defense contractors, scientific installations, key industrial plants and El Al, the national airline. A third paramilitary police force is the Yamas, a super-secret special operations unit that serves under the Shin Bet and is tasked with complex counter-terror missions involving high degrees of risk.[27]

In its operations, the Israeli police and security forces do not separate policing related to Palestinian anti-occupation efforts from street crime. For them, the "Arabs" represent both a political and armed opposition and a disenfranchised underclass with criminal tendencies. Former Shin Bet director and then Minister of Internal Security Avi Dichter, speaking before 10,000 police officers attending the International Association of Chiefs of Police in Boston, used the term "crimiterrorists" to underscore "the intimate connection between fighting criminals and fighting terrorists." "Crime and terror are two sides of the same coin," he asserted.[28]

This helps explain the militarized securitization that characterizes the approach of the Israeli police in their training of foreign police and security forces in tactics and the use of weaponry. It embodies a degree of aggressiveness not formally accepted into police work in other core countries, mainly because their own processes of militarization have been slowed and even opposed by public opinion and the reluctance of (some) lawmakers to compromise the civilian character of domestic security and its oversight. To be sure, the Israeli approach to securitization, as laid out by Arie Perlinger and Ami Pedahzur, mixes the aggressiveness of the war and criminal justice models with more "defensive" ones emphasizing preventive efforts, intelligence gathering, response involving all the relevant authorities and preparing the public to deal with attacks and effective crisis management.[29] (Pedahzur, by the way, is an Israeli academic in security studies from Haifa University who brought his TIGER Lab—Terrorists, Insurgents, and Guerrillas in Education and Research—to the University of Texas, Austin, which he intends to make the US's "state of the art research lab on terrorism."[30] Perlinger, also an Israeli-trained academic and Pedazhur's former student, today serves as the Director of Terrorism Studies at West Point's Combating Terrorism Center. Thus do Israeli methods and concepts of securitization enter core militaries, government agencies and security discourse.)

Assertiveness and the aura of effectiveness that military securitization broadcasts is nevertheless essential if only because it underlies the credibility Israel's brand of hard-headed "security." "Why Israel?" asks the Israel Export and International Cooperation Institute on its website marketing homeland security services. The answer:

What grew out of a direct military need with a high-tech edge has developed into a core element of the Israeli economy and placed Israel at the forefront of the global security and HLS industry. For a small country, Israel has conceived, developed, and manufactured military projects greatly disproportionate to its size, including satellites, the Kfir fighter aircraft, UAVs, Merkava tank, Uzi submachine gun, Galil and Tavor assault rifles, missiles, and many more. With the military providing a fertile breeding ground for future generations of engineers and entrepreneurs, many non-defense-related, high-quality technologies and solutions have been developed.[31]

It is this which sets off the "Israel model" from the others and makes it marketable.

Keeping in mind this political and behavioral context, we can proceed to consider the three broad tasks that comprise Israeli police and security operations and how they contribute to domestic pacification in the core countries and those of the semi-periphery; namely, prevention and interdiction, responses during an attack, and responses following an attack.[32]

Prevention and Interdiction: "Policing Terrorism"

A major part of Israeli counter-terror and security operations revolve around preventing attacks or other unwanted manifestations of security threats, but also extend to interdiction and the weakening infrastructures of resistance, crime, or terrorism. The Israeli approach, then, begins with teaching the public how to be vigilant (it is said that 80 percent of attempted terrorist attacks in Israel are foiled by citizens),[33] together with intelligence designed to both monitor various settings and identify potential threats. It also employs two other tactics adopted from the world of counter-terrorism: interactive intelligence and ethnic profiling. Livne, in laying out the Israeli model for airport security, stresses repeated verbal interaction and eye contact with highly trained, intelligent security personnel, since "the hardest thing for terrorists to get right is not to get nervous in any way," combined with an explicit and heavy reliance on profiling of all sorts: "If you are an Israeli Jew, your life through security will tend to be easy. If you are a Muslim, expect to spend more time through the process."[34]

This combination of innovative high-tech with a readiness to provide services to any customer and in a technical manner that ignores or minimizes individual privacy or human rights reflects the Israeli reality in which "security" trumps all else. Practices that are illegal or problematic in other core countries—ethnic profiling, for instance[35]—are the basis of Israeli security doctrines. Protections against arbitrary arrest or imprisonment—*habeus corpus* in particular—are lacking in Israel. Although the Israeli Supreme Court banned torture in 1999, it is still practiced within the loopholes provided, such as labeling suspects as "ticking bombs," or finding non-visible ways of torturing. The Israeli human rights organization B'tselem lists seven key elements of the Shin Bet's interrogation regime "harm the dignity and bodily integrity" of the detainees, harm aggravated by the fact that the interrogation process investigated by B'tselem lasted an average of 35 days. The key elements include: isolation, the use of the conditions of confinement as a means of psychological pressure, the use of the conditions of confinement as a means for weakening the detainees' physical state, tying up prisoners in painful ways, beating and degradation, threatening and intimidating.[36]

Invasive though concealed surveillance and intelligence technologies are developed and perfected on Palestinians in the Occupied Territory through joint security industry-IDF endeavors, or from technologies coming from Unit 8200. In 2014, 43 ex-soldiers from the elite intelligence unit sent a letter to their superiors and the prime minister refusing to do future reserve duty. Not only has our military service "taught us that intelligence is an integral part of Israel's military occupation over the territories," they wrote, but the information that is gathered and stored in the army's systems "harms innocent people [as it] is used for political persecution and to create divisions within Palestinian society by recruiting collaborators and driving parts of Palestinian society against itself."[37] Nonetheless, many executives and programmers of the country's security and high-tech industries that, with exports valued at $18.4 billion in 2013, account for more than 45 percent of the total, are graduates of Unit 8200. The long-time president and co-founder of NICE Systems, a major Israeli security company, served as a lieutenant-colonel in Unit 8200, as did Yehuda and Zonhar Zisapel, who have sold and floated a dozen companies worth hundreds of millions of dollars, and Gil Schwed, founder of Check Point.[38] The ability to develop invasive (if concealed) systems gives Israeli companies like NICE, Verint, Check Point, Narus, Amdocs and hundreds of others that grew out of the IDF a distinct edge on the market, the acceptability of their products limited only by the laws of their clients' countries.[39]

Regular Israeli police units also engage in prevention and interdiction, collaborating routinely with the Border Police, the Shin Bet and the IDF, and this may be a key attraction for core police forces seeking to learn from Israel's experiences in counter-terrorism. No police department has a stronger working relationship with Israel that New York's NYPD. Since 9/11, New York has been considered the prime target of terrorist attacks, and counter-terrorism a prime focus of its police department. Over the years, the NYPD's Intelligence Division has engaged in aggressive domestic intelligence activities that exceed the legal limits allowed by the federal government, particularly in its targeting of ethnic communities.

In a step reminiscent of Israeli tactics in the West Bank, the NYPD carved up the city into more than a dozen zones, assigning undercover officers to monitor each, "looking for potential trouble." These zones can then be monitored by surveillance devices or patrolled; again, the Israeli tactic of keeping tabs on what is happening "on the ground," intimidating the local population and disrupting the planning of attacks is to be "in your face" with patrols and a constant, active military/police presence, punctuated by periodic but unpredictable raids. Movement in and out of the zones is monitored and controlled, as the Israeli checkpoints and Separation Barrier do, and the zones can be locked down when necessary.[40]

The NYPD then took another page from Israel's manual on counter-terrorism: intelligence as the key to prevention and interdiction. It established a secret "Demographic Unit" that sent undercover officers, known as "rakers," to map the "human terrain" of targeted minority neighborhoods—"modeled, according to an NYPD source, "on how Israeli authorities operate in the West Bank." Informants known as "mosque crawlers" monitored sermons and mosque activities. A Terrorist Interdiction Unit followed up on their leads, and yet another squad, the Special Services Unit, conducts undercover work—illegally in some cases—outside of New York City.[41] In 2012, the NYPD even opened an Israeli office, located in the Sharon District Police Headquarters in Kfar Saba, in order "to cooperate on a daily basis with the Israel Police."[42] "If a bomber blows himself up in Jerusalem, the NYPD rushes to the scene," said Michael Dzikansky, an NYPD officer who served in Israel. "I was there to ask the New York question: 'Why this location? Was there something unique that the bomber had done? Was there any pre-notification. Was there a security lapse?'" Dzikansky subsequently co-authored a book, *Terrorist Suicide Bombings: Attack Interdiction, Mitigation, and Response*, another example of how Israeli security practices enter into US law enforcement.[43]

Among other practices followed by the NYPD that evoke those of the Israelis is the use of collaborators. As with the Palestinians, the NYPD searches for vulnerable individuals who could be turned into informants. It recruits in prisons, for example, promising better living conditions and help or money on the outside for Muslim prisoners who will work with them, or they run down Pakistani cab drivers who might have attained their licenses fraudulently, and are thus susceptible to pressure to collaborate. Field Interrogation Officers "debrief" people arrested from target communities.[44]

In 2013, Israeli National Police Chief Yochanan Danino visited the NYPD, the result being the establishment of several joint tasks forces, and the next year NYPD Commissioner Bill Bratton, accompanied by the deputy commissioner of intelligence, delivered the keynote address at the National Conference on Personal Security in Jerusalem. Taking prevention and interdiction to the extreme, Bratton asserted:

> Now, with the huge amounts of information that we can gather and analyze, both with human assets as well as algorithms and computer capabilities, we are fast approaching a time where many crimes can be detected before they occur. We will be able, with a certain degree of probability, to predict: In this geographic area and in this time frame, a crime will occur, unless you put a police source in there to prevent it. It sounds kind of like science fiction but that is the reality of the world we are going into. With regard to terrorism, the main focus is about trying to put all those dots together to predict where they are going to strike next. In many respects nobody does it better than the Israelis ... .[45]

It is in this interstice between counter-insurgency and counter-terrorism that Israel has found a niche among security and police forces. Kaplan points to the gap in American security thinking between Vietnam, when counter-insurgency doctrine was largely banished from the US military playbook, until General Petraeus and others issued the US Army and Marine Corps new Field Manual on counterinsurgency in late 2006.[46] In that vacuum, argues Niva, Israeli technologies, tactics and even strategic doctrines became a "default paradigm" and source of emulation, accelerating with American involvement in Arab and Muslim lands after 9/11.[47] It would appear that that paradigm seeped into domestic American security and police practices as well. Blumenthal describes in detail how "the Israelification of America's security apparatus, recently unleashed in full force against the Occupy Wall Street Movement, has taken place at every level of law enforcement."[48] Cathy Lanier, chief of the Washington DC police, who once stated "No experience in my life has had more of an impact on doing my job than going to Israel," authorized checkpoints in the troubled northeast

DC neighborhood of Trinidad to monitor and control street violence and the illegal narcotics trade.[49]

When it comes to prevention, deterrence and interdiction of attacks, a clear set of operational assumptions and practices runs from the Matrix of Control through Israeli methods of "policing terrorism," an "Israeli model" for export. The pieces of the puzzle are many, but police tactics taught by Israel closely replicate the military and security tactics we found in the Matrix of Control—simply adjusted and toned-down to fit police rather than military operations. In a roughly operational order, they include:

- Proactive and interactive intelligence gathering by a wide variety of means;
- Recruiting public vigilance;
- Interrogation bordering on torture;
- Close "horizontal" cooperation among the various military, security and police forces;
- Cumulative deterrence and preemptive raids against "infrastructure" of terrorism;
- In-your-face patrolling in hostile terrain;
- Use of aggressive and disproportionate force, including against targets' families;
- Aerial control;
- Targeted assassinations and impunity towards those deemed "enemies," be they non-combatants or not;
- Preventive measures such as physical barriers, checkpoints, lock-downs and layered security;
- Preventive measures such as establishing security zones, ethnic profiling and employing bureaucratic modes of monitoring or preventing movement;
- Administrative detention and mass arrests;
- Aggressive crowd control;
- "Aggressive" house-to-house searches, demoralization; and
- The pursuit of "lawfare."

Let us see how they operate as a system of securitization.

Responses During an Attack

Once the attack has been launched, the Israeli response is essentially a military one, the police generally taking a back seat to IDF units, although still playing a central and coordinated role. Responses follow the pattern we have discussed above: isolating, locking down and securing the site of the attack, issuing focused alerts to those in the immediate vicinity, and aggressively dealing with the perpetrators. Since the safety of the first responder officer comes first, a disproportionate use of force is permitted, depending, of course, on whether there are hostages or imperiled civilians.

The aggressive nature of the Israeli response is partly displayed in the confrontational, "shoot-to-kill" (and aim at the head so as not to set off any explosives) tactics of the police and security forces, justified as necessary to prevent the attackers from carrying out their mission, especially if they threaten to use body-explosives.[50] The attitude and method is explained by an officer in the Memphis Police Department who received Israeli Combative Pistol Training:

> The first point which separates the Israeli Combative Method from other teachings is the mindset with which it is employed. While American ideals on the Use of Force revolve around using the least amount of force in a conservative, defensive manner, the Israeli method is opposite this ideal. In the Israeli method, the intent is to bring the maximum amount of force into play in an offensive manner. The intent is to "attack the attacker", to be more aggressive than the aggressor, to "explode" and overwhelm the initial aggressor with violence of action. Three words that I use to describe this mindset are Aggressive, Offensive, and Decisive … The intent is to shoot until there is no longer a threat … .
>
> Israeli combative pistol training contains elements of Krav Maga, the Israeli hand-to-hand/martial arts system. Krav Maga is the only martial art in the world that does not have some form of competition associated with it, as it is not a sport. If you consider that the intent of Krav Maga is to allow un-armed combatants to successfully take down armed terrorists, including those armed with grenades and suicide bombs, then its serious nature becomes evident. To understand how Israeli pistol training is an extension of this, consider the following: Most gunfights are at extremely close range, with many being at "contact distance." If you are fighting with an assailant and your pistol malfunctions or goes empty at such distances, and the fight is still going on, then it is totally reasonable in the Israeli system to use the empty pistol itself as a "battering" tool to beat the assailant into submission![51]

An American security officer relates what he learned during his time in Israel with a Yamam Special Police Unit:

> When it came to shooting, the major difference between Israel and America training is our philosophy on close-quarter or urban combat. The biggest difference between what the Israelis did and what we Americans were trained to do was that they would oftentimes suggest going almost headlong at an enemy position while firing through whole magazines. It usually took a matter of seconds to burn through a magazine, so fast reloads factored heavily into one's success. In training, we would advance by increments of 40 or 50 meters at a time in urban settings, all the while firing on full-automatic. Back in the States, the attack is more controlled. We were taught to perhaps squeeze off rounds in three-second bursts and then seek cover. This is not the way of Israeli security apparatus and though it may be too bold in every circumstance, in the right scenario, I cannot think of a more effective way to gain ground.[52]

And in fact Krav Maga ("contact combat" in Hebrew) is an Israeli martial arts that perfectly expresses the shoot-to-kill aggressiveness of Israeli police tactics.[53] Coming out of the IDF, it is based on the principle of counter-attacking as soon as possible or pre-emptively, targeting the adversary's most vulnerable body parts. The "Israelization" of American, British and other core police forces has not gone without criticism. The fact that officers in the different police forces dealing with the Ferguson protests, who chose a confrontational approach backed up by heavy military equipment, were trained in Israel has led to a feeling that the people of Ferguson have been "Palestinianized."[54] By the same token, Operation Kratos, the aggressive tactics for dealing with suicide bombers partly adopted by the London Metropolitan Police from Israeli methods, notably firing shots to the head without warning, was apparently the cause of the shooting of Jean Charles de Menezes in the London Underground in 2005.[55]

Responses After an Attack

After an attack, and sometimes even as it is occurring, attention shifts to crisis management: management of the scene in terms of preventing second attacks, effective coordination of emergency medical personnel, issuing prompt statements to the press in order to calm public fears and quickly reconstructing the physical damage so as to remove all traces of the attack. Since terrorist violence aims to undermine the personal security of civilians, to sow fear and trepidation, and to sap public morale in order to pressure decision makers to make political concessions, the immediate goal of the response is to "preserve the psychological resilience of the civilian population" while, in the longer term, to insulate the public as if terrorism doesn't exist.[56]

Still, after an attack, the perpetrators must pay. "Zero tolerance" had characterized Israeli military and police operations for years before it became a common expression. Perpetrators are either killed on the scene or hunted down, where they may be killed or arrested. Certainly they, their accomplices, their families and the wider community are squeezed and intimidated for all the information that can be milked from the attack. In many cases, the homes of the perpetrators and their families are demolished.[57]

The Political Economy of Securitization

Indeed, Israel has become the world's No. 2 exporter of cyber products and services after the US, a clear case of the overlap and mutual fostering of military and civilian applications. There are two hundred homegrown cybersecurity companies in Israel, alongside dozens of joint research-and-development ventures. They produce about $3 billion in exports annually, or about 5 percent of the $60 billion global market in products designed to keep hackers from crashing systems or siphoning data with viruses, malware and purloined passwords.[58] Lockheed Martin recently opened a cyber-focused subsidiary in Beer Sheva.[59]

Some 416 Israeli companies specialize in homeland security, comprising 21 percent of the high-tech sector, most having to do with surveillance.[60] Although the precise revenues of Israel's homeland security/surveillance industry are impossible to determine due to the dual civilian/military use of many products, it is reasonable to assume that its revenues are comparable to and perhaps even surpass those of the military industry. Twenty-one Israeli homeland security companies are traded on NASDAQ.[61] Overall, Israel can be considered "a global homeland security capital."[62]

In its Homeland Defense Directory, SIBAT, the marketing arm of the Ministry of Defense, lists 40 categories of homeland security applications offered by Israeli companies.[63] In connecting Israel's homeland security industry to the technologies of control arising from Israel's security situation, particular Israeli "specialties" stand out, border security technologies prominent among them, as they have become hubs of hyper-surveillance. The use of UAVs for surveillance, perimeter defense and access controls, threat detection systems for cargoes, sensors, "biometric borders" in airports, smart-card IDs, credit cards and passports—all these technologies of control merge with wider applications of social sorting and monitoring such as NICE System's video cameras with image identification capabilities. The ability to surveil under adverse circumstances has long challenged securitization tasks, so the ability of Israeli firms to "borrow" electro-optical, laser and infrared applications from military reconnaissance and avionics applications, together with such military-based technologies as data mining and intelligence gathering, confer distinct advantages.[64] "Israeli capital, with considerable support from the US and Israeli governments," comments Graham, "has taken its skills, expertise and products beyond the more obvious markets surrounding urban warfare, and expertly projected them towards the much broader and ever-extensible arena of global securitization, securocratic war, 'homeland security' and counterterrorism."[65]

As in the Matrix of Control and the "Israeli model" of policing, Israel offers not only specific "solutions" but also comprehensive programs of surveillance and monitoring that draw upon the Israeli security community's rich experience "on the ground," military, security and policing being so interwoven with the country's private sector. The "Safe Cities" program sold to metropolitan police forces of the core and semi-periphery provides a graphic example.

A "Safe City" refers to an intersection between different elements of communication, command and control, sensors, biometrics, IT connectivity, cyber security and more. Israeli-made systems and devices of video surveillance and civil security air surveillance maintain public safety and security during routine times and emergency situations. In order for a project to constitute a Safe City, however, it must integrate all of the security-relevant information on a cross-cutting IT platform. Thus public safety information coming in from video surveillance, sensors, biometrics and access control is combined with information providing a clear situational picture city-wide via command, control and communications networks—all displayed on digital maps and GIS for quick and effective emergency response.[66]

NICE Systems, which the International Directory of Company Histories calls an "Israeli intelligence spinoff," offers a prime example of how Israeli military-based surveillance systems find ready markets in both government security agencies and the private sector. "Its Big Brother-like capabilities," writes Stacy Perman in *Spies, Inc.: Business Innovation from Israel's Masters of Espionage*, "include the ability to identify, locate, monitor, and record transmissions from various sources and the ability to monitor Internet traffic such as emails, web chats, instant messaging, and voice over IP."[67] NICE provides wiretapping and surveillance products to spy agencies, the military, police forces and private corporations in 150 countries. It counts among its clients dozens of police departments; in fact, all incoming phone calls to the Los Angeles and New York City police departments are recorded on NICE technology.[68] At the core of the NICE Safe City program (or "solution" as security companies like to call it) is the Situator, the command-and-control system that displays a Common Operating Picture (COP) "so that everyone in the operational chain knows what is happening and what to do."[69]

Safe Cities programs like NICE's not only install video surveillance cameras throughout a city or facility, but they deliver "strategic insights" by capturing and analyzing mass quantities of structured and unstructured data from phone calls, mobile apps, emails, chat, social media and video.[70] NICE's surveillance cameras employ advanced image processing for detecting vehicles or locating people—a practice of "social sorting" by which, without our knowledge, we are enabled or prevented access to particular places or events, our movements and even consumer patterns are followed, or we can be detained.[71] By having the police, intelligence agencies, or even corporate employers collect and pre-sort images of citizens or employees, its video analytics can instantly identify targets by their body image, features, textures and colors, instead of having to waste valuable time watching recordings from thousands of cameras scattered throughout a city. Linked to other surveillance systems, the program automatically marks the targets route on a map and indicates where they are headed.

So much for the publicly available promotional information. In promotional videos "for police eyes only," NICE presents other, more worrying scenarios. In one, reported by the IT watchdog *The Register*, NICE has a frightened old lady peeking out of her window at a group of youths below. "There's a gang outside in the street. I really don't like the look of them. I'm sure they're up to no good," she tells the police operator. The operator's extreme intelligence software leaps into action, plugging him into the street's CCTV cameras and reckoning that the youths must indeed be up to no good. They seem to be hanging around, they are wearing hoods (*à la* Trayvon Martin), they look shifty. The computer labels their behavior for the police record that will be shown in court: "Crowd accumulation" and "loitering." An armed unit is dispatched—and from there the situation escalates. The youths commandeer a car ("What more proof do you need?" asks *The Register* sardonically. "Any innocent citizen, with a crack troop of armed police bearing down on them, would stay put and stick their hands up. British armed police are renowned for their judgment and restraint.") The youths' car is tracked by a variety of ground-based, air-based and satellite-based systems, and they are apprehended. The NICE ad ends: "Policing with a more human face."[72]

Another confidential NICE video, noted in *Rolling Stone*, shows how its products can be used in the event of a political protest:

> "The NICE video analytic suite alerts on an unusually high occupancy level in a city center," a narrator says as the camera zooms in on people chanting and holding signs that read "clean air" and "stop it now." The video then shows authorities redirecting traffic to avoid a bottleneck, and promises that all audio and video from the event will be captured and processed almost immediately. "The entire event is then reconstructed on a chronological timeline, based on all multimedia sources," says the narrator.[73]

In far-away Central Asia, Privacy International investigated how the autocratic governments of Tajikistan, Kyrgyzstan, Turkmenistan, Uzbekistan and Kazakhstan managed to monitor human rights activists, journalists and other citizens within and outside their countries, revealing the most intimate details of their personal lives. "Central Asian governments installed advanced surveillance systems that included centers that could monitor all communications within the country," reads the report. "These systems were set up thanks to foreign companies who provided the equipment and services that enable these regimes to spy on their people." Sound like Safe Cities? "The biggest players," concluded Human Rights Watch, "are multinationals with offices in Israel—NICE Systems and Verint."[74]

Brazil represents the countries in Latin America and Asia—and beyond, the human-security states of the larger semi-periphery—for whom a militarized homeland security fits domestic needs more than a military geared to fighting inter-state wars. It is also a state on Israel's "far periphery." This is especially evident when one looks at Brazil's campaign of securitization between the 2011 Military World Games, through the 2014

World Cup, and on to the 2016 Olympics. Such mega-events are truly places in sore need of security. Johnson points out that

> ... over 9,000 homeless persons, primarily ethnic minorities, were arrested during the 1996 Olympic Games in Atlanta. 720,000 residents were evicted from their homes in Seoul to make way for the 1988 Olympics. Over 1.25 million people were displaced due to urban redevelopment for the 2008 Beijing Olympics. Hundreds of Roma were displaced in Athens prior to the 2004 Olympics. More recently many thousands were evicted in Cape Town, Johannesburg, Durban and elsewhere prior to the 2010 World Cup in South Africa. Since February of this year demolitions have begun in Rio de Janeiro favelas in the run-up to the 2014 World Cup and 2016 Olympics.[75]

As Brazil sends its Pacification Police Unit to pacify more than a hundred *favelas* in proximity to Olympic sites, 170,000 people are likely to be evicted from their homes and communities.[76] Given the need to pacify and control the *favelas*, monitor and control the drug and criminal gangs, keep angry populations of the working class and poor at bay alongside the displaced indigenous peoples, while still protecting the millions of tourists and sports fans on the scene, Brazil will spend more than $3 billion on security: "Israel's decades of experience in the combating of Palestinian resistance to dispossession, armed and unarmed, have made it the 'go-to' destination for the necessary expertise."[77]

In October 2010, the president of Brazil's Olympic Committee paid a visit to Israel, and in December 2010, Defense Minister Ehud Barak signed an agreement with Brazil's minister of intelligence whereby IAI will sell to Brazil's Federal Police a number of "homeland security products": UAVs, radars and sensors, unmanned vehicles, electronic fences, optics and satellite technology. The Israeli company International Security and Defense Systems (ISDS), which specializes in pacifying cities, "advised" IAI and the Federal Police in putting together the agreement. In Brazil, IAI's CEO Yitzhak Nissan said that his company's line of UAVs and other security technologies would also deal effectively with other security problems facing Brazil, namely guerrilla organizations and smugglers in the vast region of the Amazon. Under the deal, IAI will supply a range of UAV systems to the Brazilian police, as well as ground radar systems, electronic fences, optical equipment, sensors, unmanned vehicles and satellite technology, mainly to secure the World Cup and the 2016 Olympics. Fifteen agents of the

Brazilian Federal Police are already training in Israel to use the UAVs. IAI will also open a factory in Brazil for manufacturing UAVs.[78]

In 2011, Israel-based Magal Security Systems won a contract of $35.5 million to install its Fortis surveillance system for the African Cup of Nations football championships. The contract covered a surveillance and intrusion detection systems developed for and deployed at several Israeli West Bank settlements, the Separation Barrier and the border with Gaza, then exported to Equatorial Guinea before finally being installed in Johannesburg.[79]

In what is described as "an unprecedented Israeli achievement," ISDS was selected to manage and coordinate the security of the Rio 2016 Olympics, the first time an Israeli company will serve in this capacity. In a deal worth an estimated $2.2 billion, ISDS's operations will range from consulting to supplying security systems. According to ISDS's vice president,

> ... this is a rare opportunity to provide a platform for Israeli companies to take part in securing the games. We very much want to take this platform and integrate Israeli and international technologies that address the specific issues—from intelligence to perimeter security, crowd control and so forth. It will be a technology hotbed of Israeli security solutions.[80]

ISDS secures off-shore drilling rigs at sea, civilian nuclear reactors in Mexico, the US, Brazil and elsewhere, as well as merchant ships and other HLS projects.

In order to implement the contract, ISDS will work opposite dozens of Brazilian organizations and the world's leading companies. Leo Gleser, ISDS founder, said in an interview with *Israel Defense* that "the entire purpose of the security effort is to effectively support the flow of the event, establish deterrence where necessary and uphold security in the most discrete manner." To accomplish that, he will endeavor to incorporate as many Israeli companies and technologies as possible into the security for the Olympic Games:

> We had very serious backing from the Israeli Ministry of Economy, from the Defense Export & Defense Cooperation Division (SIBAT) at IMOD, from the Israel Export & International Cooperation Institute and even from the President's Residence. Former Israeli President Shimon Peres did his best to facilitate our selection during his visits to Brazil ... [But] as far as HLS is concerned, [the Brazilians] seek Israeli help, owing to

our experience … Everyone knows that Israel is a global leader in this field. We prove it every day.[81]

In fact, the choice of ISDS to secure the 2016 Olympics did not come out of the blue. In 2008, the company was hired to train Chinese security personnel in the run-up to the 2008 Beijing Olympics (for which, tellingly, the US blocked Israeli defense firms from submitting security tenders).[82] ISDS "was asked to provide know-how and situation reports about international terror, mainly regarding threats of extremist Muslim groups in Asia"—which in the Chinese context means Uighur nationalism. China was also concerned with other kinds of protest; by Tibetans, of course, but also by the 1.25 million people forcibly displaced to build the Olympic infrastructure, by millions living in new cities with little infrastructure or employment, by dissidents, and others. To this end, Israeli police were brought in to train members of China's police force in a six-week course that included, as reported in *Ha'aretz*, "how to deal with a crowd that riots on the playing field, and how to protect VIPs and remove demonstrators from main traffic arteries." The article noted, "Although the main focus of the training was to give the Chinese police the tools necessary to handle terrorist attacks, they also learned how to handle mass civilian demonstrations."[83]

Indeed, crowd control is yet another homeland security "niche" coming out of Israel's suppression of innumerable Palestinian demonstrations and uprisings. Beit Alfa Technologies (BAT), located on the Beit Alfa kibbutz in northern Israel, specializes in riot control vehicles. It sells to more than 35 countries, including the notorious Mugabe regime in Zimbabwe, which purchased 30 of the vehicles for $10 million. The vehicles, which the BAT website boasts have been "proven in combat" worldwide, are in fact widely deployed by the IDF, and particularly the Border Police. Its "sophisticated" riot control gear, including an accurate jet pulse water cannon capable of shooting water, pepper spray, tear gas, dyes and other "chemical additives" for "dangerous inmate situations" can be mounted on a wide variety of ballistic armored chasses.[84] Zimbabwe received armored vehicles and crowd control systems.[85]

Water cannons sound innocuous. "As long as they are using water with food color, instead of live ammunition, I'm happy," the general manager of BAT is quoted as saying.[86] But a report on crowd control technologies reveals that a pulse jet cannon system such as BAT employs actually turns small quantities of water—as little as 5 liters—into shells or bullets of water as they are shot out at high pressure. This has made water cannon effective in breaking up protests, and often result in serious injuries. To increase the effectiveness of the water cannon, chemical agents are added, generally the tear agents CS or CN, while dye can be used to mark out individuals for later identification and snatch squad capture.[87]

BAT's water cannons can also shoot "Skunk," a non-lethal, malodorous riot control solution produced by an Israeli company Odortec and "in operational use by the Israeli National Police and the IDF since 2008," says the Odortec website:

> The success of Odortec Ltd. is due to the joint effort of our multifaceted team and external consultants. Our scent research and development experts have over 20 years of experience in the field. And our management team includes command-level police officers with extensive field experience, alongside successful entrepreneurs with rich business and academic backgrounds.[88]

Skunk, a nauseating, sewage-smelling liquid that lingers on bodies and in homes for days and weeks, is sold to "law enforcement agencies, agriculturalists and environmental protection organizations in Israel, Europe and South America."

And, indeed, weekly demonstrations against the Separation Barrier in the West Bank town of Bil'in, held since 2005, and elsewhere in the Occupied Territory (including the Aida refugee camp in Bethlehem and in Hebron) have provided testing grounds for a wide variety of violent crowd control measures, including highly toxic and deadly gas, sprays and liquids.[89] A report on crowd control weapons by the Israeli group Who Profits quotes David Ben Harosh, head of the Technological Development Department of the Israel Police, that developed Skunk along with Odortec, admitting that Skunk was piloted in West Bank villages:

> In Bil'in and Ni'lin, there were two monitored exercises ... I was there. I accompanied the experiment. All the professionals accompanied it. After each spraying an observation of the area was conducted, to check if there were casualties, to see how the demonstrators reacted.

So the substance is first tested in labs, then in 'monitored exercises" conducted on human beings—Palestinians, Israelis and foreign citizens demonstrating in West Bank villages—then, after these experiments and the proper certification, the manufacturer markets the product, as having been "field tested and proven to disperse even the most determined of violent protests." The report concludes: "The occupied Palestinian territories are being used as a lab for testing new civil oppression weapons on humans, in order to label them as 'proven effective' for marketing abroad." BAT riot control vehicles are most commonly those used to fire the spray.[90]

Finally (though we're barely scratching the surface), besides its growing military ties, Israel has made a concerted push to carve out a share of India's domestic security budget, which currently stands at more than $1 billion. Since the 2008 attacks in Mumbai, its involvement with internal Indian security has deepened significantly.[91] The two countries drafted a plan in which Israeli commando forces would conduct specialized counter-terrorism exercises for Indian troops in various environments: jungles, mountains and densely populated urban areas. The Indian forces will undergo intense close quarter combat training. The Indian Army is also taking a keen interest in the homeland security operations, armaments and surveillance devices used by Israeli troops.[92]

For its part, NICE Systems installed for the Bangalore Metro Rail Corporation Limited (BMRCL) a version of its Simulator Control and Command system, joining similar deployments in India's Parliament House, the Beijing Metro, Shanghai Pudong International Airport and other "global icons," such as the Eiffel Tower and the Statue of Liberty.[93]

Alan Feldman describes securocratic war within core societies as a kind of meta-war: "wars of dystopia that assume that 'perfected' liberal democracies are threatened by an invisible, infiltrating menace ... demonized border-crossing figures and forces, including drug dealers, terrorists, asylum seekers, undocumented immigrants and microbes." Intended to secure a "specific internal hegemony" rather than fight an identifiable enemy or take territory, securocratic wars are "de-territorialized wars of public safety."[94] Although the term "public safety" denotes internal security and policing, securocratic wars know no such internal-external distinctions. Hence they are truly de-territorialized and universalized, less focused on actual enemies than on menaces, threats, challenges and sources of contamination, be they political, social and physical, and less concerned with "winning" than with prevailing in the sense of ensuring permanent hegemony. To the degree that "the Israel model" addresses these pervasive fears instilled in the public and contributes to the pacification project of the world's human-security states—"globalizing Palestine"—it effectively advances Israeli security politics.

Conclusions:
Challenging Hegemony
and Resisting Pacification

My journey into the shadow world of securocratic warfare has been both rewarding and terrifying. I began knowing virtually nothing about what I was writing and, as anthropologists do when encountering a little-documented field of study, have had to figure a lot of things out for myself, to fit the pieces of the puzzle into a coherent whole. It's not that the military/security/policing realm itself lacks documentation—the "Military History" section of major bookstores is packed with literature—or even that critical studies of the MISSILE Complex and its ongoing impact on our lives are not available. The problem I faced—and that I tried to address in this work—was a lack of a theoretical framework through which I could approach these interrelated aspects of war and securitization. Lacking that, I faced a welter of information that I could not integrate into a coherent and useful whole—certainly not one that activists who needed to be both informed themselves and then to inform and mobilize others could readily use. There was neither a Big Picture nor any way to convey the information holistically to the lay public. I also suspected that the military does not figure more prominently in public discussion because we all know so little about it, which is why I dwelt at length on describing various weapons systems and deciphering the jargon of contemporary warfare.

Since this book is aimed primarily at raising securocratic "warfare amongst the people" and the totalizing power of emerging military and surveillance technologies onto the progressive agenda, I adopted a five-fold strategy in attempting to make the information more accessible to activists and more translatable into popular campaigns. First, I put my analysis within the loose framework of world-systems analysis. Within this approach to the workings of the transnational capitalism, securitization plays a key role in perpetuating the hegemonic relationships through which the world-system operates, promoting a certain social order while also ensuring the smooth flow of capital.

Second, I focused on pacification, the ultimate goal of securitization. Reappropriating this term, which had become somewhat obscure and even outdated, focuses attention on the pointed questions raised in the book: *Who* is being pacified, and *by whom? Why* are they being pacified and *what* are they resisting—or are perceived as resisting? *Whose interests* are being served by pacification and to what ends? And *in what ways* are we being pacified? The study of pacification is holistic, all the instruments of social control—militaries, security agencies, police forces, courts and prisons in all their international and domestic forms, the MISSILE Complex— are seen as interrelated and commonly directed towards eliminating any source of counter-hegemony.

Third, the question with which I began this book—How does Israel get away with it?—focused attention particularly on a less visible manifestation of international relations, what I called "security politics." Rather than a mere export commodity, trade in military and security products constitute a resource whereby a country converts its military prowess into political clout. Weapons diplomacy, as Klieman terms it, reveals constellations of alliances (as between Israel and the conservative Arab states, Israel and China, or Israel's ability to recruit the support of American defense corporations in Congress), emerging fault-lines (as between Israel and the US over the former's military/security ties to China) and subtle shifts in policy (Nigeria failing to support the Palestinians in the Security Council because of Israel's military assistance in fighting Boko Haram), alliances not evident in the normal course of international relations.

Fourth, in order to specify even more precisely the dangers of pacification, I focused on two main aspects of "full-spectrum domination and control": securocratic war and the high-tech power of contemporary and emerging weaponry. I suspect that one reason why the MISSILE Complex is so absent from the progressive agenda, as well as from critical analysis from Marxism through world-system analysis, is that most of us come from the social sciences and humanities. Not only are we put off by (or at best not interested in) military and security matters, we are unfamiliar with the technologies and thinking underlying them. For that reason, and so we may be sensitized to what we are up against, I delved (apologetically) into the nitty-gritty of weapons systems and their use, including the Matrix of Control. There is still much to learn—someone asked me recently whether

Israel uses its satellites to direct its drones, for which I had no answer—but I feel that I've helped open up an area of inquiry and action for activists that has been largely missing from the left's agenda.

Finally, I chose Israel rather than a major core power like the US, Britain, or Germany as my vehicle for exploring security politics and securitization for several reasons. One was Israel's pivotal position along key axes: having fought conventional wars yet embroiled in a century of "war amongst the people" and securitization; its role as an agent for identifying major "niches" in the securocratic needs of the world's hegemons and filling them, and its ability to apply the most advanced technologies to field-based tasks of pacification. I went so far as to argue that in terms of the breadth of its military relations across the globe and the depth of its involvement in countries' internal security operations, Israel has an unparalleled degree of securocratic reach throughout the world-system.

So the question "How does Israel get away with it?" goes beyond the specifics of the Israeli case and usefully illuminates not only the wider shadow world of security politics and pacification, but also its interconnectedness with the other "scapes" that comprise the "landscape" of the world system (see Figure C.1).[1]

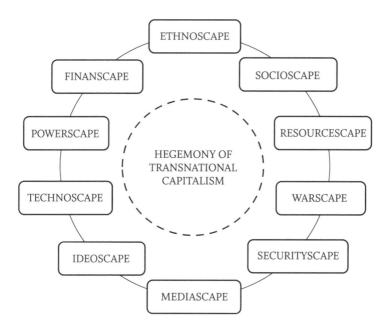

Figure C.1   The global "scapes"

Resisting Pacification

The task before progressives today is to raise activism to the level of effective counter-hegemony. "Activism" tends to target particular problems or issues. When, as the head of the Israeli Committee Against House Demolitions, I stand in front of a bulldozer sent by the Israeli authorities to demolish a Palestinian home, that is activism. So, too, is writing an article about Israel's occupation policies, or testifying before the UN Human Rights Council. For progressives, "counter-hegemony," by contrast, aims to reorder the entire social order so as to bring about a new constellation of hegemons that, ideally, would promote more egalitarian, inclusive and sustainable societies, whether locally or throughout the world-system. Attempting to parlay the home demolition issue into a broader critique of Israel's Occupation, formulating a just alternative and forming effective coalitions to end the Occupation and replace it with a new system based on equal rights of all the inhabitants of Palestine/Israel—this is localized counter-hegemony. Linking the struggle for equal rights in Palestine/Israel to movements throughout the world in order to bring about fundamental social, political, economic and environmental change throughout the world-system—represented, for example, by the World Social Forum, in which I often participate—constitutes a movement towards counter-hegemony on a global scale.

Seeking to overthrow the capitalist world-system in its entirety out of a evaluation that it is inherently exploitative, unequal and unsustainable is what is meant by "anti-systemic." While people on the left generally agree that capitalism is unsustainable, if only for environmental reasons, and favor more socialistic systems, we have neither formulated nor effectively mobilized for a fundamentally new world-system. If such a truly revolutionary movement is still out of our reach, the wholesale destruction wrought by capitalism and the immense disparities of wealth and opportunity it has created, particularly in its neoliberal form, may yet trigger systemic collapse. Islamic militants and messianic Jews and Christians, among others, know exactly what system should succeed it. Hopefully, the progressive left could scramble in the event of collapse and, if not exactly proactive, manage to offer an alternative world-system of its own.

An effective anti-pacification campaign might begin with activism—that is the immediate aim of this book—but would have to assume the proportions of counter-hegemony if it truly aspired to counter the "hegemonic tasks" and profits driving militarism and securitization. One offshoot of this book will be the mounting of a website graphically mapping out weapons systems, their technologies and uses. It will place technologies of control within the context of the global arms and security trade, linking that, in turn, with current conflicts being waged throughout the world-system and what lies behind them. And it will examine ways and instances where hegemony is being enforced, be they in military conflicts, domestic campaigns of securitization or the manipulation of "consensus." In this endeavor, of course, I will link up with other critical scholars and activists, many of whose works are referenced in these pages. By helping to focus and coordinate disparate activist activities and academic studies, my hope is that an anti-pacification campaign, when linked to those of the other "scapes," may give rise to a genuinely left/progressive movement of counter-hegemony.

No campaign of counter-hegemony can succeed, of course, without an informed vision around which to mobilize. In a packed auditorium at the 2010 North American Social Forum in Detroit, Michigan, Immanuel Wallerstein spoke about the structural crisis in capitalism. Founded on the endless and increasingly competitive accumulation of capital in which everything is commodified, the present world-system survives—or rather its elites survive—thanks mainly to militarization and securitization. This reality will only intensify as the world-system begins to implode under the weight of population growth and migration, urbanization, competition for scarce resources, inequities caused by differential access to vital technologies, environmental destruction, conflicts unprecedented in their levels of violence and fought with unimaginably powerful weapons, eroding freedoms and more.

This dismal forecast took an inspiring and useful turn, however, when a young person in the audience asked him what alternative system he envisioned. Struggling a bit to formulate his answer, Wallerstein admitted he had no concrete plan, but he did offer the essential elements of a humane, inclusive, just, counter-hegemonic, counter-capitalist system. It must embody, he said, the antithesis of relentless economic growth and the exploitation of people and the environment. It must be non-hierarchical, as least in terms of flattening the huge disparities that exist between the classes worldwide, and must be able to address polarization and alienation—of people from people, from the environment, from their own lands and from their own identities. In this new world-system, militarism and the obsession over securitization would no longer have a role; pacification would be pointless. This is a vision that could well guide our movement of counter-hegemony and anti-security. Critical visionaries need to be given a more prominent place at our table.

But how could a truly just alternative be structured? Here intellectuals and academics play a key role. They provide much of the analysis upon which programs must be based—and there is a plethora of progressive analyses and programs out there, much of it unfortunately confined to academic discourse, to which most people have little access, or else it is pursued in a fragmentary way by activist groups. Community-based, participatory institutes—popular think-tanks—need to be established to ensure a mutually profitable interchange: that activists and others not associated with the university have access to critical knowledge, concepts and analyses essential for formulating effective campaigns, while activists have a way of communicating their concerns and issues to academics and professionals, thus raising the level of advocacy. Community-based think-tanks would nurture what Robert Cox calls "organic intellectuals" from the grassroots.[2] I am involved, for instance, in establishing an Institute for Strategic Activism, part of a movement to provide an infrastructure of counter-hegemony.[3]

Thus empowered, community-based organizations, linked into national, regional and global coalitions, could then formulate, organize and sustain "bottom-up" initiatives. As unsexy as it may sound, a movement for systemic change needs an infrastructure. Social Forums have played an important role in grass-roots networking and brainstorming on a regional and global scale, but with no structures to ensure follow-up, they dissipate. Each organization returns to its locale and particular set of issues, again isolated. Institutions of popular education and action-research must be established, together with community-based media, and participatory cultural and political forums, all sustained by community-based economic enterprises. And they must be linked by networks that facilitate brainstorming and envisioning, the sharing of analyses, materials and initiatives and on to engendering collective endeavors that span the various "scapes."

If this work has helped "arm" us with a broad picture of the global pacification system and has thus helped define an agenda for the forces of anti-security and counter-hegemony, then it will have achieved its purpose. War amongst the people is in fact war against the people, and we must use that realization to mobilize against pacification and the world-system it supports. After all, who wants to be pacified?

Notes

Introduction

1. Noam Chomsky, "The Real Reasons the U.S. Enables Israeli Crimes and Atrocities." *Alertnet* interview, 2010. Retrieved at: <http://www.alternet.org/story/147865/noam_chomsky%3A_the_real_reasons_the_u.s._enables_israeli_crimes_and_atrocities>.
2. The Iraq Study Group Report, 2006, pp. 7, 33. Retrieved at: <http://bakerinstitute.org/media/files/news/8a41607c/iraqstudygroup_findings.pdf>.
3. Ali Abunimah, "When Former CIA Chief David Petraeus Enraged the Israel Lobby." *Electronic Intifada*, November 10, 2012. Retrieved at: <http://electronicintifada.net/blogs/ali-abunimah/when-former-cia-chief-david-petraeus-enraged-israel-lobby>.
4. Small Arms Survey, *Civilian Inventories*, 2013. Retrieved at: <http://www.smallarmssurvey.org/de/weapons-and-markets/stockpiles/civilian-inventories.html>.
5. Peter Evans, "Counterhegemonic Globalization: Transnational Social Movements in the Contemporary Global Political Economy," in Thomas Janoski (ed.), *Handbook of Political Sociology: States, Civil Societies, and Globalization.* Cambridge: Cambridge University Press, 2005, pp. 444–50.

Chapter 1

1. Alan Freeman and Boris Kagarlitsky (eds.), "Introduction: World Empire – or a World of Empires?" *The Politics of Empire: Globalisation in Crisis.* London: Pluto, 2004, p. 8.
2. Mike Davis, *Planet of Slums.* London: Verso, 2006.
3. World-systems analysis has been developed over the years by Immanual Wallerstein, Samir Amin, Beverly Silver, Giovanni Arrighi, Terence Hopkins, Andre Gunder Frank, Christopher Chase-Dunn, Waldon Bello and others. See also Gary Gereffi and Manual Korzeniewicz (eds.), *Commodity Chains and Global Capitalism.* Westport, CT: Greenwood, 1994.
4. Jim O'Neil, "Who You Calling a BRIC?" *Bloomberg News*, November 12, 2013. Retrieved at: <http://www.bloomberg.com/news/articles/2013-11-12/who-you-calling-a-bric->.
5. David Harvey, *Brief History of Neo-Liberalism.* Oxford: Oxford University Press, 2005, p. 145.
6. Evans, "Counterhegemonic Globalization," p. 657; Harvey, *Brief History*, pp. 64–86; 152–82.
7. Mark Neocleous, " 'A Brighter and Nicer New Life': Security as Pacification," *Social Legal Studies* 20(2): 24, 2011.

8. S.P. Reyna, "Deadly Developments and Phantasmagoric Representations," in S.P Reyna and R.E. Downs (eds.), *Deadly Developments: Capitalism, States and War*. Amsterdam: Gordon and Breach, 1999, pp. 16, 23–67; Eric Wolfe, *Europe and the People Without History*. Berkeley: University of California Press, 1982.

9. Mark Neocleous, "Security as Pacification," in Mark Neocleous and George S. Rigakos (eds.), *Anti-Security*. Ottawa: Quill Books, 2010, pp. 24–56.

10. Virilio, Paul and Sylvere Lotringer, *Pure War*. New York: Semiotext(e), 1983.

11. Mark Duffield, *Development, Security and Unending War: Governing the World of Peoples*. Cambridge: Polity Press, 2007; Paul Amar, *The Security Archipelago: Human-Security States, Sexuality Politics, and the End of Neoliberalism*. Durham, NC: Duke University Press, 2013; Stephen Graham, *Cities Under Siege: The New Military Urbanism*. London: Verso, 2010; Ross Glover, "The War on _____," in John Collins and Ross Glover (eds.). *Collateral Language: A User's Guide to America's New War*. New York: NYU Press, 2002, pp. 155–73.

12. Allen Feldman, "Securocratic Wars of Public Safety: Globalized Policing as Scopic Regime." *Interventions* 6(3): 330–50, 2004; Graham, *Cities*.

13. Rupert Smith, *The Utility of Force: The Art of War in the Modern World*. New York: Vintage Books, 2005.

14. Michael T. Klare, *Resource Wars*. New York: Henry Holt, 2001; William Tabb "Resource Wars." *Monthly Review* 58(8): 32–42, 2007.

15. Martin van Creveld, *The Changing Face of War: Lessons of Combat, from the Marne to Iraq*. New York: Ballantine, 2006.

16. Neocleous, "Brighter"; Mark Neocleous, George Rigakos and Tyler Wall (eds.), "On Pacification: Introduction to the Special Issue." *Socialist Studies* 9(2): 1–31, 2013, among others.

17. George Rigakos, "'To Extend the Scope of Productive Labour': Pacification as a Police Project," in Mark Neocleous and George S. Rigakos (eds.). *Anti-Security*. Ottawa: Quill Books, 2011, pp. 62.

18. Ibid., p. 64.

19. Neocleous, "Brighter," p. 26; Rigakos, "To Extend the Scope," pp. 62, 63.

20. Brad Evans, "Foucault's Legacy: Security, War and Violence in the 21st Century." *Security Dialogue* 41: 413–33, 2012; Marcus Kienscherf, "A Programme of Global Pacification: US Counterinsurgency Doctrine and the Biopolitics of Human (In) security." *Security Dialogue* 42: 517–35, 2011. Retrieved at: <http://sdi.sagepub.com/search?author1=Markus+Kienscherf&sortspec=date&submit=Submit>; Thomas Lemke, *Foucault, Governmentality, and Critique*, 2000. Retrieved at: <http://www.andosciasociology.net/resources/Foucault$2C+Governmentality$2C+and+Critique+IV-2.pdf>.

21. Robert Cox, "Gramsci, Historical Materialism and International Relations," in Stephen Gill (ed.). *Gramsci, Historical Materialism and International Relations*. Cambridge: Cambridge University Press, 1993, pp. 43–4.

22. John Agnew, *Hegemony: The New Shape Of Global Power*. Philadelphia, PA: Temple University Press, 2005; Joseph Nye, Jr., *Soft Power: The Means to Success in World Politics*. New York: Public Affairs, 2004.

23. Carl Conetta, *An Undisciplined Defense: Understanding the $2 Trillion Surge in US Defense Spending*. Project on Defense Alternatives Briefing Report #20, January 18, 2010. Cambridge, MA: Commonwealth Institute, p. 43.

24. US Department of Defense, "Hagel Outlines Budget Reducing Troop Strength, Force Structure," 2014. Retrieved at: <http://www.defense.gov/news/news article.aspx?id=121703>.

25. Dinah Walker, "Trends in Military Spending." *Council on Foreign Relations*, 2014. Retrieved at: <http://www.cfr.org/defense-budget/trends-us-military-spending/ p28855>.

26. Conetta, *Undisciplined Defense*, p. 43; Richard F. Grimmett, *Conventional Arms Transfers to Developing Nations, 2001–2008*. Washington, DC: CRS Report for Congress.

27. UK Department of Defence, *Strategic Defence Review*, 1998. Retrieved at: <http://fissilematerials.org/library/mod98.pdf>.

28. Robert Gates, US Department of Defense, 2008. Retrieved at: <http://www. defense.gov/qdr/gates-article.html>.

29. *Quadrennial Defense Review (QDR)*, Department of Defense, Washington, DC, p. iv. Retrieved at: <http://www.defense.gov/qdr/qdr%20as%20of%20 29jan10%201600.pdf>.

30. Rick Rozoff, "America's Imperial Design. Prompt Global Strike: World Military Superiority Without Nuclear Weapons." *Global Research*, April 11, 2010. Retrieved at: <http://www.globalresearch.ca/america-s-imperial-design-prompt-global-strike-world-military-superiority-without-nuclear-weapons/18595>.

31. *QDR*, 2006, p. 29.

32. Office of the Secretary of Defense, *Military and Security Developments Involving the People's Republic of China: 2011*. Washington, DC: Department of Defense, 2011.

33. SIPRI (Stockholm International Peace Research Institute), *Military Expenditure Database, 2015*. Retrieved at: <http://www.sipri.org/research/armaments/milex/ recent-trends>.

34. Office of the Secretary of Defense, *China*.

35. *QDR* 2006, pp. 28-29; SIPRI, *Database, 2015*.

36. SIPRI, *Database, 2015*.

37. Meredith Reid Sarkees and Frank Whelon Wayman, *Resort to War: A Data Guide to Interstate, Extra-State, Intra-state, and Non-State Wars, 1816–2007*. Washington, DC: CQ Press, 2010; List of interstate wars retrieved at: <http:// www.correlatesofwar.org/COW2%20Data/WarData_NEW/ListInterstateWars. pdf>.

38. van Creveld, *Changing Face*, p. 187.

39. William K. Carroll, "Hegemony, Counter-hegemony, Anti-hegemony." *Studies in Social Justice* 1:1 (2007): 12.

40. Noam Chomsky, *The New Military Humanism: Lessons From Kosovo*. Monroe, ME: Common Courage Press, 1999.

41. Michael Ignatieff, *Empire Lite: Nation-Building in Bosnia, Kosovo and Afghanistan*. Toronto: Penguin, 2003.

42. Duffield, *Development*, p. 126.

43. van Creveld, *Changing Face*, p. 187.

44. Mary Kaldor, *New and Old Wars: Organized Violence in a Global Era*. Cambridge: Polity Press, 2006.

45. Tabb, "Resource Wars."

46. Kaldor, *New Wars*, p. 107.

47. *QDR* 2006, p. 9.

48. *QDR* 2006, p. v.

49. US Joint Forces Command, quoted in Russell W. Glenn, "Thoughts on 'Hybrid' Conflict." *Small Wars Journal*, March 2, 2009. Retrieved at: <http://smallwarsjournal.com/jrnl/art/thoughts-on-hybrid-conflict>.

50. SIPRI, *Database, 2015*; Matthew Bodner, "Why Russia Ended its Ban on Selling Advanced Air Defense Systems to Iran." *The Moscow Times*, April 14, 2015. Retrieved at: <http://www.themoscowtimes.com/business/article/putin-acts-to-grab-iran-arms-market-for-russia/519105.html>.

51. Patrick Cockburn, "Iraq Crisis: How Saudi Arabia Helped Isis Take Over the North of the Country." *The Independent*, July 13, 2014. Retrieved at: <http://www.independent.co.uk/voices/comment/iraq-crisis-how-saudi-arabia-helped-isis-take-over-the-north-of-the-country-9602312.html>.

52. SIPRI, *SIPRI Military Expenditure Database*, 2015.

53. *QDR* 2006; Klare, *Resource Wars*.

54. Davis, *Planet*, pp. 203, 205

55. James N. Mattis, "Future Warfare: The Rise of Hybrid Wars." *Proceedings Magazine* 132(11): 1, 233, 2007. Retrieved at: <http://milnewstbay.pbworks.com/f/MattisFourBlockWarUSNINov2005.pdf>.

56. Smith, *Utility*, p. 19.

57. Graham, *Cities*, p. xiii.

58. Duffield, *Development*; Amar, *Archipelago*; Giorgio Agamben, *Homo Sacer: Sovereign Power and Bare Life*. Stanford, CA: Stanford University Press, 1998.

59. Duffield, *Development*, p. 28.

60. van Creveld, *Changing Face*, p. 268.

61. Neocleous, Rigakos and Wall, *Socialist Studies*; Neocleous, "Brighter."

62. Amar, *Archipelago*.

63. Graham, *Cities*, pp. xiii, XV, 96.

64. Colin Crouch, *The Strange Non-Death of Neo-Liberalism*. Cambridge: Polity Press, 2011; P.W. Singer, *Wired for War: The Robotics Revolution and Conflict in the 21st Century*. New York: Penguin, 2003; Solomon Hughes, *War on Terror, Inc.: Corporate Profiteering from the Politics of Fear*. London: Verso, 2007; S. Perlo-Freeman and E. Sköns, "The Private Military Services Industry," SIPRI Research Paper 001, 2008.

65. Naomi Klein *The Shock Doctrine: The Rise of Disaster Capitalism*. New York: Henry Holt, 2007, p. 15; Market and Markets 2013, *Global Home Security and Emergency Management Market, 2013–2018*. Retrieved at: <https://www.academia.edu/3520288/Homeland_Security_Market_-_Global_Forecast_-_2018>.

66. Klein, *Shock Doctrine*, p. 14.

67. Fred Kaplan, *David Petraeus and the Plot to Change the American Way of War*. New York: Simon and Schuster, 2013, p. 71.

68. Ibid.

69. Michael Dillon and Julian Reid, *The Liberal Way of War: Killing to Make Life Live*. Routledge: London, 2009, p. 87.

70. US Department of Defense, *Dictionary of Military and Associated Terms*. Washington, DC: Department of Defense, 2004, p. 64.

71. Christopher Bowie, Robert P. Hafa, Jr. and Robert E. Mullins, "Trends in Future Warfare." *Joint Force Quarterly* (Summer), 2003, p. 132.

72. Colin Gray, *Another Bloody Century: Future Warfare.* London: Phoenix, 2005, pp. 169–70.

73. Graham, *Cities*, p. xv.

74. Neocleous, Rigakos and Wall, *Socialist Studies*, pp. 8–9.

Chapter 2

1. Andrew Feinstein, *The Shadow World: Inside the Global Arms Trade.* Johannesburg: Jonathan Ball, 2011.

2. Jeremy Scahill, *Dirty Wars: The World is a Battlefield.* New York: Nation Books, 2013.

3. Thomas C. Schelling, *Arms and Influence.* New Haven, CT: Yale University Press, 2008.

4. Yehezkel Dror, *Israeli Statecraft: National Security Challenges and Responses.* London: Routledge, 2011.

5. Jacob Abadi, *Israel's Quest for Recognition and Acceptance in Asia: Garrison State Diplomacy.* London: Frank Cass, 2004.

6. Victor Perera, "Uzi Diplomacy: How Israel Makes Friends and Enemies Throughout the World." *Mother Jones* 10(6) (1985): 40–48.

7. Aaron Klieman, *Israel's Global Reach: Arms Sales as Diplomacy.* Oxford: Brassey's, 1985.

8. INSS (The Institute for National Security Studies), *Strategic Survey for Israel, 2014–15,* 2015, pp. 170–71. Retrieved at: <www.inss.org.il/ uploadImages/ systemFiles/INSS2014-15Balance_ENG%20(2).pdf>; SIPRI, *Background Paper on SIPRI Military Expenditure Data, 2011,* 2012. Retrieved at: <http://www.sipri. org/media/pressreleases/press-release-translations-2012bgeng.pdf>.

9. SIPRI, *Military Expenditure Database,* 2010.

10. Ze'ev Maoz, *Defending the Holy Land: A Critical Analysis of Israel's Security & Foreign Policy.* Ann Arbor: University of Michigan Press, 2006, pp. 5, 231.

11. Bonn International Center for Conversion 2014, *The Global Militarisation Index (GMI),* p. 5. Retrieved at: <https://www.bicc.de/uploads/tx_bicctools/141209_ GMI_ENG.pdf>.

12. Uri Ben-Eliezer, *The Making of Israeli Militarism.* Bloomington: Indiana University Press, 1998, pp. x, 7–8.

13. Ibid., pp. 194–5.

14. Yoram Peri, *Generals in the Cabinet Room: How the Military Shapes Israeli Policy.* Washington, DC: United States Institute of Peace Press, 2006, p. 19; Baruch Kimmerling, "Patterns of Militarism in Israel." *European Journal of Sociology* 34 (1993): 196–221.

15. Ben-Eliezer, *Israeli Militarism,* pp. 13–14, 194; Joyce Robbins and Uri Ben-Eliezer, "New Roles or "New Times"? Gender Inequality and Militarism in Israel's Nation-in-Arms." *Social Politics: International Studies in Gender, State & Society* 7(3) (2000): 309–42.

16. Ben-Eliezer, quoted in Peri, *Generals,* p. 22.

17. Ben Eliezer, *Militarism,* p. 195.

18. Shlomo Gazit, *Trapped Fools: Thirty Years of Israeli Policy in the Territories.* London: Frank Cass, 2003, pp. 8–11, 20–22.

19. Stewart Reiser, *The Israeli Arms Industry: Foreign Policy, Arms, Transfers, and Military Doctrine of a Small State.* New York: Holmes & Meier, 1989.

20. Maoz, *Defending*, p. 5.

21. Ibid., pp. 40–41.

22. Peri, *Generals*, pp. 217–18.

23. Reiser, *Industry*, pp. 31–77.

24. Ibid., pp. 43–5; Avraham Ben Zvi, *John F. Kennedy and the Politics of Arms Sales to Israel.* London: Frank Cass, 2002.

25. Donald Neff, "Israel's Technology Transfers to China." *Washington Report on Middle East Affairs*, June/July, 1997: 70.

26. Klieman, *Global Reach*, p. 175.

27. Reiser, *Industry*, p. 132.

28. Ibid., p. 135.

29. Ibid., pp. 135–6.

30. Ibid., p. 132.

31. Ibid., p. 160.

32. Gordon, "Working Paper," p. 20.

33. Charles D. Freilich, *Zion's Dilemmas: How Israel Makes National Security Policy.* Ithaca, NY: Cornell University Press, 2012.

34. Martin van Creveld, *The Sword And The Olive: A Critical History Of The Israeli Defense Force.* New York: Public Affairs, 1998, p. 17.

35. Ibid., p. 17; Rashid Khalidi, *Palestinian Identity: The Construction of Modern National Consciousness.* New York: Columbia University Press, pp. 105–11; Benny Morris, *Righteous Victims: A History of the Zionist-Arab Conflict, 1881–1949.* New York: Knopf, 1999, pp. 59–63.

36. Maoz, *Defending*, p. 232; Morris, *Victims*, p. 53; Yigal Allon, *The Making of Israel's Army.* London: Valentine, 1970, p. 4.

37. Morris, *Victims*; Ilan Pappe, *The Ethnic Cleansing of Palestine*, Oxford: One World Publications, 2007.

38. Morris, *Victims*, pp. 260, 269–328.

39. Israel Shahak, *Israel's Global Role: Weapons for Repression.* Belmont, MA: Association of Arab-American University Graduates, 1982.

40. Steve Goldfield, *Garrison State: Israel's Role in U.S. Global Strategy.* New York: EAFORD, 1985.

41. Bishara Bahbah, *Israel and Latin America: The Military Connection.* New York: St. Martin's Press, 1986.

42. Milton Jamail and Margo Gutierrez, *It's No Secret: Israel's Military Involvement in Central America.* Belmont, MA: Association of Arab-American University Graduates, 1986.

43. Benjamin Beit-Hallahmi, *The Israeli Connection: Whom Israel Arms and Why.* New York: Pantheon, 1987.

44. Andrew Cockburn and Leslie Cockburn, *Dangerous Liaison: The Inside Story of the U.S.-Israeli Covert Relationship.* New York: HarperCollins, 1991.

45. Baylis Thomas, *The Dark Side of Zionism: Israel's Quest for Security Through Dominance.* Lanham, MD: Lexington Books, 2009.

46. IJAN (International Jewish Anti-Zionist Network), *Israel's Worldwide Role in Repression*, 2012. Retrieved at: <http://israelglobalrepression.files.wordpress. com/2012/12/israels-worldwide-role-in-repression-footnotes-finalized.pdf>.

47. Ian Almond, "British and Israeli Assistance to U.S. Strategies of Torture and Counterinsurgency in Central and Latin America, 1967–96: An Argument Against Complexification." *Journal of Critical Globalisation Studies* (2013), 6: 57–77. Retrieved at: <http://www.criticalglobalisation.com/Issue6/57_77_BRITISH_ISRAELI_JCGS6.pdf>.

48. Shahak, *Israel's Global Role*, p. 15.

49. Beit Hallahmi, *Israel Connection*, p. xii.

50. Ya'akov Amidror, "Winning Counterinsurgency War." *Strategic Perspectives.* Jerusalem: Jerusalem Center for Public Affairs, 2008, pp. 11–14. Retrieved at <http://jcpa.org/text/Amidror-perspectives-2.pdf>.

51. Klieman, *Global Reach*, p. 30.

52. Ibid., pp. 36–46.

53. Barbara Opall-Rome, "Israel Limits Security Cooperation with Russia." *Defense News*, June 1, 2014. Retrieved at: <http://www.defensenews.com/apps/pbcs.dll/article?AID=2014306010019>.

54. Klieman, *Global Reach*, p. 36.

55. P.R. Kumaraswamy, "Israel-China Arms Trade: Unfreezing Times." *Middle East Institute*, 2012. Retrieved at: <http://www.mei.edu/content/israel-china-arms-trade-unfreezing-times>.

56. Stephen Zunes, *The Israel Lobby: How Powerful is it Really?* Washington, DC: Foreign Policy in Focus, May 16, 2006.

57. Klieman, *Global Reach*, p. 46.

58. Ibid., p. 41.

59. Bahbah, *Latin America*, p. 98.

60. Klieman, *Global Reach*, p. 38.

61. Ibid., p. 38; See also Alvite Singh Ningthoujam, "Return of Israel's Arms Sales Diplomacy?" *Jerusalem Post*, June 24, 2013.

62. Klieman, *Global Reach*, pp. 29–30, 45–46; Maoz, *Defending*, pp. 8–9; Daniel Bar-Tal, Dan Jacobson and Aharon Klieman, *Security Concerns: Insights from the Israeli Experience*. Stamford, CT: JAI Press, 1998, pp. 8–88; Shay Shabtai, "Israel's National Security Concept: New Basic Terms in the Military-Security Sphere." *Strategic Assessment* (2010) 13(2): 7–18.

63. Avraham Ben-Zvi, *Lyndon B. Johnson and the Politics of Sales to Israel*. London: Frank Cass, 2004.

64. Neff, "Transfers," p. 70.

65. Jeremy M. Sharp, *U.S. Foreign Aid to Israel*. Washington, DC: CRS Report for Congress, 2014. Retrieved at: <https://fas.org/sgp/crs/mideast/RL33222.pdf>, Summary.

66. Adam Gonn, "Israeli Arms Industry a Major Economic Engine." *Xinhuanet*, 2011. Retrieved at: <http://news.xinhuanet.com/english2010/world/2011-06/20/c_13938425.htm>.

67. Clyde Mark, *Israel: Foreign Assistance*. Washington, DC: CRS Issue brief for Congress, 2005, p. 5. Retrieved at: <http://fas.org/sgp/crs/mideast/IB85066.pdf>.

68. <http://www.gpo.gov/fdsys/pkg/PLAW-110publ429/html/PLAW-110publ429. htm>.

69. Sharp, *Foreign Aid*, p. 3.

70. SIPRI, *The SIPRI Military Expenditure Database, 2014*, p. 260. Retrieved at:<http://www.sipri.org/research/armaments/milex_database>; QCEA (Quaker Council for European Affairs), *Security Cooperation Between the EU and Israel*, 2011. Retrieved at: <http://www.qcea.org/wp-content/uploads/2011/04/bp-mideast-secresearch-en-mar-2011.pdf>.

71. Richard F. Grimmett and Paul K. Kerr, *Conventional Arms Transfers to Developing Nations, 2004–2011*. Washington, DC: CRS Report for Congress, 2012, p. 4. Retrieved at <http://www.fas.org/sgp/crs/weapons/R42678.pdf>.

72. Tony Cappacio, "Gates Says Israel Gave In on Saudi Arms After F-35 Pledge." *Bloomberg News*, January 9, 2014. Retrieved at: <http://www.bloomberg.com/news/2014-01-09/gates-says-israel-gave-in-on-saudi-arms-after-f-35-pledge. html>; Walter Pincus, United States Needs to Reevaluate Its Assistance to Israel. *The Washington Post*, October 18, 2011.

73. Avi Lewis, "Cabinet Authorizes Purchase of 14 F-35 Fighter Jets." *Times of Israel*, December 1, 2014. Retrieved at: <www.timesofisrael.com/cabinet-authorizes-purchase-of-14-f-35-fighter-jets>.

74. Alon Ben David, "IAI Opens Production Line For F-35 Wings." *Aviation Week & Space Technology*, November 19, 2014. Retrieved at: <http://aviationweek.com/author/alon-ben-david-1>; Wendela de Vries, "F-35 Might Undercut European Arms Export Policy." *Stop Wapenhandel*, 2015. Retrieved at: <http://www. stopwapenhandel.org/node/1693>.

75. Council on Foreign Relations, *The Campaign to Ban Cluster Bombs*, 2006. Retrieved at: <http://www.cfr.org/weapons-of-mass-destruction/campaign-ban-cluster-bombs/p12060>; Global Security, *Guided Bomb Unit-28 (GBU-28)*, 2012. Retrieved at: <http://www.globalsecurity.org/military/systems/munitions/gbu-28.htm>.

76. Global Security, *F-16I Sufa (Storm)*. Retrieved at: <http://www.globalsecurity. org/military/world/israel/f-16i.htm>.

77. Sharp, *Foreign Aid, 2014*, pp. 6–7.

78. Jeremy M. Sharp, *U.S. Foreign Aid to Israel*. Washington, DC: CRS Report for Congress, 2012.

79. "Congress Triples Obama's Request on Defense Cooperation with Israel." *Times of Israel*, December 12, 2013. Retrieved at: <http://www.timesofisrael.com/congress-triples-obamas-request-on-defense-cooperation-with-israel>.

80. Ken Klippenstein and Paul Gottinger, "US Congress Passes Bill Increasing Weapons in Israel by $200 Million." *Middle East Monitor*, December 20, 2014. Retrieved at: <https://www.middleeastmonitor.com/articles/middle-east/15913-us-congress-passes-bill-increasing-weapons-in-israel-by-200-million>.

81. Naval Technology. *Eilat Class, Israel*, n.d. Retrieved at: <www.naval-technology. com/projects/saar5>.

82. Gonn, "Israeli Arms"; Yaacov Lifshitz, *The Economics of Producing Defense: Illustrated by the Israeli Case*. Boston, MA: Kluwer, 2007.

83. Bassam Haddad, "US on UN Veto: 'Disgusting', 'Shameful', 'Deplorable'", 'a Travesty' … Really?" *Jadaliyya*, February 5, 2012. Retrieved at: <http://www.jadaliyya.com/pages/index/4237/us-on-un-veto_disgusting-shameful-deplorable-a-tra>.

84. European Commission, "Dual-use Controls," 2012. Retrieved at: <http://ec.europa.eu/trade/import-and-export-rules/export-from-eu/dual-use-controls>.

85. EU Arms Export, *Thirteenth Annual Report on Exports Control of Military Technology and Equipment*, pp. 140–44. Retrieved at: <http://eur-lex.europa.eu/LexUriServ/LexUriServ.do?uri=OJ:C:2011:382:FULL:EN:PD>.

86. QCEA, *The Arms Trade between EU Member States and Israel*, 2010. Retrieved at: <http://static.qcea.org/wp-content/uploads/2011/04/bp-mideast-euisraelarms-en-dec-2010.pdf?9d7bd4>.

87. David Cronin, "France: 'Defying Rules on Arms Sales to Israel'," 2009. Retrieved at: <http://ipsnews.net/news.asp?idnews=47025>.

88. Arie Egozi, "Will IAI's Heron-TP Become NATO's MALE UAS?" *Flightglobal Blogs*, 2012. Retrieved at: <http://www.flightglobal.com/blogs/ariel-view/2012/05/will-iais-heron-tp-become-natos-male-uas.html>.

89. Global Security, *Weapons of Mass Destruction: Dolphin*, Retrieved at: <http://www.globalsecurity.org/wmd/world/israel/dolphin.htm>; Otfried Nassauer, personal communication, 2009.

90. Defense News, *Israel Completes $1B Jet Trainer Deal*, 2012. Retrieved at: <http://www.defensenews.com/article/20120719/DEFREG04/307190004/Israel-Completes-1B-Jet-Trainer-Deal>.

91. Judy Siegel-Itzkovitch, "Italy, Israel to Build Nano Lab Together." *Jerusalem Post*, May 5, 2008.

92. Saferworld, *Arms Production, Exports and Decision-Making in Central and Eastern Europe*, 2002. Retrieved at: <http://www.saferworld.org.uk/smartweb/resources/view-resource/68>.

93. Alejandro Pozo Marín, *Spain-Israel: Military, Homeland Security and Armament-Based Relations Affairs and Trends*, 2009. Barcelona: Delàs Peace Research Centre.

94. Globes, *Rafael Wins Huge Anti-Tank Missile Order from Spain*, 2007. Retrieved at: <http://archive.globes.co.il/searchgl/The%20$425%20million%20contract%20is%20part%20of%20collaboration_s_hd_1L3atE3GpN34mC30nDp4tCpokQ7HjR000.html>.

95. Bruno Jäntti, "Finnish-Israeli Arms Trade Flouts EU Regulations." *Electronic Intifada*, May 27, 2009. Retrieved at: <http://electronicintifada.net/v2/article10557.shtml>; Bruno Jäntti and Jimmy Johnson, "Finland Shopping for 'Battle-tested' Israeli Weaponry." *Electronic Intifada*. Retrieved at: <http://electronicintifada.net/content/finland-shopping-battle-tested-israeli-weaponry/9847>, January 18, 2011.

96. Defense Industry Daily, "Finland to Field Israeli Orbiter UAVs." 2012. Retrieved at: <http://www.defenseindustrydaily.com/Finland-to-Field-Israeli-Orbiter-UAVs-07380>.

97. David Cronin, *How Israeli Arms Companies Benefit from European Union Science Funds*, 2009. Retrieved at: <http://www.silviacattori.net/article1077.html>; QCEA, *Security Cooperation*.

98. Cordis News, "Israel Will Take Part in Horizon 2020." 2013. Retrieved at: <http://cordis.europa.eu/news/rcn/36298_en.html>.

99. Ben Hayes, "How the EU Subsidises Israel's Military-Industrial Complex." *Open Democracy*, 2013. Retrieved at: <http://www.opendemocracy.net/ben-hayes/how-eu-subsidises-israel%E2%80%99s-military-industrial-complex>.

100 Cronin, "France."

101. Egozi, "Heron-TP"; Rick Rozoff, *Israel: Global NATO's 29th Member*, 2010. Retrieved at: <www.australia.to/2010>.

102. Rotzoff, "Israel."

103. Jewish Telegraphic Agency, June 27, 2006.

104. Lea Landman, "US-Europe-Israeli Trilateral Relationship: The Strategic Dimension." 2010 (emphasis added). Retrieved at: <http://www.herzliyaconference.org/_Uploads/3058Trilateral_partnership.pdf>.

105. Reiser, *Industry*, p. 129.

106. Ibid., pp. 129–31.

107. Ibid., pp. 132–4.

108. Maoz, *Defending*. p. 15.

109. Reiser, *Industry*, p. 234.

110. Maoz, *Defending*, p. 12.

111. Stuart Cohen, *Israel and Its Army: From Cohesion to Confusion*. London: Routledge, 2008; Seymour Hersh, *The Samson Option: Israel's Nuclear Arsenal and American Foreign Policy*. New York: Random House, 1991; Hans M. Kristensen and Robert S. Norris, "Israeli Nuclear Weapons, 2014." *Bulletin of the Atomic Scientists* (2014) 70(6): 97–115.

112. Neff, "Transfers."

113. Frederik Stakelbeck, Jr., "The Israel-US Bilateral Relationship Needs to be Mended." *The National Interest* (2005). Retrieved at: <http://nationalinterest.org/article/israel-and-china-2746>.

114. Sudha Ramachandran, "US Up in Arms Over Sino-Israel Ties." *Asia Times*, December 21, 2004; Kumaraswamy, "India-China."

115. Naser al-Tamimi, "The Uncertain Future of China-Israel Relations." *Al Arabiya News*, April 4, 2014.

116. Klieman, *Global Reach*, p. 26.

117. Arms Control Association 2012 *Nuclear Weapons: What Has What at a Glance*. Retrieved at: <http://www.armscontrol.org/factsheets/Nuclearweaponswhohaswhat>.

118. Klieman, *Global Reach*, pp. 38, 39.

119. Uzi Eilam, *Defense Export Control in 2007: State of Affairs*. The Institute for National Security Studies, 2007, p. 59. Retrieved at: <http://www.inss.org.il/uploadImages/systemFiles/AdkanEng9_4_Eilam.pdf>.

120. Aluf Benn, "Who Does Israel Sell Arms To? The Defense Ministry Won't Tell." *Ha'aretz*, January 9, 2014. Retrieved at: <http://www.haaretz.com/news/diplomacy-defense/1.567696>; Itay Mack, personal communication.

121. Klieman, *Global Reach*, p. 45.

122. Beit Hallahmi, *Israel Connection*, pp. 243–8.

123. Klieman, *Global Reach*, pp. 39–40.

124. Ibid., p. 63; Jane Hunter, *Israeli Foreign Policy: South Africa and Central America*. Boston, MA: South End Press, 1987; SIPRI, *Military Expenditure*, 2014.

125. Defense Update, *David's Sling – Israel's Extended Air and Missile Defense*, 2010. Retrieved at: <http://defense-update.com/products/d/david_sling_271009.html>.

126. Grimmett and Kerr, *Arms Transfers*, p. 80; HIS/Jane's Press Room, *Peak Defence on Horizon as US, UK & Europe Erodes Competitive Edge*. Retrieved at: <http://press.ihs.com/press-release/country-industry-forecasting/peak-defence-horizon-us-uk-europe-erodes-competitive-edge>.

127. SIPRI, *Military Expenditure*, 2014.

128. *Israel High-Tech and Investment Report*, September 2004. Retrieved at: <http://www.ishitech.co.il/0904ar4.htm>.

129. Ran Dagoni, "Defense Exports Fall 10%." *Globes*, December 10, 2008. Retrieved at: <http://www.globes.co.il/en/article-1000406070>.

130. Klieman, *Global Reach*, pp. 53–69.

131. SIPRI, *Military Expenditure*, 2014.

132. Ibid.

133. Israeli Ministry of Industry and Trade 2010. Retrieved at: <http://www.moital.gov.il/NR/rdonlyres/3725F17F-5A8C-4B53-BBBD-69AC5AD8CC4B/0/epicosisrael2010.pdf>; Neve Gordon, "Working Paper III: The Political Economy of Israel's Homeland Security/Surveillance Industry." Kingston: Surveillance Study Centre at Queen's University, 2009. Retrieved at: <http://www.sscqueens.org/sites/default/files/The%20Political%20Economy%20of%20Israel's%20Homeland%20Security.pdf >.

134. Jimmy Johnson, "Israel's Export of Occupation Police Tactics." *Electronic Intifada*, October 9, 2009. Retrieved at: <http://electronicintifada.net/content/israels-export-occupation-police-tactics/8485>.

Chapter 3

1. Chalmers Johnson, *The Sorrows of Empire: Militarism, Secrecy and the End of the Republic*. New York: Metropolitan Books, 2004, pp. 151–85.

2. IDF website, *International Commando Teams Train with the IDF in Israel*, 2010. Retrieved at: <http://dover.idf.il/IDF/English/News/today/10/01/2603.htm>.

3. Richard A. Bitzinger, "Introduction: Challenges Facing the Global Arms Industry in the 21st Century," in Richard A. Bitzinger (ed.). *The Modern Defense Industry: Political, Economic and Technological Issues*, 2009. Santa Barbara, CA: Greenwood, pp. 1–9.

4. Maoz, *Defending*, p. 5.

5. Eliot A. Cohen, Michael Eisenstadt and Andrew Bacevich, *Knives, Tanks and Missiles: Israel's Security Revolution*, 1998. Washington, DC: The Washington Institute for Near East Policy, pp. 89–92.

6. David E. Johnson, Jennifer D.P. Moroney, Roger Cliff, M. Wade Markel, Laurance Stallman and Michael Spirtas, *Preparing and Training for the Full Spectrum of Military Challenges: Insights from the Experiences of China, France, the United Kingdom, India and Israel*. Santa Monica, CA: RAND Corporation, 2009, p. xv.

7. Ibid., p. xv; Johnson, *Sorrows*; Andrew J. Bacevich, *American Empire: The Realities and Consequences of U.S. Diplomacy*, 2002. Cambridge, MA: Harvard University Press.

8. Graham, *Cities*, p. 259.

9. Andrew C. Smith, "Americanization of Israeli Defense and Weapons Industry," 2010. Retrieved at: <http://andrewcsmith.blogspot.com/2010/09/americanization-of-israeli-defense-and.html>.

10. Department of Defense, *Joint Vision 2010*. Washington, DC, 1996. Retrieved at: <http://www.dtic.mil/jv2010/jv2010.pdf>; Department of Defense, *Joint Vision 2020: America's Military – Preparing for Tomorrow*. Washington, DC, 2000, p. 58. Retrieved at: <http://www.fraw.org.uk/files/peace/us_dod_2000.pdf>.

11. Department of Defense, *Joint Vision 2020*, p. 4.

12. Graham, *Cities*, p. 31; Tim Blackmore, *War X: Human Extensions in Battlespace*. Toronto: University of Toronto Press, 2005; William A. Owens, *Dominant Battlespace Knowledge*. Honolulu, HI: University Press of the Pacific, 2002.

13. Yiftah Shapir, "Trends in Military Buildup in the Middle East," in Shlomo Brom and Anat Kurz (eds.). *Strategic Survey for Israel 2009*. Tel Aviv: The Institute for National Security Studies, 2009, pp. 112.

14. Amy F. Woolf, Conventional Prompt Global Strike and Long-Range Ballistic Missiles: Background and Issues, Washington, DC: Congressional Research Service, 2015, p. 3. Retrieved at: <https://fas.org/sgp/crs/nuke/R41464.pdf>.

15. Andrew Feickert, *Missile Survey: Ballistic and Cruise Missiles of Foreign Countries*. Washington, DC: Congressional Research Service, 2004. Retrieved at: <http://www.au.af.mil/au/awc/awcgate/crs/rl30427.pdf>.

16. *Joint Vision 2010*, p. 23.

17. Gray, *Bloody Century*, pp. 199–210.

18. Smith, *Utility*, pp. 19–20.

19. Department of Defense, *The Long War*, *Quadrennial Defense Review (QDR 2006)*, 2006, pp. 9, 14. Retrieved at: <www.defense.gov/qdr/report/Report20060203.pdf>.

20. Smith, *Utility*, pp. 18–19.

21. Graham, *Cities*, pp. 96; Duffield, *Development*; Radley Balko, "A Decade After 9/11, Police Departments Are Increasingly Militarized." *Huffington Post*, 2011. Retrieved at: <http://www.huffingtonpost.com/2011/09/12/police-militarization-9-11-september-11_n_955508.html>.

22. Laura K. Donohue, *The Cost of Counterterrorism*. New York: Cambridge University Press, 2008, p. 184; Tony Platt, and Cecilia O'Leary, "Patriot Acts." *Social Justice* (2003), 30(1): 5–21.

23. Defense Logistics Agency, *About the 1033 Program*, 2014. Retrieved at: <http://www.dispositionservices.dla.mil/leso/pages/default.aspx>.

24. Robert Mandel, "Exploding Myths About Global Arms Transfers." *Journal of Conflict Studies* (1998), 18(2). Retrieved at: <http://journals.hil.unb.ca/index.php/JCS/article/view/11694/12446>.

25. Balko, *Warrior*, pp. 174–5.

26. Ibid., pp. 263, 307.

27. Quoted in John W. Whitehead, *A Government of Wolves: The Emerging American Police State*. New York: Select Books, 2013, p. 209.

28. Rita Taureck, "Securitization Theory and Securitization Studies." *Journal of International Relations and Development*, 2006, 9: 54.

29. David Keen, *Useful Enemies: When Waging Wars is More Important Than Winning Them*. New Haven, CT: Yale University Press, 2012.

30. Lawfare Project, *Lawfare: The Use of Law as a Weapon of War*, 2010 (original emphasis). Retrieved at <http://www.thelawfareproject.org/what-is-lawfare.html>.

31. Whitehead, *Wolves*, pp. 187, 609.

32. Naomi Darom, "Meet the Biggest PR firm in the Middle East: IDF Spokesman's Unit." *Ha'aretz*, January 1, 2015. Retrieved at: <http://www.haaretz.com/news/diplomacy-defense/.premium-1.644692>.

33. Avihai Mandelbit, "Lawfare: The Legal Front of the IDF." *Military and Strategic Affairs* (2012), 4(1): 51–7.

34. Jeff Halper, "Globalizing Gaza: How Israel Undermines International Law Through 'Lawfare.'" *Counterpunch*, August 18, 2014. Retrieved at: <www.counterpunch.org/2014/08/18/globalizing-gaza>.

Chapter 4

1. Yaacov Lifshitz, "Strategic and Economic Roles of Defense Industries in Israel." BESA Center Perspectives Paper No. 164, February 13, 2012. Retrieved at: <http://www.biu.ac.il/SOC/besa/docs/perspectives164.pdf>.

2. Gordon, "Working Paper," pp. 19–32.

3. Quoted in Reiser, *Industry*, p. 106.

4. Shapir, "Trends," pp. 116–17.

5. Michael Eisenstadt and David Pollock, *Asset Test: How the United States Benefits from Its Alliance with Israel*. Washington, DC: The Washington Institute for Near East Policy, 2012.

6. Sharon Sadeh, "Israel's Defense Industry in the 21st Century: Challenges and Opportunities." *Strategic Assessment*, 2004, 7(3): 32.

7. Nassauer, personal communication.

8. SIBAT, *Israel Defense Sales Directory, 2009–10*. Tel Aviv: Israeli Ministry of Defense, p. 6.

9. Gordon, "Working Paper," p. 14.

10. D. Dvir and A. Tishler, "The Changing Role of the Defense Industry in Israel's Industrial and Technological Development." *Defense Analysis*, 2000, 16(1): 33–52.

11. David Lewis, "Diversification and Niche Market Exporting: The Restructuring of Israel's Defense Industry in the Post-Cold War Era," in Sean DiGiovanna, Ann Markusen and Michael C .Leary (eds.), *From Defense to Development? International Perspectives on Realizing the Peace Dividend*. London: Routledge, 2003, pp. 121–50.

12. Reiser, *Industry*.

13. Aharon Klieman and Reuven Pedatzur, *Rearming Israel: Defense Procurements Through the 1990s*. Boulder, CO: Westview Press, 1991.

14. Lewis, "Diversification," p. 181.

15. Jason Sherman, "Niche Carving: Subsystem Upgrades Catapult Israeli Defense Industry To New Heights." *Armed Forces Journal International*, 1997, 134(12): 34–7.

16. Klieman, *Global Reach*, p. 127.

17. Yoram Ettinger, "The Mutually-Beneficial Bottom-Up US-Israel Relations." *The Ettinger Report*, 2011. Retrieved at: < http://www.theettingerreport.com/OpEd/General/The-Mutually-Beneficial-Bottom-Up-US-Israel-Relati.aspx >.

Chapter 5

1. Dennis J. Reimer, "Dominant Maneuver and Precision Engagement." *JFQ Forum* (Winter, 1997): 14,16.
2. E.L. Zorn, "Israel's Quest for Satellite Intelligence." *Studies in Intelligence* (2001), 10: 33–8.
3. Defense Update, "Miniaturizing the Aerial Weapons," 2011. Retrieved at: < http://defense-update.com/features/2010/december/31122010_miniature_weapons.html >.
4. Aviel Magnezi, "Experts: Ofek 9 will detect Iranian activity." *Ynet*, June 24, 2010. Retrieved at: < http://www.ynetnews.com/articles/0,7340,L-3909935,00.html >.
5. *Defense Review Asia*, "Israel's Advanced Capability," 2010. Retrieved at: < http://www.defencereviewasia.com/articles/45/Israel-s-advanced-capability >.
6. ImageSat International website: < www.imagesatintl.com >.
7. *UPI*, "Israel Lines Up $1.8 Billion India Deal," 2011. Retrieved at: < http://www.upi.com/Business_News/Security-Industry/2011/03/29/Rafael-lines-up-18-billion-India-deal/UPI-51661301420599 >.
8. Israeli Aeronautics Industry (IAI), "TECSAR-SAR Technology Demonstration Satellite." Retrieved at: < http://www.iai.co.il/Sip_Storage//FILES/8/36838.pdf >; *Global Security*, TecSAR/Polaris/Ofeq 8, 2014 Retrieved at: < http://www.globalsecurity.org/space/world/israel/techsar.htm >.
9. Ninan Koshi, *India and Israel Eye Iran*. Washington, DC: Foreign Policy In Focus, February 12, 2008.
10. Israeli Ministry of Science, Technology and Space, "International Cooperation." Retrieved at: < http://www.most.gov.il/english/space/international/Pages/default.aspx >.
11. Strategy Page, *Intelligence: Israeli Satellites Guide Arab Warplanes Over Iraq*, 2014. Retrieved at: < http://www.strategypage.com/htmw/htintel/20141017.aspx >.
12. Rafael, "Iron Dome: Defense System Against Short-Range Artillery Rockets," 2009. Retrieved at: < http://www.rafael.co.il/marketing/SIP_STORAGE/FILES/6/946.pdf >; Alon Ben David, "Iron Dome Blunts 90% of Enemy Rockets." *Aviation Week & Space Technology*, September 1, 2014. Retrieved at: < http://aviationweek.com/defense/iron-dome-blunts-90-enemy-rockets >.
13. Defense Update, "David's Sling."
14. Arie Egozi, "From Iron Dome to Arrow-3." *Defense Review Asia*, 2012. Retrieved at: < http://www.defencereviewasia.com/articles/184/From-Iron-Dome-to-Arrow-3 >; David Fulghum, "Higher-Altitude Arrow Design To Show Its Potential.", *Aviation Week*, September 3, 2012. Retrieved at: < http://aviationweek.com/awin/higher-altitude-arrow-design-show-its-potential >.
15. Israeli Ministry of Defense, *Story of the Arrow Weapon System*. Retrieved at: < http://www.mod.gov.il/pages/homa/bg.htm >.
16. Ibid.
17. Israeli-Weapons.com, *Heron*. Retrieved at: < http://www.israeli-weapons.com/weapons/aircraft/uav/heron/Heron.html >.

18. Kenneth Munson, *World Unmanned Aircraft*, London: Jane's, 1988, p. 8.

19. Terraviva United Nations, *Drone Technology Takes Off*, 2012. Retrieved at: < http://www.ipsterraviva.net/UN/news.asp?idnews=107258 >; Stephen J. Zaloga, *Unmanned Aerial Vehicles: Robotic Air Warfare 1917–2007*. Oxford: Osprey Publishing, 2008.

20. Elizabeth Bone and Christopher Bolkcom, *Unmanned Aerial Vehicles: Background and Issues for Congress*. Washington, DC: Congressional Research Service, 2003, p. 2.

21. P.W. Singer, *Wired for War: The Robotics Revolution and Conflict in the 21st Century*. New York: Penguin Books, 2009, p. 57.

22. Israeli-Weapons.com, *Heron*.

23. Israeli-Weapons.com, *Hermes 450*. Retrieved at: < http://www.israeli-weapons. com/weapons/aircraft/uav/hermes_450/Hermes_450.html >; Spacewar, "Israel's New UAV Can Reach Iran," 2009. Retrieved at: < http://www.spacewar. com/reports/Israels_new_UAV_can_reach_Iran_999.html >.

24. Elbit, *Hermes 900*, 2012. Retrieved at: < http://elbitsystems.com/Elbitmain/ files/HERMES_900.pdf >; Elbit, *Hermes 900 – Multi-Role, Medium Altitude Long Endurance*, 2014. Retrieved at: < http://62.0.44.103/elbitmain/area-in2. asp?parent=3&num=31&num2=31 >; Airforce-Technology, *Hermes 900, Israel*, 2011. Retrieved at: < http://www.airforce-technology.com/projects/hermes-900 >.

25. Defense Update, "Switzerland Selects the Israeli Hermes 900 for its Future Drone," 2014. Retrieved at: < http://defense-update.com/20140606_hermes-900-switzerland.html#.VJ6GjACAQ >.

26. Defense Review Asia, "Asian Region UAV Capability on the Rise," 2012. Retrieved at: < http://www.defencereviewasia.com/articles/195/Asian-region-UAV-capability-on-the-rise >.

27. Israeli Air Force website, *The First UAV Squadron*. Retrieved at: < http://www. iaf.org.il/4968-33518-en/IAF.aspx >.

28. Free Snowden, "Transcript: ARD Interview with Edward Snowden," January 26, 2014. Retrieved at: < https://www.freesnowden.is/2014/01/27/video-ard-interview-with-edward-snowden >.

29. Nicky Hager, "Israel's Omniscient Ears." *Le Monde Diplomatique*, September 4, 2010. Retrieved at: < http://mondediplo.com/2010/09/04israelbase >.

30. Ibid.

31. Gil Zohar, "Lifting the Veil of Secrecy." Tel Aviv University publication, 2008, p. 9. Retrieved at: < http://www.aftau.org/site/DocServer/lifting_secrecy. pdf?docID=5601 >.

32. Yoav Limor, "Bringing Intelligence to the Field." *Israel Hayom*, September 25, 2012. Retrieved at: < http://www.israelhayom.com/site/newsletter_article. php?id=5891 >.

33. Richard A. Clark, *Cyber War*. New York: HarperCollins, 2010.

34. Ken Berry, "New Weapons Technology." International Commission on Nuclear Non-proliferation and Disarmament, 2011, p. 3. Retrieved at: < icnnd.org/ Documents/New_Weapons_Technology.rtf >.

35. Jeffrey Carr, *Inside Cyber Warfare: Mapping the Cyber Underworld*. Sebastopol, CA: O'Reilly Media, 2012.

36. David Fulghum, Robert Wall and Amy Butler, "Israel Shows Electronic Prowess." *Aviation Week*, November 25, 2007.

37. David Sanger, "Obama Order Sped Up Wave of Cyberattacks Against Iran." *New York Times*, June 1, 2012.

38. Richard Engel, and Robert Windrem, "Israel Teams with Terror Group to Kill Iran's Nuclear Scientists, U.S. Officials Tell NBC News, February 8, 2012. Retrieved at: <http://rockcenter.msnbc.msn.com/_news/2012/02/08/10354553-israel-teams-with-terror-group-to-kill-irans-nuclear-scientists-us-officials-tell-nbc-news>; Eli Lake, "Has Israel Been Killing Iran's Nuclear Scientists?" *The Daily Beast*, January 13, 2012. Retrieved at: <http://www.thedailybeast.com/articles/2012/01/13/has-israel-been-killing-iran-s-nuclear-scientists.html>; Irving Lachow, "The Stuxnet Enigma: Implications for the Future of Cybersecurity." *Georgetown Journal of International Affairs*. Special Edition (November, 2011): 118–26.

39. *Washington Post*, June 20, 2012; *The New York Times*, June 20, 2012.

40. Stacy Perman, *Spies Inc., Business Innovation from Israel's Master's of Espionage*. Englewood Cliffs, NJ: Prentice Hall, 2004, pp. 172–3.

41. SIBAT, *Israel Defense Sales Directory, 2009–10*. Tel Aviv: Israeli Ministry of Defense, p. 79.

42. Ocnus.Net, "Israel Now Flying New Phalcon AWACS," 2006. Retrieved at: <http://www.ocnus.net/cgi-bin/exec/view.cgi?archive=102&num=26121>.

43. Amy L. Fletcher, "Robo-SEAL: Constructing the Soldier-as-Cyborg on the Nanotechnological Front." Paper presented at the 1st Conference on Advanced Nanotechnology: Research, Applications, and Policy, 2004. Retrieved at: <http://www.foresight.org/Conferences/AdvNano2004/Abstracts/Fletcher/index.html>.

44. ISN (Institute for Soldier Nanotechnologies), 2014. Retrieved at: <http://web.mit.edu/isn/aboutisn/index.html>.

45. Ray Kurzweil, *The Singularity is Near: When Humans Transcend Biology*. New York: Viking, 2005, p. 200; Singer, *Wired*.

46. SIBAT, *Sales Directory*, p. 124.

47. Ibid., p. 131; Elbit/Dominator. Retrieved at: <http://elbitsystems.com/Elbitmain/files/Dominator.pdf>.

48. G3 Defense, "Elbit Systems Dominator® Concept Enables Forces to Dominate the Battlefield," 2012. Retrieved at: <http://www.g3defence.co.uk/blog/elbit-systems-dominator-concept-enables-forces-to-dominate-the-battlefield>.

49. Slippery Brick, "Xaver 800 Device Sees Through Walls," 2007. Retrieved at: <http://www.slipperybrick.com/2007/01/device-sees-through-walls>; Camero, n.d. *Xaver 800*. Retrieved at: <http://satellite.bfioptilas.com/objects/8_2_1312347358/Camero_Xaver800.pdf>; Camero. Retrieved at: <http://defense-update.com/directories/companies/c/camero.html>.

50. Kurzweill, *Singularity*; Jurgen Altmann, *Military Nanotechnology: Potential Applications and Preventive Arms Control*. London: Routledge, 2006. Retrieved at: <https://www.academia.edu/9918729/Military_Nanotechnology>; Jurgen Altmann, "Critical Analysis of New Weapons Technologies." *Peace Review* (2006), 21(2): 144–54; ETC Group, *BANG*, 2003. Retrieved at: <http://www.etcgroup.org/issues/bang>; Mihail C. Roco and William Sims Bainbridge (eds.), *Converging Technologies for Improving Human Performance: Nanotechnology,*

Biotechnology, Information Technology And Cognitive Science. Dordrecht: Kluwer Academic Publishers, 2002.

51. Altmann, *Nanotechnology*, pp. 5–6.
52. NYACT (New Yorkers Against the Cornell-Technion Partnership), 2012. Retrieved at: <http://nyact.net/links/about-the-technion>.
53. TASP, "Technion Autonomous Systems Program." Retrieved at: <http://tasp.technion.ac.il/index.php/en>.
54. Ofer Petersberg, "Israel's Secret New Weapon?" *Y-Net Magazine*, 2010. Retrieved at: <http://www.ynetnews.com/articles/0,7340,L-3919257,00.html>.
55. Berry, *New Weapons*; Fletcher, "Robo-SEAL"; Singer, *Wired*; Lester Martinez-Lopez, "Biotechnology Enablers for the Soldier System of Systems." *The Bridge* (2004), 34(3) 17–25; NRC (National Research Council), *Opportunities in Biotechnology for Future Army Applications*. Washington, DC: National Academies Press, 2003; DARPA website. Retrieved at: <http://www.darpa.mil/default.aspx>.
56. SIBAT, *Sales Directory*, pp. 231–48.
57. Elbit, *WINBMS: Advanced Networked Battle Management*. Retrieved at: <http://elbitsystems.com/Elbitmain/files/winbms%20%20[2011].pdf>; Elbit, *Battle Management Systems*. Retrieved at: <https://www.elbitsystems.com/elbitmain/area-in2.asp?parent=4&num=41&num2=41>.

Chapter 6

1. International Institute of Strategic Studies, *The Military Balance 2014*. London: IISS, 2014.
2. Duncan Lennox, (ed.), "Arrow 2 (Israel), Defensive Weapons." *Jane's Strategic Weapon Systems* (2009), 50, pp. 253–6; Spiegel Online International, *Operation Samson: Israel's Deployment of Nuclear Missiles on Subs from Germany*, 2012. Retrieved at: <http://www.spiegel.de/international/world/israel-deploys-nuclear-weapons-on-german-built-submarines-a-836784.html>; SIPRI, *Military Expenditure, 2013*, p. 321.
3. NTI, "Israel: Missile." Retrieved at: <http://www.nti.org/country-profiles/israel/delivery-systems>.
4. Ibid.; Feikert, *Missile Survey*.
5. NTI, "Israel: Missile"; *Jane's*, pp. 85–6.
6. Abdullah Toukan and Anthony H. Cordesman, *Study on a Possible Israeli Strike on Iran's Nuclear Development Facilities*. Center for Strategic and International Studies, March 4, 2009. Retrieved at: <http://csis.org/files/media/csis/pubs/090316_israelistrikeiran.pdf>.
7. Abraham Rabinovich, "Escape from Cherbourg." *Jerusalem Post Magazine*, December 24, 2009.
8. *Gabriel*, Retrieved at: <http://en.wikipedia.org/wiki/Gabriel_(missile)#Users>.
9. Defense Industry Daily, "India & Israel's Barak-8 SAM Development Project(s)," March 2, 2015. Retrieved at: <http://www.defenseindustrydaily.com/india-israel-introducing-mr-sam-03461/>; Globes, "Barak-8 Success Reflects Close Israel-India Defense Ties," November 11, 2014. Retrieved at: <http://www.globes.co.il/en/article-barak-8-success-reflects-close-israel-india-defense-ties-1000985694>.

10. Rafael/Python. Retrieved at: <http://www.rafael.co.il/marketing/SIP_STORAGE/FILES/1/921.pdf>.

11. Army-Technology.com/Spyder, Retrieved at: <http://www.army-technology.com/projects/spyder>.

12. *Defense Industry Daily*, "India Buys Israeli 'Spyder' Mobile Air Defense System," August 19, 2009. Retrieved at: <Army-Technology.com/Spyder, Retrieved at: <http://www.army-technology.com/projects/spyder>.

13. Max Defense, "Israeli SPYDER Air Defense Missile System for the Philippines - A Good Choice," 2013. Retrieved at: <http://maxdefense.blogspot.co.il/2013/06/israeli-spyder-air-defense-missile.html>.

14. Defense Industry Daily, "Peru's Next-Generation Air Defenses," 2012. Retrieved at: <http://www.defenseindustrydaily.com/perus-next-generation-air-defenses-07339>.

15. SIPRI, *Arms Transfer Database*, 2014. Retrieved at: <http://armstrade.sipri.org/armstrade/page/trade_register.php>.

16. Defense Industry Daily, "If Necessary, Alone: The Shield of Poland," 2014. Retrieved at: <http://www.defenseindustrydaily.com/if-necessary-alone-the-shield-of-poland-022785>.

17. Israel Export Institute <http://www.export.gov.il>.

18. Joe Tuzara, "Israel's EMP Attack Can Send Iran Back to the Stone Age." *Arutz Sheva*, 2012. Retrieved at: <http://www.israelnationalnews.com/Articles/Article.aspx/12017#.VHmqD76fvdk>.

19. Defense Review Asia, "Elbit Systems of America Awarded Two Contracts to Upgrade Marine Corps AH-1W Attack Helicopters," 2014. Retrieved at: <http://www.defencereviewasia.com/articles/333/Elbit-Systems-of-America-Awarded-Two-Contracts-to-Upgrade-Marine-Corps-AH-1W-Attack-Helicopters>.

20. Rafael/Litening, "Advanced Targeting Pod." Retrieved at: <http://www.rafael.co.il/marketing/SIP_STORAGE/FILES/7/477.pdf>.

21. Israel Defense, "Rafael's Mini-Spike," 2012. Retrieved at: <http://www.israeldefense.com/?CategoryID=411&ArticleID=1314>.

22. Defense Update, "Delilah – the IAF's Loitering Missile," 2009. Retrieved at: <http://defense-update.com/newscast/0609/news/delilah_140609.html>; SIBAT, *Sales Directory*, p. 65; Israeli Airforce website, "Delilah's Secrets." Retrieved at: <http://www.iaf.org.il/5642-35312-en/IAF.aspx>.

23. SIBAT, *Sales Directory*, p. 69.

24. SIBAT, *Sales Directory*, p. 69; "Rafael/Spice." Retrieved at: <www.rafael.co.il/marketing/SIP_STORAGE/FILES/4/924.pdf>; Arie Egozi, "The Israeli Defense Industries." *Defense Review Asia*, 2013. Retrieved at: <http://www.defencereviewasia.com/articles/230/The-Israeli-Defence-Industries>.

25. SIBAT, *Sales Directory*, p. 65; IMI/MPR-500, "MPR-500: Multi-Purpose Rigid Bomb." Retrieved at: <http://www.imi-israel.com/home/doc.aspx?mCatID=66598>.

26. IMI/IFB-500, "IFB-500 – Improved Fragmentation Bomb." Retrieved at: <http://www.imi-israel.com/home/doc.aspx?mCatID=66597>; Business Library, "IMI Unveils Miniature Smart Submunition," 2004. Retrieved at: <http://findarticles.com/p/articles/mi_6712/is_8_224/ai_n29136110>.

27. SIBAT, *Sales Directory*, p. 332.

28. Sandra Erwin, "Directed-Energy Weapons Promise 'Low Cost Per Kill.'" *National Defense Magazine*, 2001. Retrieved at: < http://www.nationaldefensemagazine. org/archive/2001/September/Pages/Directed-Energy6955.aspx >.

29. Gad Nahshon, "Dr. Oded Amichai: 'SkyGuard will Defend Israel.'" *Jewish Post*, 2011. Retrieved at: < http://www.jewishpost.com/news/Dr-Oded-Amichai-SkyGuard-will-Defend-Israel.html >.

30. Defense Update, "RAFAEL Develops a New High Energy Laser Weapon," 2014. Retrieved at: < http://defense-update.com/20140119_rafael-develops-new-high-energy-laser-weapon.html#.VAmLTFYY6zA >.

31. Israeli-Weapons.com, "HARPY." Retrieved at: < http://www.israeli-weapons. com/weapons/aircraft/uav/harpy/HARPY.html >.

32. Barbara Opall-Rome, "Israel AF Hones Manned-UAV Mix." *Defense News*, 2008. Retrieved at: < http://www.defensenews.com >.

33. Defense Industry Daily, "Israel is Hermes 900 UAV Launch Customer, as IDF Expands Fleets," 2010. Retrieved at: < http://www.defenseindustrydaily. com/Israel-is-Hermes-900-UAV-Launch-Customer-as-IAF-Expands-its-fleets-06363 >.

34. Egozi, "Israeli Defence."

35. Spencer Ackerman, "41 Men Targeted But 1,147 People Killed: US Drone Strikes – The Facts on the Ground." *The Guardian*, November 24, 2014. Retrieved at: < http://www.theguardian.com/us-news/2014/nov/24/-sp-us-drone-strikes-kill-1147 >.

36. INSS, "Challenges of Warfare in Densely Populated Areas: Conference Proceedings." *Military and Strategic Affairs*, April 2014. Retrieved at: < http:// d26e8pvoto2x3r.cloudfront.net/uploadImages/systemFiles/MASAApril2014 Eng_3.pdf >.

37. SIBAT, *Sales Directory*, p. 326.

38. Yaakov Katz, "Security and Defense: 'The Tank is One of the Most Technologically Advanced Platforms Around,'" *Jerusalem Post*, August 13, 2009. Retrieved at: < http://www.jpost.com/Features/Front-Lines/Security-and-Defense-The-tank-is-one-of-the-most-technologically-advanced-platforms-around >.

39. Opall-Rome, "Israel Blurs Roles, Missions in Ground War Concept." *Defense News*, 2010. Retrieved at: < http://www.defensenews.com/apps/pbcs.dll/ article?AID=201010250306 >.

40. Israel Defense, "Barak Promotes Deals in Colombia," 2012. Retrieved at: < http://www.israeldefense.com/?CategoryID=474&ArticleID=1170 >.

41. Defense Update, "LIC Modeled Merkava Mk-3 Baz/Mk 4." 2006. Retrieved at: < http://www.defense-update.com/products/m/merkava-lic.htm >.

42. Defense Update, "Enter the Namer." Retrieved at: < http://defense-update.com/ features/2010/june/namer_merkava_update_09062010.html >.

43. Strategy Page, "The Ultimate IFV." Retrieved at: < http://www.strategypage. com/htmw/htarm/articles/20070720.aspx >.

44. Global Security, "Nagmachon." Retrieved at: < http://www.globalsecurity.org/ military/world/israel/nagmachon.htm >.

45. SIBAT, *Sales Directory*, p. 184; "Rafael/Samson RWS." Retrieved at: < http://www. rafael.co.il/Marketing/402-990-en/Marketing.aspx >; Army Guide, "Achzarit." Retrieved at: < http://www.army-guide.com/eng/product1004.html >; NIMDA, "Achzarit HAPC." Retrieved at: < http://www.nimda.co.il/199098/Achzarit >.

46. Thomas, *Dark Side*.

47. Haim Barzilay, "Growth of Defensive Exports of Israel in the Decade 1998–2007." *Journal of National Defense Studies* (2010), 8: 127–60 (in Hebrew).

48. SIBAT, *Sales Directory*, p. 150; Defense Update, "Iron Fist Active Protection System APC," 2009. Retrieved at: < http://www.defense-update.com/products/i/iron-fist.htm >.

49. SIBAT, *Sales Directory*, p. 160; "Rafael/Trophy." Retrieved at: < http://www.rafael.co.il/Marketing/349-963-en/Marketing.aspx >.

50. Defense Update, "Trophy Active Protection System," 2007. Retrieved at: < http://www.defense-update.com/products/t/trophy.htm >.

51. SIBAT, *Sales Directory*, p. 124.

52. DefenseTech, "U.S. Gets Explosive Armor From Israel," 2004. Retrieved at: < http://defensetech.org/2004/05/19/u-s-gets-explosive-armor-from-israel >.

53. SIBAT, *Sales Directory*, p. 158.

54. Arutz Sheva, "Israel Looks to Expand Navy to Protect Gas Interests," 2011. Retrieved at: < http://www.israelnationalnews.com/News/News.aspx/148917#.T9jqzHhldS0 >.

55. Federation of American Scientists (FAS), "Popeye Turbo." Retrieved at: < http://fas.org/nuke/guide/israel/missile/popeye-t.htm >.

56. Global Security, "Weapons of Mass Destruction: Dolphin." Retrieved at: < http://www.globalsecurity.org/wmd/world/israel/dolphin.htm >.

57. Robert Bechhusan, "Israel's Quiet Doomsday Submarines Almost Are Ready," 2014. Retrieved at:< https://medium.com/war-is-boring/israels-quiet-killer-submarines-are-almost-ready-3adff7c1279f >.

58. Yaakov Katz, "Navy Bolsters Its Amphibious Presence." *Jerusalem Post*, September 22, 2009; "Security & Defense: Sailing on Stormy Seas." *Jerusalem Post*, July 29, 2011.

59. Israel News Agency, "Israel Defense Forces Navy Unleashes Death Shark Against Terrorism," 2005. Retrieved at: < http://www.israelnews agency.com/navyterrorismisraelidfweapons481020.html >; "Rafael/Protector." Retrieved at: < http://www.rafael.co.il/marketing/SIP_STORAGE/FILES/3/633.pdf >.

60. Debkafile, "New Israeli Unmanned Wonder Boat Deployed in Persian Gulf," 2009. Retrieved at: < http://www.debka.com/search/?search_string=wonder+boat&x=45&y=14 >.

61. Defense Update, *Silver Marlin*, 2006. Retrieved at: < http://defense-update.com/products/s/silver-marlin.htm >; Defense Update, *Stingray*, 2006. Retrieved at: < http://defense-update.com/products/s/stingray.htm >.

62. Defense Review Asia, "Israeli Company Showcases Manned/Unmanned Patrol Boat," 2014. Retrieved at: < http://www.defencereviewasia.com/articles/392/Israeli-company-showcases-manned-unmanned-patrol-boat >.

63. SIBAT, *Sales Directory*, p. 197; G-nius, "Guardium Mk-1." Retrieved at: < http://g-nius.co.il/unmanned-ground-systems/guardium-ugv.html >; Defense Update, "Enguard!" 2009. Retrieved at: < http://defense-update.com/products/g/guardium.htm >.

64. Charles Levinson, "Israeli Robots Remake Battlefield." *Wall Street Journal*, January 13, 2010.

65. SIBAT, *Sales Directory*, p. 124.

66. Defense Update, "Elbit Systems Unveils VIPeR a Portable Combat Robot," 2007. Retrieved at: <http://defense-update.com/newscast/0307/news/080307_viper.htm>.

67. Yaakov Katz, "IDF Using 'James Bond' Gadgetry." *Jerusalem Post*, February 17, 2009. Retrieved at: <http://www.jpost.com/Israel/IDF-using-James-Bond-gadgetry>.

68. Hanan Greenberg, "IDF Robots to be Used During Raids." *Y-Net*, June 6, 2009. Retrieved at: <http://www.ynetnews.com/articles/0,7340,L-3739422,00.html>.

69. Defense Update, *Miniature Aerial Vehicles*, 2004. Retrieved at: <http://defense-update.com/features/du-2-04/feature-mav.htm>.

70. SIBAT, *Sales Directory*, p. 30.

71. Ibid., p. 315.

72. Ibid., pp. 321, 322.

73. IAI, "Unmanned Air Systems: The Panther Family." Retrieved at: <http://www.iai.co.il/2013/35673-en/BusinessAreas_UnmannedAirSystems_PantherFamily.aspx>.

74. IAI – Ghost, "IAI to Unveil 'Ghost', A Rotary Mini UAV System At AUVSI's Unmanned Systems North America," 2011. Retrieved at: <http://www.iai.co.il/32981-43072-en/MediaRoom_News.aspx>.

75. Flightglobal, "IAI Unveils Mosquito UAV for Ground Support Concept," 2009. Retrieved at: <http://www.flightglobal.com/news/articles/picture-iai-unveils-mosquito-uav-for-ground-support-331780>; IAI – Jumper, *IAI Presents JUMPER – Autonomous Artillery for the Ground Forces – at Eurosatory*, 2010. Retrieved at: <http://www.iai.co.il/35490-41113-en/Eurosatory_2010_Homepage.aspx>.

76. RT News, "Spy-Butterfly: Israel Developing Insect Drone for Indoor Surveillance," 2012. Retrieved at: <http://www.rt.com/news/israel-drone-indoor-butterfly-672>.

77. Reuters, "Israel Developing Anti-Militant 'Bionic Hornet,'" November 17, 2006. Retrieved at: <http://www.reuters.com/article/2006/11/17/us-mideast-weapons-idUSL175109120061117>.

78. Itamar Eichner, "A Bionic Hornet and a Steve Austin Glove." *Yediot Ahronot*, November 17, 2006 (in Hebrew).

79. TASP (Technion Autonomous Systems Program), "Research Projects," 2014. Retrieved at: <http://tasp.technion.ac.il/index.php/en/research-projects>.

80. Barbara Frank, and Amanda Jaffe-Katz. "Snake Robots." Mechanical Engineering, Technion. Retrieved at: <http://meeng.technion.ac.il/Biorobotics>.

81. Asaf Shtull-Trauring, "In an Israeli Lab, the World's Smallest Drone." *Haaretz*, April 9, 2012. Retrieved at: <http://www.haaretz.com/misc/iphone-article/in-an-israeli-lab-the-world-s-smallest-drone-1.423298>.

82. Zohar, "Lifting the Veil," p. 7.

83. Luca Petricca and Per Ohlckersa, "Micro- and Nano-Air Vehicles: State of the Art." *International Journal of Aerospace Engineering*, 2011. Retrieved at: <http://www.hindawi.com/journals/ijae/2011/214549/#B3>; Debbie Kedar and Shlomi Arnon, "Optical Wireless Communication in Distributed Sensor Networks." *SPIE Newsroom*, 2006. Retrieved at: <https://spie.org/documents/Newsroom/Imported/55_228_0_2005-11-16/55_228_0_2005-11-16.PDF>.

84. Zohar, "Lifting the Veil," p. 8.

85. SIBAT, *Sales Directory*, pp. 186-187; Army-Technology.com/Atmos, "Atmos 2000 155mm Self-Propelled Artillery System, Israel." Retrieved at: <http://www.army-technology.com/projects/atmos>; Defence Update, "ATHOS 2025 Autonomous, Towed Howitzer 155mm," 2004. Retrieved at: <http://defense-update.com/products/a/athos.htm>; Army-Technology.com, "Rascal 155mm Light Self-Propelled Howitzer, Israel." Retrieved at: <http://www.army-technology.com/projects/rascal>.

86. Defense Update, "LORA Surface Attack Missile," 2005. Retrieved at: <http://www.defense-update.com/products/l/lora.htm>; IAI – LORA, "LORA Artillery Weapon System." Retrieved at: <http://www.misile-iai.com/34225-36447-en/Groups_SystemMissileandSpace_MLM_Products_PrecisionStrikingSystems.aspx?btl=1>.

87. Elbit, "Artillery: Soltam Spear." Retrieved at: <http://elbitsystems.com/Elbitmain/files/SPEAR.pdf>.

88. Yaakov Lappin, "Elbit Unveils Mortar-Launching System." *Jerusalem Post*, May 20, 2014. Retrieved at: <http://www.jpost.com/Defense/Elbit-unveils-mortar-launching-system-352774>.

89. IWI Israel Weapon Industry, "TAVOR Models," 2005. Retrieved at: <http://www.israel-weapon.com/default.asp?catid={BE33B6E6-080B-45B8-AD85-C4E1E40D0422}>; World Guns, "Tavor TAR 21." Retrieved at: <http://world.guns.ru/assault/isr/tavor-tar-21-e.html>; Defense Update, "Micro Tavor," 2006. Retrieved at: <http://defense-update.com/20061018_micro-tavor.html.>.

90. Thomas P. Ehrhart, *Increasing Small Arms Lethality in Afghanistan: Taking Back the Infantry Half-Kilometer*. Fort Leavenworth, KS: School of Advanced Military Studies United States Army Command and General Staff College, 2009.

91. IWI Israel Weapon Industry, "X95." Retrieved at: <http://www.israel-weapon.com/files/brochure_2012/IWI_X95_Family.pdf>.

92. IWI Israel Weapon Industry, "Negev NG7." Retrieved at: <http://www.israel-weapon.com/?catid=%7B19D5D496-ADA9-4A2E-BD7C-69B598FE4002%7D>; Israel-Weapon/Negev NG7>.

93. Defense Review, "Israel Weapon Industries IWI NEGEV NG7 LMG/LMG SF Belt-Fed 7.62mm NATO 'Light Machine Gun,'" 2012. Retrieved at: <http://www.defensereview.com/israel-military-industries-iwi-negev-ng7-light-machine-gun-lmg-lightweight-and-highly-mobile-select-fire-7-62mm-natomedium-machine-gungeneral-purpose-machine-gun-mmggpmg-for-military-infan>.

94. Defence Update, "Silver Shadow Unveils a Production Ready Version of Gilboa Assault Pistol Rifle (APR)," 2011. Retrieved at: <http://defense-update.com/20111031_silver-shadow-unveil-production-ready-version-of-gilboa-assault-pistol-rifle-apr.html>; Gilboa, "The New Assault Rifle Made in Israel." Retrieved at: <http://www.gilboa-rifle.com>.

95. Defense Review Asia, "Israel Military Industries Multi-Purpose Rifle System," 2010. Retrieved at: <http://www.defencereviewasia.com/articles/26/ISRAEL-MILITARY-INDUSTRIES-MULTI-PURPPOSE-RIFLE-SYSTEM>.

96. "Corner Shot." Retrieved at: <http://www.cornershot.com/About%20Us/index.html>.

97. Moriya Ben-Yosef, "Barak Rifle Upgraded." *Israeli Defense*, 2014. Retrieved at: <http://www.israeldefense.com/?CategoryID=485&ArticleID=1832>.

98. "M337 HE-MP-T." Retrieved at: <http://defense-update.com/products/digits/120m337.htm>.

99. Meron Rapoport, "Italian Probe: Israel Used New Weapon Prototype in Gaza Strip." *Washington Report on Mideast Affairs*, December, 2006. Retrieved at: <http://www.wrmea.org/2006-december/italian-probe-israel-used-new-weapon-prototype-in-gaza-strip.html>.

100. James Brooks, "Warfare of the Future, Today? The DIME Bomb: Yet Another Genotoxic Weapon." *Grassroots Peace*, 2006. Retrieved at: <http://www.grassrootspeace.org/israel_dime_bombs_121206.pdf>; Michele Esposito, "The Israeli Arsenal Deployed Against Gaza During Operation Cast Lead." *Journal of Palestine Studies* (229), 28(3): 175–91; Peoples Geography-Reclaiming Space, "The Wounds of Gaza." Retrieved at: <http://peoplesgeography.com/2009/01/30/the-wounds-of-gaza-2009>.

101. Quoted in Brooks, "Warfare of the Future."

102. Landmine and Cluster Munition Monitor, *Israel*. Mines Action Canada, 2014. Retrieved at: <http://www.the-monitor.org/custom/index.php/region_profiles/print_profile/910>.

Chapter 7

1. The Fletcher Forum of World Affairs, *An Interview with Laleh Khalili*, Tufts University, November 20, 2014. Retrieved at:<http://www.fletcherforum.org/2014/11/20/khalili>.

2. Boaz Ganor, *The Counter-Terrorism Puzzle: A Guide for Decision Makers*, New Brunswick, NJ: Transaction, 2005, Kindle locs 5581–646.

3. Kaplan, *Petraeus*, p. 20.

4. US Marine Corps, *Counterinsurgency Field Manual*. Chicago, IL: University of Chicago Press, 2007.

5. Ganor, *Puzzle*, loc 5686.

6. Laleh Khalili, *Time in the Shadows: Confinement in Counterinsurgencies*. Stanford, CA: Stanford University Press, 2013.

7. Nir, quoted in Peri, *Generals*, p. 125.

8. Amidror, *Winning*.

9. Ephraim Inbar and Eitan Shamir, "'Mowing the Grass': Israel's Strategy for Protracted Intractable Conflict." *Journal of Strategic Studies* (204), 37(1): 70, 73. Retrieved at: <http://besacenter.org/wp-content/uploads/2014/02/Mowing-the-Grass-English.pdf>.

10. Klein, *Shock Doctrine*, p. 442.

11. Tera Herivel and Paul Wright, *Prison Nation: The Warehousing of America's Poor*. New York: Routledge, 2003.

12. Moshe Ya'alon, "Introduction: Restoring A Security-First Peace Policy," in Dan Diker (ed.). *Israel's Critical Security Requirements for Defensible Borders: The Foundation for a Viable Peace*. Jerusalem: Jerusalem Center For Public Affairs, 2011, pp. 12–21.

13. Lisa Stampnitzky, *Disciplining Terror: How Experts Invented "Terrorism."* Cambridge: Cambridge University Press, 2013.

14. Benjamin Netanyahu, *Fighting Terrorism: How Democracies Can Defeat the International Terrorist Network*. New York: Farrar, Strauss and Giroux, 1995, p. 8.

15. Ganor, *Puzzle*, loc 589.

16. Ibid., loc 604.

17. William Booth, "Israeli Strike Kills Four Children on a Gaza Beach," *Washington Post*, July 16, 2014.

18. Israel Defense Forces (IDF), "Spokesperson of the Chinese Ministry of National Defense Arrives in Israel for Visit," March 22, 2010. Retrieved at:<http://www.idfblog.com/blog/2010/03/22/spokesperson-of-the-chinese-ministry-of-national-defense-arrives-in-israel-for-visit-22-mar-2010>.

19. Ze'ev Jabotinsky, *The Iron Wall*. Retrieved at:<https://www.jewishvirtuallibrary.org/jsource/Zionism/ironwall.html>.

20. Eligar Sadeh, "Militarization and State Power in the Arab-Israeli Conflict: Case Study of Israel, 1948–1982". Dissertation.com, 1994.

21. Mark A. Heller, *Continuity and Change in Israeli Security Policy. The International Institute for Strategic Studies*, Oxford: Adelphi Paper (2000), 335: p. 49; Defense News, "Israeli Brass, Experts Differ in Strategic Diagnosis," 2014. Retrieved at: <http://www.defensenews.com/article/20140203/DEFREG04/302030015/Israeli-Brass-Experts-Differ-Strategic-Diagnosis>.

22. "A fence, but not a solution on the Israel-Egypt border." *Ha'aretz*, January 12, 2010.

23. Israel Ministry of Foreign Affairs, Address by Acting PM Ehud Olmert to the 6th Herzliya Conference. Retrieved at: <http://www.mfa.gov.il/mfa/pressroom/2006/pages/address%20by%20acting%20pm%20ehud%20olmert%20to%20the%206th%20herzliya%20conference%2024-jan-2006.aspx>.

24. B'tselem, *Land Grab: Israel's Settlement Policy in the West Bank*, 2002. Retrieved at: <http://www.btselem.org/download/200205_land_grab_eng.pdf>.

25. Sharon Rotbard, "Wall and Tower", in Philipp Misselwitz and Tim Rieniets (eds.). *City of Collision: Jerusalem and the Principles of Conflict Urbanism*. Basel: Birkhauser, 2006, pp. 102–12.

26. Eyal Weizman, *Hollow Land: Israel's Architecture of Occupation*. London: Verso, 2007, pp. 9–10.

27. Almond, "British and Israeli", pp. 67–8.

28. Eyal Weizman, "Strategic Points, Flexible Lines, Tense Surfaces and Political Volumes: Ariel Sharon and the Geometry of Occupation." *The Philosophical Forum* (2004), 35(2): 176–7, 181).

29. PASSIA, "Land & Land Confiscation." *PASSIA Diary*. Jerusalem: Palestinian Academic Society for the Study of International Affairs, 2011, p. 335.

30. PCHR/IDMC (Palestinian Center for Human Rights, Internal Displacement Monitoring Centre), *Under Fire: Israel's Enforcement of Access Restricted Areas in the Gaza Strip*. Geneva: IDMC, 2014. Retrieved at: <http://www.pchrgaza.org/files/2014/palestine-under-fire-report-en.pdf>.

31. UNEP (United Nations Environment Programme), *Environmental Assessment of the Gaza Strip Following the Escalation of Hostilities in December 2008–January 2009*. Nairobi, 2009: UNEP. Retrieved at:<http://www.unep.org/pdf/dmb/unep_gaza_ea.pdf>.

32. Doron Almog, "Lessons of the Gaza Security Fence for the West Bank." *Jerusalem Issue Brief*. Jerusalem Center for Public Affairs, 2004. Retrieved at: <http://www.jcpa.org/brief/brief004-12.htm>.

33. Jonathan Cook, "Remote-Controlled Killing." *Counterpunch*, July 13, 2010. Retrieved at: <http://www.counterpunch.org/2010/07/13/remote-controlled-killing>.

34. Amira Hass, "2,279 Calories Per Person: How Israel Made Sure Gaza Didn't Starve." *Ha'aretz*, October 17, 2012. Retrieved at: <http://www.haaretz.com/news/diplomacy-defense/2-279-calories-per-person-how-israel-made-sure-gaza-didn-t-starve.premium-1.470419>.

35. Jonathan Cook, "Israel's Starvation Diet for Gaza." *Electronic Intifada*, October 24, 2012. Retrieved at: <http://electronicintifada.net/content/israels-starvation-diet-gaza/11810>.

36. COGAT, *Food Consumption in the Gaza Strip – Red Lines Presentation*, 2012. Retrieved at: <http://www.haaretz.com/resources/Pdf/red-lines.pdf>.

37. Gisha, "'Red Lines' Presentation: New Details About the Old Policy, While the Current Policy Remains Shrouded in Secrecy," 2012. Retrieved at: <http://gisha.org/updates/1825>.

38. Doron Almog, "Cumulative Deterrence and the War on Terrorism." *Parameters* (2012), 34: 4–19.

39. NBC News, "US Employs Israeli Tactics in Iraq: Urban Warfare Methods Adapted to Fight Insurgency," 2003. Retrieved at: ttp://www.nbcnews.com/id/3702655/ns/world_news-mideast_n_africa/t/us-employs-israeli-tactics-iraq/#.U9YTIFYY6zA>.

40. B'tselem, "Restrictions of Movement: Checkpoints, Physical Obstructions, and Forbidden Roads," 2014. Retrieved at: <http://www.btselem.org/freedom_of_movement/checkpoints_and_forbidden_roads>.

41. Who Profits, *Technologies of Control: The Case of Hewlett Packard*, 2011. Retrieved at: <http://www.whoprofits.org/sites/default/files/hp_report-_final_for_web.pdf>.

42. Ben-Eliezer, *Militarism*, pp. 19–20.

43. Gazit, *Fools*, p. 4; David Kretzmer, *The Occupation of Justice: The Supreme Court of Israel and the Occupied Territories*. Albany: State University of New York Press, 2002, pp. 32–3.

44. Israel Law Resource Center, "Israeli Military Orders." Retrieved at: <http://www.israellawresourcecenter.org/israelmilitaryorders/israelimilitaryorders.htm>.

45. Israel Law Resource Center. "Israel Military Order No. 947 Concerning the Establishment of a Civilian Administration." Retrieved at: <http://www.israellawresourcecenter.org/israelmilitaryorders/fulltext/mo0947.htm>.

46. Jeff Halper, *An Israeli in Palestine: Resisting Dispossession, Redeeming Israel*. London: Pluto Press, 2010.

47. Amir Cheshen, Bill Hutman and Avi Melamed, *Separate and Unequal: The Inside Story of Israeli Rule in East Jerusalem*. Cambridge, MA: Harvard University Press, 1999; Meir Margalit, *Seizing Control of Space in East Jerusalem*. Jerusalem: Sifrei Aliat Gag, 2010, pp. 31–6.

48. B'tselem, *Detained Without Trial: Administrative Detention in the Occupied Territories Since the Beginning of the Intifada*. Jerusalem, 1992.

49. Addameer, *Palestinian Political Prisoners in Israeli Prisons*, January 2014. Retrieved at: <http://www.addameer.org/files/Palestinian%20Political%20Prisoners%20in%20Israeli%20Prisons%20(General%20Briefing%20

January%202014).pdf>; B'tselem, *Statistics on Palestinians in the Custody of the Israeli Security Forces.* May 15, 2015. Retrieved at: <http://www.btselem.org/statistics/detainees_and_prisoners>.

50. Barton Gellman, "Palestinians Await Release of Prisoners." *Washington Post,* October 3, 1995.

51. *Fédération Internationale des ligues des Droits de l'Homme* (FIDH), "Palestinian Prisoners in Israel: The Inhuman Conditions Being Suffered by Political Prisoners," July 13, 2003. Retrieved at: <https://www.fidh.org/International-Federation-for-Human-Rights/north-africa-middle-east/israel-occupied-palestinian-territories/Palestinian-Prisoners-in-Israel>.

52. Addameer, *Latest Quarterly Update on Palestinian Prisoners (July to September, 2014).* Retrieved at: <http://www.addameer.org/files/Quart%20Newsletter%20 2014%203%20QTR.pdf>.

53. Helga Tawil-Souri, "Colored Identity: The Politics and Materiality of ID Cards in Palestine/Israel." *Social Text* (2011), 29(2): 78.

54. Amnesty International, "New Israeli Military Order Could Increase Expulsions of West Bank Palestinians," April 28, 2010; Amira Hass, "IDF Order Will Enable Mass Deportation from West Bank." *Ha'aretz,* April 11, 2010. Retrieved at: <http://www.haaretz.com/print-edition/news/idf-order-will-enable-mass-deportation-from-west-bank-1.780>.

55. Andrew Stevens, "Surveillance Policies, Practices and Technologies in Israel and the Occupied Palestinian Territories: Assessing the Security State." The New Transparency Project, November, Working Paper IV, 2011.

56. B'tselem, *The Prohibition on Family Unification in the Occupied Territories.* Jerusalem, 2011.

57. Internal Displacement Monitoring Centre, "Occupied Palestine: Displacement as of October 2014," 2014. Retrieved at: <http://www.internal-displacement.org/middle-east-and-north-africa/palestine/2014/syria-displacement-in-occupied-palestine-as-of-october-2014>.

58. Ben-Eliezer, *Militarism,* pp. 7–8.

59. Peri, *Generals,* p. 58.

60. Ministry of Public Security, "The Israel Police: Public Security." Retrieved at: <http://mops.gov.il/english/policingeng/police/pages/default.aspx>.

Chapter 8

1. Jonathan Tucker, "Strategies for Countering Terrorism – Lessons from the Israeli Experience." *COIN Central: The Counterinsurgency Journal,* 2003. Retrieved at: <http://coincentral.wordpress.com/2008/06/04/strategies-for-countering-terrorism-lessons-from-the-israeli-experience>.

2. RP Defense, "Upgrading Intelligence Collection In Urban Warfare (Israel)," 2011. Retrieved at: <http://rpdefense.over-blog.com/article-upgrading-intelligence-collection-in-urban-warfare-israel-89698564.html>.

3. Nadav Morag, *Homeland Security in Israel (Part 3): Counterterrorism Strategies.* Naval Post-Graduate School: Center for Homeland Defense and Security, 2009. Retrieved at: <https://www.chds.us/coursefiles/comp/lectures/comp_HS_in_israel_pt3/player.html>; Avi Dichter and Daniel L. Byman, "Israel's Lessons For Fighting Terrorists and Their Implications for the United States." Analysis Paper

#15. Washington, DC: Saban Center for Middle East Policy, 2006; Weizman, *Hollow Land*, p. 242.

4. Almog, "Lessons," p. 4.

5. Center for Research and Documentation of Palestinian Society, Interview with Dr. Salah Abdul Jawad, Bir Zeit University, 1996. Retrieved at: <http://mouv4x8. perso.neuf.fr/11Sept01/A9999_5_Abdul_Jawad_Palestine.pdf>; Jonathan Cook, "Israel's Dark Art of Ensnaring Palestinian Collaborators." *Anti-War.Com*, 2008. Retrieved at: <http://www.antiwar.com/cook/?articleid=13450>; B'tselem, *Collaborators in the Occupied Territories: Human Rights Abuses and Violations*, Jerusalem, 1994.

6. Saleh Abdel-Jawad, "Collaboration." *Media Monitors Network*, 2002. Retrieved at: <http://www.mediamonitors.net/salehabdeljawad2.html>.

7. Yitzhak Be'er and Saleh 'Abdel-Jawad, *Collaborators in the Occupied Territories: Human Rights Abuses and Violations*: Jerusalem: B'tselem, 1994.

8. Cook, "Dark Art."

9. Aaron Cohen, *Brotherhood of Warriors*. New York: Harper Collins, 2008; Amira Hass, "In the Name of Security, But Not for Its Sake." *Ha'aretz*, September 20, 2006. Retrieved at: <http://www.haaretz.com/print-edition/opinion/in-the-name-of-security-but-not-for-its-sake-1.197668>.

10. Sergio Catignani, "The Strategic Impasse in Low-Intensity Conflicts: The Gap Between Israeli Counterinsurgency Strategy and Tactics During the Al-Aqsa Intifada." *Journal of Strategic Studies* (2005), 28(1): 63.

11. Catignani, "Impasse," p. 63; Maoz, *Defending*, pp. 231–3.

12. Catignani, "Impasse," p. 65.

13. Almog, "Lessons," p. 6.

14. Ahron Bregman, *Israel's Wars: A History Since 1947*. London: Routledge, 2010, p. 50; Benny Morris, *Israel's Border Wars, 1949–1956: Arab Infiltration, Israeli Retaliation and the Countdown to the Suez War*. Oxford: Oxford University Press, 1993, pp. 260, 269–80; David Rodman, "Israel's National Security Doctrine: An Appraisal of the Past and a Vision of the Future." *Israel Affairs* (2003), 9(4): 117.

15. Morris, *Border Wars*, pp. 258–9; Maoz, *Defending*, pp. 232–68.

16. Anthony H. Cordesman, *Peace and War: The Arab-Israeli Military Balance Enters the 21st Century*. Westport, CT: Praeger, 2002, p. 229.

17. Reuven Pedatzur, "More Than a Million Bullets." *Ha'aretz*, June 29, 2004.

18. B'tselem, *10 Years to the Second Intifada – Summary of Data*, September 27, 2010. Retrieved at: <http://www.btselem.org/press_releases/20100927>.

19. Tsadok Yeheskeli, "I made them a stadium in the middle of the camp." *Yediot Aharonot*, "7 Days" Supplement, May 31, 2002; Graham, *Cities*, p. 226.

20. Akiva Eldar, "The constructive destruction option." *Ha'aretz*, October 25, 2002.

21. "Israeli Military Operations Against Gaza, 2000–2008." *Journal of Palestine Studies* (Spring, 2009), 38(3): 122–38. Retrieved at: <http://www.palestine-studies.org/sites/default/files/uploads/files/Israeli%20Military%20Attacks%20on%20Gaza%202009.pdf>; B'tselem, "Disproportionate Force Suspected in Northern Gaza Strip," October 18, 2004. Retrieved at: <http://www.btselem.org/press_releases/20041018>.

22. PCATI (Public Committee Against Torture), *No Second Thoughts: The Changes in the Israeli Defense Forces' Combat Doctrine in Light of "Operation Cast Lead,"*

2009. Retrieved at: <http://www.stoptorture.org.il/files/no%20second%20 thoughts_ENG_WEB.pdf>; Gabi Siboni, "Disproportionate Force: Israel's Concept of Response in Light of the Second Lebanon War." *INSS Insight*, (2008), 74, October 2, 2008. Retrieved at: <http://www.inss.org.il/index. aspx?id=4538&articleid=1964>.

23. Siboni, "Disproportionate."

24. Goldstone Report, *Report of the United Nations Fact-Finding Mission on the Gaza Conflict*, 2009, p. 48. Retrieved at: <http://www2.ohchr.org/english/bodies/ hrcouncil/docs/12session/A-HRC-12-48.pdf>.

25. Kim Sengupta and Donald MacIntyre, "Israeli Cabinet Divided Over Fresh Gaza Surge." *The Independent*, January 13, 2009. Retrieved at: <http://www. independent.co.uk/news/world/middle-east/israeli-cabinet-divided-over-fresh-gaza-surge-1332024.html>.

26. Goldstone Report, p. 48.

27. OCHA (UN Office for Coordinating Humanitarian Affairs), "Military Operations Displacing Palestinians." Retrieved at: <http://www.ochaopt.org/annual/c2/8. html>; B'tselem, "Fatalities during Operation Cast Lead." Retrieved at: <http:// www.btselem.org/statistics/fatalities/during-cast-lead/by-date-of-event>.

28. OCHA (UN Office for Coordinating Humanitarian Affairs, OPT), "Gaza Emergency," August 2, 2014. Retrieved at: <http://www.ochaopt.org/ documents/ocha_opt_sitrep_03_08_2014.pdf>.

29. Sara Leibovich-Dar, "The Hannibal Procedure." *Ha'aretz*, May 21, 2003; Sara Leibovich-Dar, "Continuation of the Hannibal Procedure." *Ha'aretz*, May 21, 2003; Anshel Pfeffer, "The Hannibal Directive: Why Israel Risks the Life of the Soldier Being Rescued." *Ha'aretz*, August 3, 2014.

30. Maoz, *Defending*.

31. Almog, "Lessons," p. 13; Morag, *Homeland Security*.

32. Almog, "Cumulative," pp. 8–9, 12.

33. Almog, "Lessons," p. 6; Almog, "Cumulative," p. 12.

34. Amidror, "Winning."

35. Maoz, *Defending*, p. 233; Robert J. Brym and Robert Andersen, *Rational Choice and the Political Bases of Changing Israeli Counterinsurgency Strategy*, 2010. Retrieved at: <http://projects.chass.utoronto.ca/soc101y/brym/BrymAndersen. pdf>.

36. Weizman, *Hollow Land*, pp. 239–40.

37. Scott Wilson, "In Gaza, Lives Shaped by Drones." *Washington Post*, December 3, 2011. Retrieved at: <http://www.washingtonpost.com/world/national-security/ in-gaza-lives-shaped-by-drones/2011/11/30/gIQAjaP6OO_story.html>.

38. Pappe, *Cleansing*, p. 19.

39. "List of Israeli Assassinations," Compiled by Wikipedia, 2014. Retrieved at: <http://en.wikipedia.org/wiki/List_of_Israeli_assassinations>; Simon Frankel Pratt, "'Anyone Who Hurts Us': How the Logic of Israel's 'Assassination Policy' Developed During the Aqsa Intifada." *Terrorism and Political Violence* (2013), 25, pp. 224–45.

40. Weizman, *Hollow Land*, p. 243.

41. Morag, *Homeland Security*.

42. Weizman, *Hollow Land*, p. 247.

43. Esposito, *Arsenal*.

44. Weizman, *Hollow Land*, pp. 246–48.

45. Laleh Khalili, "A Habit of Destruction." *Society & Space*, August 25, 2014. Retrieved at: <http://societyandspace.com/material/commentaries/laleh-khalili-a-habit-of-destruction>.

46. Thomas Henriksen, *The Israeli Approach to Irregular Warfare and Implications for the United States*. Hurlburt Field, FL: The Joint Special Operations University Press, 2007, pp. 11–12.

47. Avi Shlaim, *The Iron Wall: Israel and the Arab World*. London: Norton, 2000, pp. 410–16.

48. Weizman, *Hollow Land*, pp. 187–8; See also Graham, referenced in Weizman, pp. 186–7.

49. Yotam Feldman, "Dr. Naveh, or, How I Learned to Stop Worrying and Walk Through Walls." *Ha'aretz* Supplement, November 1, 2007.

50. Weizman, *Hollow Land*, p. 188.

51. Graham, *Cities*, p. 2.

52. Morag, *Homeland Security*.

53. Weizman, *Hollow Land*, pp. 12–16.

54. Ibid., pp. 12–16.

55. Ibid., pp. 196–7.

56. Ibid., pp. 185–201; Graham, *Cities*, p. 121; Human Rights Watch, *Jenin: IDF Military Operations*, 2002. Retrieved at: <http://www.hrw.org/reports/2002/israel3/israel0502.pdf>; Human Rights Watch, *Jenin: IDF Military Operations*, 2002. Retrieved at: <http://www.hrw.org/reports/2002/israel3/israel0502.pdf>.

57. Morag, *Homeland Security*.

58. Jabotinsky, *Iron Wall*.

59. Quoted in Shlaim, *Iron Wall*, pp. 18–19.

60. Ari Shavit, "Survival of the Fittest." *Ha'aretz*, January 8, 2004. Retrieved at: <http://www.haaretz.com/survival-of-the-fittest-1.61345>.

61. Amira Hass, "Someone Even Managed to Defecate Into the Photocopier." *Ha'aretz*, May 6, 2002. Retrieved at: <http://www.haaretz.com/print-edition/features/someone-even-managed-to-defecate-into-the-photocopier-1.46032>.

62. Weizman, *Hollow Land*, pp. 205-208; Anthony H. Cordesman, *Arab-Israeli Military Forces in an Era of Asymmetrical Warfare*. Westport, CT: Praeger, 2006, p. 73.

63. IDF Blog, "Urban Warfare Training Center – Simulating the Modern Battle-Field," 2011. Retrieved at: <http://www.idfblog.com/blog/2011/10/26/urban-warfare-training-center-simulating-the-modern-battle-field>.

64. Steve Niva, *Walling Off Iraq: Israel's Imprint on U.S. Counterinsurgency Doctrine*. Middle East Policy Council (2008), 15:3. Retrieved at: <http://www.mepc.org/journal/middle-east-policy-archives/walling-iraq-israels-imprint-us-counterinsurgency-doctrine>; Steve Niva, "US Takes Counterinsurgency Lessons From Israel." *Anti-war.com*, 2008. Retrieved at: <http://www.antiwar.com/orig/niva.php?articleid=12727>.

65. Mike Davis, "The Pentagon as Global Slumlord." *Tom's Dispatch*, April 19, 2004. Retrieved at: <http://www.tomdispatch.com/post/1386>.

66. Niva, "Walling Off."

67. Graham, *Cities*, p. xviii.

68. Jimmy Johnson, "The Pacification Industry: Apartheid Wall Contractor to Provide Security at African Cup." *Counterpunch*, June 7, 2011. Retrieved at: <http://www.counterpunch.org/2011/06/07/the-pacification-industry>.

69. Jimmy Johnson, "A Palestine-Mexico Border? Border Wars." Retrieved at: <http://superuw.org/a-palestine-mexico-border>.

70. UNCTAD, *The Palestinian War-Torn Economy: Aid, Development and State Formation.* New York: United Nations, 2006.

71. Ibid.; Raja Khalidi and Sahar Taghdisi-Rad, *The Economic Dimensions of Prolonged Occupation: Continuity and Change in Israeli Policy Towards the Palestinian Economy.* New York: UNCTAD, 2009; ARIJ and the Palestinian Ministry of the Economy, *The Economic Costs of the Israeli Occupation for the Occupied Palestinian Territory,* 2011. Retrieved at:<http://www.mne.gov.ps/pdf/EconomiccostsofoccupationforPalestine.pdf>; Shir Hever, *The Political Economy of Israel's Occupation: Repression Beyond Exploitation.* London: Pluto Press, 2010.

72. Shir Hever, *The Economy of the Occupation (Part 1): Foreign Aid to the Occupied Palestinian Territories and Israel.* Jerusalem: Alternative Information Center, 2005, p. 7.

Chapter 9

1. Grimmett, *Conventional Arms*, pp. 26–7; Grimmitt and Kerr, *Arms Transfers*, p. 41.

2. Gill Cohen, "6,800 arms exporters working in Israel, state documents reveal." *Ha'aretz*, July 15, 2013. Retrieved at: <http://www.haaretz.com/news/diplomacy-defense/.premium-1.535794>.

3. Jewish Telegraphic Agency, "Shamir Leaves on 12-day Official Visit to Argentina and Uruguay," December 12, 1982. Retrieved at: <http://www.jta.org/1982/12/13/archive/shamir-leaves-on-12-day-official-visit-to-argentina-and-uruguay>.

4. Shlaim, *Iron Wall*, p. 396; Goldfield, *Garrison*, p. 18.

5. Beit-Hallahmi, *Connection*, pp. 8–21.

6. Abadi, *Quest*, p. 419; Alexander Murinson, *The Ties Between Israel and Azerbaijan.* The Begin-Sadat Center for Strategic Studies, 2014, p. 9. Retrieved at: <http://besacenter.org/wp-content/uploads/2014/10/MSPS110-web.pdf>.

7. Bruce Maddy-Weitzman, "Israel and Morocco: A Special Relationship." *The Maghreb Review* (1996), 21(1–2): 36–48. Retrieved at: <http://www.dayan.org/commentary/ISRAEL%20AND%20MOROCCO%20A%20SPECIAL%20RELATIONSHIP.pdf>.

8. Beit-Hallahmi, *Connection*, pp. 9–11; Murinson, *Ties*, p. 13; Shlaim, *Iron Wall*, p. 196.

9. Shlaim, *Iron Wall*, p. 195; IJAN, *Repression*. Retrieved at: <http://israelglobalrepression.files.wordpress.com/2012/12/israels-worldwide-role-in-repression-footnotes-finalized.pdf>.

10. Shlaim, *Iron Wall*, p. 196; Omid Voqoufi, *The US, Israel and the Foundation of SAVAK.* Islamic Revolution Document Center, Tehran, 2012. Retrieved at: <http://www.irdc.ir/en/content/18727/default.aspx>.

11. Chomsky, *Reasons*.

12. Feinstein, *Shadow World*, pp. 378–82; Goldfield, *Garrison*, pp. 19–20.

13. Hunter, *Israeli Foreign Policy*.

14. Beit-Hallahmi, *Connection*, pp. 13–15.
15. Shlaim, *Iron Wall*, pp. 195–6; Ephraim Inbar, *The Deterioration in Israeli-Turkish Relations and Its International Ramifications*. The Begin-Sadat (BESA) Center for Strategic Studies, 2011, pp. 2–3. Retrieved at: <http://www.biu.ac.il/Besa/MSPS89.pdf>.
16. Moustapha Slieman, *The Turkish Middle East Role: Between the Arabs and Israel*. US Army War College, 2002, p. 15. Retrieved at: <www.dtic.mil/cgi-bin/GetTRDoc?AD=ada404530>.
17. Shlaim, *Iron Wall*, pp. 558–9.
18. UPI, "Turkey 'Freezes Arms Deals With Israel,'" 2010. Retrieved at: <http://www.upi.com/Business_News/Security-Industry/2010/06/18/Turkey-freezes-arms-deals-with-Israel/UPI-24011276879457>.
19. Ofra Bengio, "Surprising Ties between Israel and the Kurds." *Middle East Quarterly* (2014), 21: 3. Retrieved at: <http://www.meforum.org/3838/israel-kurds>.
20. Trita Parsi, *Treacherous Alliance: The Secret Dealings of Israel, Iran and the US*, 2007. New Haven, CT: Yale University Press; Sohrab Sobhani, *The Pragmatic Entente: Israeli-Iranian Relations, 1948–1988*. New York: Praeger, 1989, pp. 46–7.
21. Bengio, *Surprising*; Magdi Abdelhadi, "Israelis 'Train Kurdish Forces.'" *BBC News*, 2006. Retrieved at:<http://news.bbc.co.uk/2/hi/5364982.stm>.
22. Sergey Minasian, "The Israeli-Kurdish Relations." *21ˢᵗ Century* (2007) 1: 27–8. Retrieved at: <http://www.noravank.am/upload/pdf/256_en.pdf>.
23. Maddy-Weitzman, "Morocco," pp. 39–40; Shmuel Segev, *The Moroccan Connection: The Secret Relations Between Israel and Morocco*. Tel Aviv: Matar Books, 2008. (Hebrew).
24. Beit-Hallahmi, *Connection*, pp. 9–21.
25. Jimmy Johnson, "Israeli Arms Sales to Rwandan Genocidaires Should Not Be Surprising." *Jadaliyya*, 2012. Retrieved at: <http://www.jadaliyya.com/pages/index/6229/israeli-arms-sales-to-rwandan-genocidaires-should->.
26. Elizabeth Blade, "The Unspoken Alliance: Israel and the House of Saud." *Israel Today*, 2012. Part 1 retrieved at: <http://www.israeltoday.co.il/NewsItem/tabid/178/nid/23416/Default.aspx>; Part 2: <http://www.israeltoday.co.il/NewsItem/tabid/178/nid/23420/Default.aspx>.
27. Alexander Bligh, "Israel and the Arab World – From Conflict to Coexistence." Jewish Virtual Library, 2012. Retrieved at: <http://www.jewishvirtuallibrary.org/jsource/isdf/text/bligh.html>.
28. Quoted in James Dorsey, "Israel and Saudi Arabia: Forging Ties on Quicksand." *The World Post*, April 5, 2014. Retrieved at: < http://www.huffingtonpost.com/james-dorsey/israel-and-saudi-arabia-f_b_5582049.html>.
29. Aluf Benn, "Pakistan Denies Receiving Military Equipment from Israel." *Ha'aretz*, June 11, 2013. Retrieved at: <http://www.haaretz.com/news/diplomacy-defense/.premium-1.529120>.
30. Alexander Murinson, "Strategic Realignment and Energy Security in the Eastern Mediterranean," Begin-Sadat Center for Strategic Studies, January 9, 2012. Retrieved at: <http://www.biu.ac.il/SOC/besa/perspectives159.html>.
31. Gil Feiler and Kevjn Lim, *Israel and Kazakhstan Assessing the State of Bilateral Relations*. Ramat Gan: The Begin-Sadat Center for Strategic Studies, 2013, pp. 18, 21.

32. Murinson, *Ties*, p. 9.
33. Christopher Boucek, "The Impact of Israeli Foreign Policy in Central Asia: The Case of Uzbekistan." *Central Asia and the Caucasus* (2004), 4(28): 71. Retrieved at:<http://cyberleninka.ru/article/n/the-impact-of-israeli-foreign-policy-in-central-asia-the-case-of-uzbekistan>.
34. Marlène Laruelle, "Israel and Central Asia: Opportunities and Limits for Partnership in a Post-Arab Spring World." *GMF*, 2012. Retrieved at: <http://www.gmfus.org/wp-content/blogs.dir/1/files_mf/1342636966Laruelle_IsraelCentralAsia_Jul12.pdf>.
35. Murinson, *Ties*, pp. 10.
36. Mark Perry, "Israel's Secret Staging Ground." *Foreign Policy*, March 28, 2012; Michael Segall, *Iran Fears Growing Israel-Azerbaijan Cooperation.* Jerusalem Center for Public Affairs, 2013. Retrieved at:<http://jcpa.org/article/iran-fears-growing-israel-azerbaijan-cooperation>.
37. Feiler and Lim, *Kazakhstan*, p. 26.
38. Human Rights Watch, *World Report 2014: Azerbaijan*, 2014. Retrieved at: <http://www.hrw.org/world-report/2014/country-chapters/azerbaijan>; Murinson, *Ties*, pp. 10, 20.
39. Murinson, *Ties*, pp. 24–6; SIPRI, "Israeli and Russian Arms Sales to Azerbaijan." *SIPRI Arms Transfers Database*, 2011; TR Defense, "Azerbaijan Eliminated Aselsan, Selected Israeli Elbit to Upgrade Tanks," 2010. Retrieved at: <http://www.trdefence.com/2010/10/18/azerbaijan-eliminated-aselsan-to-upgrade-tanks>.
40. SIPRI: ibid.
41. Nicholas Clayton, "Drone Violence Along Armenian-Azerbaijani Border Could Lead To War." *Global Post*, October 23, 2012. Retrieved at: <http://www.globalpost.com/dispatch/news/regions/europe/121022/drone-violence-along-armenian-azerbaijani-border-could-lead-war>.
42. Murinson, *Ties*, p. 26.
43. Ibid.
44. Richard Weitz, "Azerbaijani Defense Policy and Military Power." *Second Line of Defense*, 2012. Retrieved at: <http://www.sldinfo.com/azerbaijani-defense-policy-and-military-power>; "Israel Rearms Azerbaijani Army." PanArmenian. Net, June 30, 2009. Retrieved at: <http://www.panarmenian.net/eng/world/news/33537>.
45. Murinson, *Ties*, p. 21.
46. Ami Rojkes Dombe, "Meeting in Azerbaijan." *Israel Defense*, January 2, 2014. Retrieved at: <http://www.israeldefense.com/?CategoryID=474&ArticleID=2676>.
47. Murinson, *Ties*, p. 31.
48. Human Rights Watch, *World Report 2014: Kazakhstan*, 2014. Retrieved at: <http://www.hrw.org/world-report/2014/country-chapters/kazakhstan>.
49. Feiler and Lim, *Kazakhstan*, p. 9.
50. Ibid., p. 22.
51. John Daly, "Kazakhstan, Israel Deepen Military Ties." *Eurasia Daily Monitor* (2014), 11:19. Retrieved at: <http://www.jamestown.org/regions/centralasia/single/?tx_ttnews%5Bpointer%5D=5&tx_ttnews%5Btt_news%5D=41896&tx_ttnews%5BbackPid%5D=53&cHash=a1672deddc68e51b4507cb8d04cec

a8e#.VJgusACAQ>; Erik Blackwell, "Kazakhstan, Israel Strengthen Military Cooperation." *Astana Times*, January 22, 2014. Retrieved at: <http://www. astanatimes.com/2014/01/kazakhstan-israel-strengthen-military-cooperation>.

52. Feiler and Lim, *Kazakhstan*, pp. 31–2.

53. Boucek, "Impact," p. 78.

54. Laruelle, "Central Asia."

55. Daly, "Deepen"; Feiler and Lim, *Kazakhstan*, pp. 35–6.

56. Laruelle, "Central Asia."

57. "Israeli Diplomats Nix Drone Sale to Ukraine." *Times of Israel*, September 15, 2014. Retrieved at: <http://www.timesofisrael.com/israeli-diplomats-nix-drone-sale-to-ukraine-report>.

58. Feinstein, *Shadow World*, pp. 384–5.

59. Yossi Melman, "Bloody Business in Africa." *Ha'aretz*, December 31, 2009. Retrieved at: <http://www.webguinee.net/etat/postcolonial/cndd/camara_moussa_dadis/vu_presse/israel-bloody-business-guinea.html>.

60. Michael Bishku, "Israel and Ethiopia: From a Special to a Pragmatic Relationship." *Conflict Quarterly*, Spring 1994. Retrieved at: <http://journals. hil.unb.ca/index.php/JCS/article/viewFile/15180/16249>; Stratfor Global Intelligence, *Eritrea: Another Venue for the Iran-Israel Rivalry*, 2012.

61. Naomi Chazan, *Israel and Africa: Assessing the Past, Envisioning the Future*. Tel Aviv: American Jewish Committee, 2006, p. 2.

62. Sara Leibovich-Dar, "The Israeli-African Connection: Who Are The Israelis That Pull The Strings of the Black Continent." *Liberal* (2014), 7: 47 (in Hebrew).

63. Siemon Wezeman, "Israeli Arms Transfers to Sub-Saharan Africa." SIPRI Background Paper, 2011, pp. 1–2, 5. Retrieved at: <http://www.nonproliferation. eu/documents/other/siemontwezeman4e9eb5e5806bd.pdf>.

64. Small Arms Survey, *Small Arms Transfers: Exporting States*, 2011. Retrieved at: <http://www.smallarmssurvey.org/fileadmin/docs/H-Research_Notes/SAS-Research-Note-11.pdf>.

Chapter 10

1. Amnon Barzilai, "Israel Set Up Singapore's Army, Former Officers Reveal." *Ha'aretz*, July 15, 2004; Abadi, *Quest*, pp. 171–81.

2. Arie Egosi, "Defense Exports: Strong Growth for Israel in Asia." *Defense Review Asia*, 2012. Retrieved at: <http://www.defencereviewasia.com/articles/165/Strong-growth-for-Israel-in-Asia>.

3. Gill Cohen, "India Buys $525m Worth of Missiles From Israel, Rejecting Rival U.S. Offer." *Ha'aretz*, October 25, 2014; Egosi, "Defense Exports."

4. Dinshaw Mistry, "US Arms Sales to India." *Asia Pacific Bulletin*, #271 (2014), East-West Center. Retrieved at: <http://www.eastwestcenter.org/sites/default/files/private/apb271.pdf>; Gill Cohen, "Israel Ranks as the World's Sixth Largest Arms Exporter in 2012." *Ha'aretz*, June 25, 2013. Retrieved at:<http://www.haaretz.com/news/diplomacy-defense/.premium-1.531956>; Richard A. Bitzinger, "Indian-Israeli Defence Cooperation: The Elusive Strategic Partnership – Analysis." *Eurasia Review*, April 11, 2013. Retrieved at: <http://www.eurasiareview.com/11042013-indian-israeli-defence-cooperation-the-elusive-strategic-partnership-analysis>.

5. *Defense Review Asia*, "Asian Region UAV Capability"; Efraim Inbar and Alvite Singh Ningthoujam, *Indo-Israeli Defense Cooperation in the Twenty-First Century*. Begin-Sadat Center for Strategic Studies, 2012, pp. 6–15.

6. "India & Israel's Barak-8 SAM Development Project." *Defense Review Asia*, March 2, 2015. Retrieved at: <http://www.defenseindustrydaily.com/india-israel-introducing-mr-sam-03461/>.

7. Egosi, "Defense Exports."

8. Ibid.

9. Alvite Singh Ningthoujam, *India-Israel Defense Cooperation*. Begin-Sadat Center for Strategic Studies, 2014. Retrieved at: <http://besacenter.org/perspectives-papers/india-israel-defense-cooperation>.

10. "Large Israeli Presence at Defexpo 2014." *Defense Review Asia*, 2014. Retrieved at: <http://www.defencereviewasia.com/articles/285/Large-Israeli-Presence-at-Defexpo-2014>.

11. Amit Baruah, "India may end support to Palestine at U.N." *The Hindu*, December 21, 2014. Retrieved at: <http://www.thehindu.com/news/national/india-may-end-support-to-palestine-at-un/article6713364.ece>.

12. Goldfield, *Garrison*, p. 18; Jonas Lindberg, Camilla Orjuela, Siemon Wezeman and Linda Åkerström, *Arms Trade With Sri Lanka - Global Business, Local Costs*. Stockholm: The Swedish Peace and Arbitration Society, 2011; Lakkana Nanayakkara, "How Israel Helped Sri Lanka Defeat the Tamil Tigers." *The Algemeiner*, 2012. Retrieved at: <http://www.algemeiner.com/2012/01/31/how-israel-helped-sri-lanka-defeat-the-tamil-tigers>; Shlomi Yass, "Sri Lanka and the Tamil Tigers: Conflict and Legitimacy." *Military and Strategic Affairs* (2014), 6(2): 65–82.

13. "Sri Lankan Ambassador: We Back Israel's War on Terror." *Yedioth Aharonoth*, 2010. Retrieved at: <http://www.ynetnews.com/articles/0,7340,L-3923309,00.html>; Shlomi Yass, "Sri Lanka and the Tamil Tigers: Conflict and Legitimacy." *Military and Strategic Affairs* (2014), 6(2): 65–82.

14. Ana Pararajasingham, "Sri Lanka: In the Eye of the Storm." *Defense Review Asia*, 2011. Retrieved at: <http://www.defencereviewasia.com/articles/85/Sri-Lanka-In-the-Eye-of-the-Storm>.

15. Egosi, "Defense Exports."

16. Anthony Ware, "Republic of Korea Army Selects Heron UAS." *C4ISR & Networks*, 2014. Retrieved at: <http://www.c4isrnet.com/story/military-tech/uas/2014/12/18/republic-of-korea-army-selects-heron-uas/20593589>.

17. Egosi, "Defense Exports."

18. Ibid.

19. "Elbit Systems to Upgrade Tanks for a Customer in the Asia-Pacific Region Under $290 Million Contract.", *Defense Review Asia*, 2014. Retrieved at: <http://www.defencereviewasia.com/articles/301/Elbit-Systems-to-Upgrade-Tanks-for-a-Customer-in-the-Asia-Pacific-Region-Under-290-Million-Contract>.

20. Jamail and Gutierrez, *No Secret*, p. 15; Almond, "British and Israeli," p. 65.

21. Bahbah, *Latin America*.

22. Stop the Wall Campaign, *Buying into Occupation and War: The Implications of Military Ties Between South America and Israel*, 2010, p. 8. Retrieved at:<http://stopthewall.org/downloads/pdf/buy-in2-occ.pdf>.

23. Jorge I. Domínguez, *Boundary Disputes in Latin America*. Washington, DC: United States Institute for Peace, 2003.

24. "Defense Industries Take Brazil." *Ma'ariv*, December 1, 2010.

25. "SIPRI: Latin America Military Spending Increased by 4.2 Percent in 2012." *Dialogo, Digital Military Magazine*, 2013. Retrieved at: <http://dialogo-americas.com/en_GB/articles/rmisa/features/regional_news/2013/06/17/defense-spending>. SIPRI, *Yearbook*, 2013; Stop the Wall, *Buying*, p. 21.

26. SIPRI, *Background Paper*; Stop the Wall, *Buying*, p. 21.

27. Stop the Wall, *Buying*, p. 9.

28. Ibid., pp. 16–17.

29. Yoram Gabison, "Elbit Systems Hiring Locals to Win Large Brazilian Tenders." *Ha'aretz*, November 10, 2009. Retrieved at: <http://www.haaretz.com/print-edition/business/elbit-systems-hiring-locals-to-win-large-brazilian-tenders-1.4432>.

30. Tamor Eshel, "Embraer Enters Unmanned Vehicles Market through Partnership with Elbit Systems, Santos Lab." *RP Defense*, 2011. Retrieved at: <http://rpdefense.over-blog.com/article-embraer-enters-unmanned-vehicles-market-through-partnership-with-elbit-systems-santos-lab-71660367.html>.

31. Stop the Wall, *Buying*, p. 14.

32. Elbit, "Elbit Systems Awarded Contract to Supply Brazil with Hermes 900 UAS," 2014. Retrieved at: <http://ir.elbitsystems.com/phoenix.zhtml?c=61849&p=irol-newsArticle&ID=1912412>.

33. Ibid.

34. "VBTP Guarani: A New APC for Brazil." *Defense Industry Daily*, 2014. Retrieved at: <http://www.defenseindustrydaily.com/vbtp-a-new-apc-for-brazil-06048>; Elbit, "New Achievement for Elbit Systems in Brazil: Elbit Systems Brazilian Subsidiary, Ares, Awarded Approximately $25 Million Contract to Supply 12.7/7.62mm Remote Controlled Weapon Stations," 2012. Retrieved at: <http://ir.elbitsystems.com/phoenix.zhtml?c=61849&p=irol-newsArticle&ID=1749141&highlight=>; Stop the Wall, *Buying*, p. 11.

35. AEL, "AEL Presents the Model for the First Brazilian Microsatellite for Military Applications," 2013. Retrieved at: <http://www.ael.com.br/ing/downloads/press_release_ael_apresenta_modelo_do_primeiro_microssatelite_brasileiro_para_aplicacoes_militares_ing.pdf>.

36. BDS Movement, "Elbit Systems Loses Key Brazil Deal Over Palestine Protests," 2014. Retrieved at: <http://www.bdsmovement.net/2014/elbit-systems-loses-key-brazil-Bechdeal-12878>.

37. SIBAT. *Israel at LAAD 2013: Promoting Cooperation and Partnership*, 2013. Retrieved at: <http://www.sibat.mod.gov.il/NR/rdonlyres/855A3898-5D56-41E0-8EC2-1463CE4E4342/0/SIBATIsraelPavilionLAADEnglishFinal.pdf>.

38. Stop the Wall, "Brazilians Show Their Solidarity with Palestine at the LAAD Fair in Rio," 2013. Retrieved at: <http://www.stopthewall.org/2013/04/15/brazilians-show-their-solidarity-palestine-laad-fair-rio>.

39. David Cronin, "Rotterdam Rolls Out Red Carpet For Israeli War Industry." *Electronic Intifada*, November 13, 2013. Retrieved at: <http://intifada39.rssing.com/browser.php?indx=14465053&item=21>.

40. Gabison, "Elbit."

41. Defense Update, "Following Latin-American Success, Israel's Defense Technology Innovator RAFAEL Charts Brazil Expansion," 2011. Retrieved at: <http://defense-update.com/20110405_rafael_latin_america_laad_2011_brazi. html#.VJ6JUACAQ>.

42. Sebastian Castaneda, "Mahmoud Abbas is Wasting His Time in Colombia." *Aljazeera*, 2011. Retrieved at: <http://www.aljazeera.com/indepth/opinion/20 11/10/2011103111559136471.html>.

43. Yishai Halper, "Colombian President: Proud to Be Called 'The Israel of Latin America,'" *Ha'aretz*, June 16, 2013.

44. Air Force World, "Kfir Fighter – Israel." Retrieved at: <http://www.airforceworld. com/fighter/eng/kfir.htm>; "Colombia's Defense Modernization." *Defense Industry Daily*, 2013. Retrieved at: <http://www.defenseindustrydaily.com/ colombias-defense-modernization-05273>.

45. Merco Press, "Argentina After Israeli Fighter Planes; Concern in London and Brasilia, Says Defense Expert." *Ha'aretz*, March 23, 2014.

46. Defense Update, "At 40 Years of Age, Kfir Turns into a 'Networked Fighter,'" 2013. Retrieved at: <http://defense-update.com/20131006_at-40-years-of-age-kfir-turns-into-a-networked-fighter.html#.VJ6gAACAQ>.

47. Nazih Richani, "Israel Enlists Colombian Support Against Palestinian Statehood." NACLA, 2011. Retrieved at: <https://nacla.org/blog/2011/7/18/ israel-enlists-colombian-support-against-palestinian-statehood>.

48. JTA, "Jacques Wagner Named Brazilian Minister of Defense." *Ha'aretz*, December 27, 2014. Retrieved at: <http://www.haaretz.com/jewish-world/ jewish-world-news/1.633957>.

49. Excélsior, "Militares israelíes darán clases a policías de Chiapas," May 8, 2013. Retrieved at: <http://www.excelsior.com.mx/nacional/2013/05/08/898070>.

50. Stop the Wall, *Buying*, p. 24.

51. SIPRI, *Transfers of Major Conventional Weapons, 2000–2013* <www.sipri.org/ yearbook/...>.

Chapter 11

1. Cohen, "6,800 Exporters."

2. Yossi Melman, "Why Are So Many Israelis Arrested Over Illegal Arms Deals Worldwide?" *Ha'aretz*, July 1, 2010. Retrieved at: <http://www.haaretz.com/ news/diplomacy-defense/why-are-so-many-israelis-arrested-over-illegal-arms-deals-worldwide-1.299308>.

3. Yossi Melman, "Israeli Arms Dealers Join Lieberman's Entourage to Africa." *Ha'aretz*, August 6, 2009. Retrieved at: <http://www.haaretz.com/print-edition/ features/israeli-arms-dealers-join-lieberman-s-entourage-to-africa-1.281501>.

4. Sara Leibovich-Dar, "The Israeli-African Connection: Who Are The Israelis That Pull The Strings of the Black Continent." *Liberal* (2014), 7: 40. (in Hebrew).

5. Siemon Wezeman, "Israeli Arms Transfers to Sub-Saharan Africa." SIPRI Background Paper, 2011, p. 8. Retrieved at: <http://www.nonproliferation.eu/ documents/other/siemontwezeman4e9eb5e5806bd.pdf>.

6. Human Rights Watch, *Acknowledging Genocide*, 1999. Retrieved at: <http:// www.hrw.org/reports/1999/rwanda/Geno15-8-02.htm>; see also Andrew

Wallis, *Silent Accomplice: The Untold Story of France's Role in the Rwandan Genocide*. London: I.B. Taurus, 2013, pp. 115–16.

7. Lieberman-Dar, "Israel-African," p. 40; Ilan Lor, "Israel is Sending Asylum Seekers to Rwanda Without Status, Rights." *Ha'aretz*, April 4, 2014. Retrieved at: <http://www.haaretz.com/news/national/.premium-1.583764>; "Israel Uses Refugees as "Currency" in Arms Trade With Africa." *The Real News*, 2014. Retrieved at: <http://therealnews.com/t2/index.php?option=com_content&task=view&id=31&Itemid=74&jumival=11749>; Natasha Roth, "In Israel's Trade Catalog, Arms and Asylum Seekers Are Equal Commodities." +972, December 9, 2013. Retrieved at: <http://972mag.com/for-israels-trade-catalog-arms-and-asylum-seekers-are-equal-commodities/75566>.

8. *Africa Report*, quoted in Goldfield, *Garrison*, pp. 21–2.

9. Lieberman-Dar, "Israel-African," pp. 42, 44.

10. Ibid., p. 44.

11. Yossi Melman, "Ex-IDF Top Officer Dies in Cameroon Helicopter Crash." *Ha'aretz*, November 22, 2010. Retrieved at:<http://www.haaretz.com/news/diplomacy-defense/ex-idf-top-officer-dies-in-cameroon-helicopter-crash-1.326171>.

12. Carolyn Nordstrom, *Global Outlaws: Crime, Money, and Power in the Contemporary World*. Berkeley: University of California Press, 2007, p. 58.

13. Duffield, *Development*, p. 172.

14. Michael Parenti, *Against Empire*. San Francisco, CA: City Lights, 1995.

15. "Diamonds Remain Israel's Main Export Category." *Idexmagazine* #269, 2012. Retrieved at: <http://idexonline.com/portal_FullMazalUbracha.asp?id=37256>.

16. Seán Clinton, "The Diamond Industry's Double-Standard on Israel." *Electronic Intifada*, 2011 Retrieved at: <http://electronicintifada.net/content/diamond-industrys-double-standard-israel/10102>; Seán Clinton, "Israel's Greatest Fear – Its Diamond Trade Exposed." *OpEdNews*, 2012. Retrieved at: <http://www.opednews.com/articles/Israel-s-greatest-fear--i-by-Se-n-Clinton-121027-116.html>.

17. Jimmy Johnson, "Israelis and Hezbollah Haven't Always Been Enemies." Israeli Committee Against House Demolitions (ICAHD) website, 2006. Retrieved at: <http://www.icahd.org/node/361>.

18. Yossi Melman, "A Diamond in the Rough." *Ha'aretz*, July 15, 2011. Retrieved at: <http://www.haaretz.com/weekend/week-s-end/a-diamond-in-the-rough-1.373420>; Misha Glenny, *McMafia: Seriously Organized Crime*. London: Vintage, 2009, pp. 234–5.

19. Lieberman-Dar, "Israeli-African," p. 45; Yossi Melman, "Angling in on Angola." *Ha'aretz*, January 4, 2002. Retrieved at: <http://www.haaretz.com/angling-in-on-angola-1.79089>.

20. Human Rights Watch, *Bloody Monday: The September 28 Massacre and Rapes by Security Forces in Guinea*, 2009. Retrieved at: <http://www.hrw.org/sites/default/files/reports/guinea1209web_0.pdf>.

21. Yossi Melman, "Bloody Business in Africa." *Ha'aretz*, December 31, 2009. Retrieved at: <http://www.webguinee.net/etat/postcolonial/cndd/camara_moussa_dadis/vu_presse/israel-bloody-business-guinea.html>.

22. Ibid.

23. George Ayittey, "The Worst of the Worst." *Foreign Policy*, June 15, 2010. Retrieved at: <http://foreignpolicy.com/2010/06/15/the-worst-of-the-worst-3>.

24. Lieberman-Dar, "Israeli-African," p. 45.

25. Yossi Melman, "Israelis to Train Equatorial Guinea Presidential Guard." *Ha'aretz*, June 3. 2005.

26. Ibid.

27. Yossi Melman, "Sources: Israeli Businesswoman Brokering Equatorial Guinea Arms Sales." *Ha'aretz*, November 12, 2008; Feinstein, *Shadow World*, pp. 386–7.

28. Lieberman-Dar, "Israeli-African," p. 45; Peter Maas, "A Touch of Crude." *Mother Jones*, 2005. Retrieved at: <http://www.motherjones.com/politics/2005/01/obiang-equatorial-guinea-oil-riggs>.

29. Lieberman-Dar, "Israeli-African," p. 45.

30. Yossi Melman, "Meanwhile, Back in Nigeria … ." *Ha'aretz*, September 16, 2010. Retrieved at: <http://www.haaretz.com/print-edition/features/inside-intel-meanwhile-back-in-nigeria-1.314084>. 2010.

31. Melman, "Bloody Business."

32. Nasiru L. Abubakar, "Nigeria: Govt-Israel in U.S.$25 Million Arms Deal." *All Africa*, September 9, 2009.

33. Peter Hirshberg on *Democracy Now* (2000): "Who Is Israel's Yair Klein and What Was He Doing in Colombia and Sierra Leone?" Retrieved at: <http://www.democracynow.org/2000/6/1/who_is_israels_yair_klein_and>.

34. Feinstein, *Shadow World*, pp. 98–126; Global Witness, *Glencore And The Gatekeeper*, 2014. Retrieved at: <http://www.globalwitness.org/sites/default/files/library/Glencore%20and%20the%20Gatekeeper%20May%202014.pdf>; Yossi Melman and Asaf Carmel, "Diamond in the Rough." *Ha'aretz*, March 24, 2005. Retrieved at: <http://www.haaretz.com/diamond-in-the-rough-1.153922>; Khadija Sharife and John Grobler, "Kimberley'"s Illicit Process. *World Policy Journal* (Winter 2013). Retrieved at: <http://www.worldpolicy.org/journal/winter2013/kimberleys-illicit-process>; Jason K. Stearns, *Dancing in the Glory of Monsters: The Collapse of the Congo and the Great War of Africa*. New York: Public Affairs, 2011.

35. Feinstein, *Shadow World*, p. 107.

36. Ibid.; Brandon Barrett, "Israeli Mercenary Yair Klein Trained Paramilitary 'With the Approval of the Colombian Authorities.'" *Colombia Reports*, 2012. Retrieved at: <http://colombiareports.co/israeli-mercenary-yair-klein-trained-paramilitary-with-the-approval-of-the-colombian-authorities>; Andrew Cockburn and Leslie Cockburn, *Israel: The Covert Connection* (film, 1989), PBS; Hirshberg on *Democracy Now*, "Yair Klein."

37. Almond, "British and Israeli," pp. 66–7.

38. TAR Ideal Concepts website: <http://www.tarideal.com>.

39. Wezeman, "Arms Transfers," p. 7.

40. Ibid., p. 1.

41. Global CTS website: <www.global-cst.com>.

42. Yossi Melman, "Colombia Hostage Rescue: The Israeli Angle." *Ha'aretz*, July 4, 2008. Retrieved at: <http://www.haaretz.com/print-edition/news/colombia-hostage-rescue-the-israeli-angle-1.249096>.

43. Wikileaks, Viewing Cable 09BOGOTA3483, "Colombian Defense Ministry Sours on Israeli Defense Firm," 2009. Retrieved At:<http://wikileaks.org/cable/2009/12/09BOGOTA3483.html>.

44. Ibid.

45. Ibid.

46. ISDS website: <http://www.isds.co.il>.

47. Max Security Systems website: <www.max-security.com>.

48. ISCA website: <http://www.isca.org.il/research-focus.html>.

49. SAFIRE website: <http://www.safire-project-results.eu>.

50. Golan Group Website: <http://www.golangroup.com/safeshield.html>.

51. "Foreign Armies Flock to Receive Israeli Training." *Israel Today*, January 28, 2010. Retrieved at: <http://www.israeltoday.co.il/default.aspx?tabid=178&nid=20467>.

52. SIPRI, SIPRI Database Expenditure, 2015 <www.sipri.org/research/armaments/milex...>.

53. Arms Control Association, *The Arms Trade Treaty at a Glance*, 2014. Retrieved at: <http://www.armscontrol.org/factsheets/arms_trade_treaty>;United Nations, "UN Officials Hail Entry into Force of Landmark Global Arms Trade Treaty." UN News Center, December 23, 2014. Retrieved at: <http://www.un.org/apps/news/story.asp?NewsID=49668#.VJp9KACAQ>.

54. Rebecca Shimoni Stoil, "50 Senators: UN Arms Trade Treaty Could Harm Israel." *Times of Israel*, October 20, 2013. Retrieved at: <http://www.timesofisrael.com/50-senators-un-arms-trade-treaty-could-harm-israel>.

55. Gill Cohen, "Ya'alon: Signing UN Arms-Control Treaty Puts Israel at Risk." *Ha'aretz*, May 28, 2014. Retrieved at: <http://www.haaretz.com/news/diplomacy-defense/.premium-1.595686>.

Chapter 12

1. Graham, *Cities*, pp. xiii–xiv.

2. Weizman, *Hollow Land*.

3. John Collins, *Global Palestine*. London: C. Hurst, 2011.

4. Graham, *Cities*, p. xxii.

5. From the AIPAC website. Retrieved at: <http://www.aipac.org/search-results?query=trip%20to%20israel%202013&pageSize=5&page=145>.

6. Balko, *Warrior*, pp. 61–2, 144.

7. Suzanne Goldenberg, quoted in Graham, *Cities*, p. 112.

8. Jason Vest, "The Men From JINSA and CSP." *The Nation*, September 2, 2002.

9. Law Enforcement Exchange Program (LEEP), JINSA website: <http://www.jinsa.org/events-programs/law-enforcement-exchange-program-leep/all>.

10. ADL (Anti-Defamation League), "ADL Holds A Milestone Twentieth Advanced Training School Session," 2011. Retrieved at: <http://archive.adl.org/learn/adl_law_enforcement/ats_counterterrorism_training_20.html?LEARN_Cat=Training&LEARN_SubCat=Training_News#.VKwjS77YqfQ>.

11. ADL, "ADL and Law Enforcement: Fighting Terror before 9/11 and Beyond," 2011. Retrieved at: <http://archive.adl.org/learn/adl_law_enforcement/911_adl_law_enforcement.html?LEARN_Cat=Train#.VKwgdb7YqfR>.

12. JINSA website.

13. *A Clean Break: A New Strategy for Securing the Realm*, 1996. Retrieved at: <http://www.informationclearinghouse.info/article1438.htm>.

14. Stephen Zunes, *Why the U.S. Supports Israel*. Washington, DC: Foreign Policy in Focus, 2002.

15. Graham, *Cities*, p. 58.

16. Makram Khoury-Machool, "Losing the Battle for Arab Hearts and Minds." *Open Democracy*, May 2, 2003. Retrieved at: <https://www.opendemocracy.net/media-journalismwar/article_1202.jsp>.

17. Graham, *Cities*; Ilan Berman, "New Horizons for the American-Israeli Partnership." *NATIV Online*, 2004. Retrieved at: <http://www.acpr.org.il/english-nativ/04-issue/berman-4.htm>.

18. Graham, *Cities*, p. 259.

19. Ibid., pp. 259–60.

20. Ibid., p. 260.

21. The Israeli Export and International Cooperation Institute, *Israel: Homeland Security Industry*, 2013. Retrieved at: <http://studyexport.org/docs/all_low%20rez.pdf>.

22. Michel Chossudovsky, "The Canada-Israel 'Public Security' Agreement: Ottawa & Tel Aviv Collaborate In Counter-Terrorism & Homeland Security." *Global Research*, 2008. Retrieved at <http://www.globalresearch.ca/PrintArticle.php?articleId=8530>.

23. Ben-Eliezer, *Militarism*; Baruch Kimmerling, "Patterns of Militarism in Israel." *European Journal of Sociology* (1993), 34: 196–221.

24. Badi Hasisi and Ronald Weitzer, "Police Relations with Arabs and Jews in Israel." *British Journal of Criminology* (2007), 47(5): 735–6; Sammy Smooha, "The Model of Ethnic Democracy: Israel as a Jewish and Democratic State." *Nations and Nationalism* (2002), 8(4): 478. Retrieved at: <http://soc.haifa.ac.il/~s.smooha/download/TheModelofDemIsraelasJewDeminNN.pdf>.

25. B'tselem, *Defense (Emergency) Regulations*. Retrieved at: <http://www.btselem.org/legal_documents/emergency_regulations>.

26. Website of the Israeli Police/Internal Security: <www.mops.gov.il>.

27. Ministry of Public Security, *The Israel Police*, 2014. Retrieved at: <http://mops.gov.il/English/PolicingENG/Police/Pages/default.aspx>.

28. Max Blumenthal, "From Occupation to 'Occupy': The Israelification of American Domestic Security." *Al-Akhbar English*, 2011. Retrieved at: <http://english.al-akhbar.com/node/2178>.

29. Arie Perlinger and Ami Pedahzur, "Coping with Suicide Attacks: Lessons from Israel." *Public Money and Management* (2006), 26(5): 281–6. Retrieved at: <https://www.academia.edu/247728/Coping_with_Suicide_Attacks_Lessons_from_Israel>.

30. University of Texas, *Terrorists, Insurgents and Guerillas: Professor Provides Data to Help Fight Terrorism*. Retrieved at: <http://repositories.lib.utexas.edu/bitstream/handle/2152/14215/13Life_Letters_terrorists.pdf?sequence=14>.

31. The Israeli Export and International Cooperation Institute, *Israel*.

32. Perliger and Pedahzur, "Coping," p. 283; David Weisburd, Jonathan Tal and Simon Perry, "The Israeli Model for Policing Terrorism: Goals, Strategies, and Open Questions." *Criminal Justice and Behavior* (2009), 36(12): 1259–78.

33. Raphael Ron, quoted in Jonathan Tucker, "Strategies for Countering Terrorism – Lessons from the Israeli Experience." *COIN Central: The Counterinsurgency Journal* (2003). Retrieved at: <http://coincentral.wordpress.com/2008/06/04/strategies-for-countering-terrorism-lessons-from-the-israeli-experience>.

34. Yair Livne, "What is the Israeli Model for Airport Security?" *Quora*, 2012. Retrieved at: <http://www.quora.com/What-is-the-Israeli-model-for-airport-security>.

35. Ron, "Lessons;" Philip Giraldi, "Homeland Security Made in Israel." *Global Research*, August 24, 2013. Retrieved at: <http://www.globalresearch.ca/homeland-security-made-in-israel/5346796>.

36. B'tselem, *The ISA Interrogation Regime: Routine Ill-Treatment*, 2011. Retrieved at: <http://www.btselem.org/torture/interrogation_regime>.

37. Gill Cohen, "Reservists from Elite IDF Intel Unit Refuse to Serve Over Palestinian 'Persecution,'" *Ha'aretz*, September 12, 2014. Retrieved at: <http://www.haaretz.com/news/diplomacy-defense/1.615498>.

38. COAT (Canadians Opposed to the Arms Trade), "NICE Systems." *Press for Conversion!* (2012), 67: 24–5. Retrieved at: <http://coat.ncf.ca/P4C/67/24-25.pdf>.

39. Hu Quan Hei, "Spies in the Ointment: The Israeli Espionage of Global Communications." *Conspiracy Central Blog*, 2007. Retrieved at: <https://conspiracycentral.wordpress.com/category/computer-security>.

40. Uzi Eilam, *Multi-Layered Defense and Initiated Attack in Defending the Homeland*. Institute of National Security Studies, 2013. Retrieved at: <http://i-hls.com/2013/01/multi-layered-defense-and-initiated-attack-in-defending-the-homeland-2/#sthash.XXxTVAAc.dpbs>.

41. Matt Appuzo and Amy Goldman, "NYPD CIA Anti-Terror Operations Conducted In Secret For Years." *Huffington Post*, August 24, 2011. Retrieved at: <http://www.huffingtonpost.com/2011/08/24/nypd-cia-terrorism_n_934923.html>.

42. "NYPD Opens Branch in Kfar Saba." *Times of Israel*, September 7, 2012. Retrieved at: <http://www.timesofisrael.com/nypd-opens-local-branch-in-kfar-saba>.

43. Appuzzo and Golman, "NYPD."

44. Appuzzo and Golman, "NYPD"; "21st Century Policing: An Interview with America's Top Cop." Israeli Ministry of Public Security, 2013, p. 48. Retrieved at: <http://mops.gov.il/Documents/Publications/InformationCenter/Innovation%20Exchange/Innovation%20Exchange%2017/21st%20Century%20Policing.pdf>.

45. Ali Abunimeh, *The Battle for Justice in Palestine*. Chicago, IL: Haymarket Books, 2014, p. 18; "21st Century Policing".

46. Kaplan, *Petraeus*, p. 24.

47. Niva, "Walling Off."

48. Max Blumenthal, "Occupation to 'Occupy'".

49. Jimmy Johnson, *Export Occupation*.

50. Sari Horwitz, "Israeli Experts Teach Police On Terrorism." *Washington Post*, June 12, 2005. Retrieved at: <http://www.washingtonpost.com/wp-dyn/content/article/2005/06/11/AR2005061100648.html>.

51. Marlan Ingram, *Israeli Combative Pistol Training*, 2012. Retrieved at:<http://www.israelicombattraining.com/training_article.pdf>.

52. John Elliot, "Shoot Like the Jews: Israel's Uzi Powered CQC Techniques." *Guns.*
    Com, 2011. Retrieved at: <http://www.guns.com/2011/12/20/shoot-like-the-
    jews-israels-uzi-powered-cqc-techniques>.

53. David Kahn, *Krav Maga Weapon Defenses*. Retrieved at: <http://ymaa.com/files/
    KravMagaPreview.pdf>.

54. Mark LeVine, "Ferguson is Not Gaza ... Yet." *Electronic Intifada*, August 18, 2014.
    Retrieved at: <http://america.aljazeera.com/opinions/2014/8/ferguson-police-
    violenceisraeliandusmilitarizedpolicies.html>.

55. Graham, *Cities*, pp. 258–9.

56. Ami Pedahzur, *The Israeli Secret Services & the Struggle Against Terrorism*. New
    York: Columbia University Press, 2009; Boaz Ganor, "A New Strategy Against
    the New Terror." *Policy View*, No. 10 (January); Tucker, *Strategies*, p. 1; Weisburd,
    Tal and Perry, *Israeli Model*.

57. Jeff Halper, "Revenge Devoid of Purpose: Punitive Demolitions of Palestinian
    Homes." *Hamishpat*, 2014. (in Hebrew).

58. Gordon, "Working Paper," pp. 11–12; Israeli Ministry of the Economy: "Business
    Sectors: Homeland Security." Retrieved at: <http://www.investinisrael.gov.il/
    NR/exeres/7C2F6937-A259-4A4A-9C29-DE351032B87A.htm>.

59. "Lockheed Martin Opens New Office In Israel." Lockheed Martin website:
    <http://www.lockheedmartin.com/us/news/press-releases/2014/april/0409hq-
    israel.html>.

60. Gordon, "Working Paper, p. 10.

61. Ibid., p. 12.

62. Ibid., p. 6.

63. SIBAT, *Israel Homeland Defense Sales Directory, 2012–13*. Tel Aviv: Israeli Ministry
    of Defense, 2013 Retrieved at: <http://www.sibat.mod.gov.il/sibatmain/Catalog/
    homeland-defense/home-defense.html>.

64. Gordon, "Working Paper," pp. 33–5.

65. Graham, *Cities*, p. 253.

66. i-hls, "It is Better to be Smart than Safe – The Growing Buzz Surrounding Safe
    Cities," 2013. Retrieved at:<http://i-hls.com/2013/06/it-is-better-to-be-smart-
    than-safe-the-growing-buzz-surrounding-safe-cities>.

67. Perman, *Spies*.

68. Gordon, "Working Paper," p. 6.

69. NICE, *Company Overview*. Retrieved at: <www.nice.com>.

70. NICE, *NICE Suspect Search*, 2014. Retrieved at: <http://www.nice.com/find-
    right-now/files/NICE_Suspect_Search.pdf>.

71. David Lyon (ed.), *Surveillance as Social Sorting: Privacy, Risk and Digital
    Discrimination*. London: Routledge, 2003.

72. "NICE Video Shows Policing of the Future." *The Register*, 2006. Retrieved at:
    <http://www.theregister.co.uk/2006/06/25/future_policing>.

73. "Meet the Private Companies Helping Cops Spy on Protesters." *Rolling Stone*,
    2014. Retrieved at:<http://www.rollingstone.com/politics/news/meet-the-
    private-companies-helping-cops-spy-on-protesters-20131024>.

74. Oded Yaron, "Israeli High-Tech Companies Helping Central Asian Regimes Spy
    on Citizens, Report Says." *Ha'aretz*, November 20, 2014. Retrieved at: <http://
    www.haaretz.com/news/features/.premium-1.627524>.

75. Johnson, "Pacification Industry."

76. Flavie Halais, "Rio's Favela Residents Fight Mega-Event Eviction." *Open Security*, February 14, 2013. Retrieved at: <https://www.opendemocracy.net/opensecurity/flavie-halais/rios-favela-residents-fight-mega-event-eviction>.

77. Johnson, "Pacification Industry;" Dave Zirin, "'Exporting Gaza': The Arming of Brazil's World Cup Security." *The Nation*, June 30, 2014. Retrieved at: <http://www.thenation.com/blog/180465/exporting-gaza-arming-brazils-world-cup-security#>.

78. *Ma'ariv*, "Take Brazil"; Globes, "Israeli Defense Industry Substitutes Brazil for Turkey," 2011. Retrieved at: <http://www.globes.co.il/en/article-1000637682>; IAI, Avionics, "IAI's Partner, Enters the Brazilian UAVs Market With the Cacador," March 21, 2015. Retrieved at: <http://www.iai.co.il/2013/32981-46414-en/MediaRoom_News.aspx>.

79. "Magal S^3 Signs a $35.5 Million Contract to Supply an Integrated Security System for the 2012 African Cup of Nations." Magal S^3 website, 2011. Retrieved at: <http://www.magal-s3.com/53969.html>.

80. "Exclusive Exposure: Israeli Company Selected as the Security Coordinator of Rio 2016 Olympics." *Israel Defense*, 2014. Retrieved at: <http://www.israeldefense.com/?CategoryID=475&ArticleID=3178>.

81. Ibid.

82. Yitzhak Shichor, "The U.S. Factor In Israel's Military Relations With China." *China Brief.* The Jamestown Foundation, 2007. Retrieved at <http://www.jamestown.org/single/?no_cache=1&tx_ttnews%5Btt_news%5D=3044>.

83. Yossi Melman, "Israeli Security Expert Takes Pride in His Role at the Olympics." *Ha'aretz*, August 8, 2008. Retrieved at: <http://www.haaretz.com/print-edition/news/israeli-security-expert-takes-pride-in-his-role-at-the-olympics-1.251402>; Jimmy Johnson, "China Imports Israel's Methods of Propaganda and Repression." *Electronic Intifada*, December 28, 2010. Retrieved at: <http://electronicintifada.net/content/china-imports-israels-methods-propaganda-and-repression/9160>.

84. "Riot Control Vehicles." Beit Alfa Technologies (BAT). Retrieved at: <http://www.bat.co.il/products1.htm>; Ben Lynfield, "Israeli Riot-Gear Sale to Mugabe Fuels Concern." *Christian Science Monitor*, August 23, 2001. Retrieved at: <http://www.csmonitor.com/2001/0823/p6s1-wome.html>.

85. "ZIMBABWE: Israel to Sell Heavy Riot Control Vehicles to Mugabe Government," *SADOCC*, May 15, 2002. Retrieved at: <http://www.sadocc.at/news2002/2002-163.shtml>.

86. Lynfield, "Riot-Gear."

87. Omega Research Foundation, *Crowd Control Technologies*, 2000, pp. xxviii. Retrieved at: <http://www.omegaresearchfoundation.org/assets/downloads/publications/19991401a_en.pdf>.

88. "Skunk." *Odortec*. Retrieved at: <http://www.skunk-skunk.com>.

89. "Deadly Experiments: Israel's Murderous Testing Ground for 'Less-Lethal' Weapons." *Corporate Watch*, 2011. Retrieved at: <http://www.corporatewatch.org/?lid=3866>.

90. "Proven Effective: Crowd Control Weapons in the Occupied Palestinian Territories." *Who Profits*, 2014, p. 31. Retrieved at <http://www.whoprofits.org/sites/default/files/weapons_report-8_1.pdf>.

91. Alvite Singh Ningthoujam, *India-Israel Defense Cooperation*. Begin-Sadat Center for Strategic Studies, 2014. Retrieved at: <http://besacenter.org/perspectives-papers/india-israel-defense-cooperation>.

92. Vvek Raghuvanshi, "Israeli Troops to Train Indians in Counterterrorism." *Defense News*, September 9, 2009. Retrieved at: <http://www.defensenews.com/story.php?i=3714649>.

93. "NICE Security Solutions Deployed at Bangalore's 'Namma Metro' to Secure Millions of Passengers on India's Rapid Transit Rail System." *NICE*, 2012. Retrieved at: <http://mayafiles.tase.co.il/RPdf/763001-764000/P763263-00.pdf>.

94. Feldman, *Securocratic Wars*, p. 331.

Conclusions

1. Arjun Appadurai, *Modernity at Large: Cultural Dimensions of Globalization*. Minneapolis: University of Minnesota Press, 1996, pp. 27–47.

2. Robert Cox, Gramsci, Historical Materialism and International Relations in Stephen Gill (ed.). *Gramsci, Historical Materialism and International Relations*. Cambridge: Cambridge University Press, 1993, pp. 49–66.

3. Anyone interested in this project of strengthening the "infrastructure" of the left, what we are calling The People Yes! Network, is welcome to contact me for further information <jeff@icahd.org>.

Online Resources

AntiWar.Com	www.antiwar.com
Arms Control Association	www.armscontrol.org
B'tselem	http://www.btselem.org
Centre for Analysis of World Arms Trade	armstrade.org/english.shtml
Committee Against the Arms Trade (CAAT)	www.caat.org.uk
Control Arms	controlarms.org/en
Critical Military Studies	www.criticalmilitarystudies.org
DCSC	www.dcsc.ws
Defense News	www.defensenews.com
Defense Tech	defensetech.org
Defense Update	www.defense-update.com
Federation of American Scientists (FAS)	fas.org
G2mil, The Magazine of Future Warfare	www.g2mil.com
Geographical Imaginations	geographicalimaginations.com/author/derekjgregory
Global Security	www.globalsecurity.org
Ha'aretz newspaper	www.haaretz.com
Hamushim (a Hebrew website)	https://hamushim.wordpress.com
IDF website	www.idfblog.com
i-hls (Israeli Homeland Security)	http://i-hls.com
The [Israeli] Institute for National Security Studies	www.inss.org.il
Institute for Soldier Nanotechnologies	web.mit.edu/isn/aboutisn/index.html
Israel Defense	www.israeldefense.com
The Israeli Committee Against House Demolitions (ICAHD)	www.icahd.org
Military Embargo	military-embargo@lists.bdsmovement.net
New Profile	http://www.newprofile.org/english
Police State USA	www.policestateusa.com
PRIO, The Peace Research Institute Oslo	www.prio.org
Small Wars Journal	smallwarsjournal.com
Stockholm International Peace Institute (SIPRI)	www.sipri.org
Strategy Page	www.strategypage.com/default.asp
Tom Dispatch	www.tomdispatch.com
War is Boring	medium.com/war-is-boring
War Profiteers' News	www.wri-irg.org/publications/war_profiteers
Who is Arming Israel?	disarmtheconflict.wordpress.com
Who Profits	www.whoprofits.org
+972	972mag.com

Index